WE 830 WYN

88

2704

 Scarborough Health Au--

WE
68S
WYN

D1391574

REHABILITATION OF THE HAND

REHABILITATION OF THE HAND

Fourth Edition

C. B. WYNN PARRY
MBE, MA, DM, FRCP, FRCS, DPhysMED

Director of Rehabilitation and Consultant Rheumatologist,
Royal National Orthopaedic Hospital, London;
Honorary Consultant in Applied Electrophysiology,
National Hospital for Nervous Diseases, Queen Square, London;
Civil Consultant in Rehabilitation and Rheumatology to the
Royal Air Force;
Sometime Consultant and Adviser in Rehabilitation and
Rheumatology to the Royal Air Force

assisted by

MAUREEN SALTER
MCSP
Superintendent Physiotherapist,
Medical Rehabilitation Unit,
Royal Air Force, Chessington

and

DORIS MILLAR
MAOT
Superintendent Occupational Therapist,
Medical Rehabilitation Unit,
Royal Air Force, Chessington

with a contribution from

IAN FLETCHER
MRCS, LRCP
Senior Medical Officer,
DHSS Limb Fitting Centre,
Roehampton;
Assistant Surgeon in Chief,
St John Ambulance Brigade

Butterworths
London   Boston   Durban   Singapore   Sydney   Toronto   Wellington

All rights reserved. No part of this publication may be reproduced or transmitted in any form or by any means, including photocopying and recording, without the written permission of the copyright holder, application for which should be addressed to the Publishers. Such written permission must also be obtained before any part of this publication is stored in a retrieval system of any nature.

This book is sold subject to the Standard Conditions of Sale of Net Books and may not be re-sold in the UK below the net price given by the Publishers in their current price list.

First published 1958
Second edition 1966
Third edition 1973
Reprinted 1977
Fourth edition 1981
Reprinted 1986

©Butterworth & Co (Publishers) Ltd., 1981

British Library Cataloguing in Publication Data

Wynn Parry, Christopher Berkeley
Rehabilitation of the Hand. – 4th ed.
1. Hand – Wounds and injuries
2. Hand – Diseases
I. Title   II. Salter, Maureen   III. Miller, Doris
617′.575   RD559   80-41761

ISBN 0-407-38502-9 (Cased)
ISBN 0-407-38503-7 (PPC)

Typeset by Butterworths Litho Preparation Department
Printed by Butler & Tanner Ltd, London and Frome

Foreword to the Second Edition

Successful treatment of the hand affected by injury or disease rests upon wise assessment, skilful operative technique and good after-care. This book deals with the principles and details of assessment and physical treatment. When the first edition appeared in 1958 it was greeted with acclamation for many had felt the need for such a work. We were not disappointed and there can be few surgeons, physiotherapists and occupational therapists concerned with the improvement of hand function who do not turn to this book for advice. All will be delighted that a new edition with its additional sections has now appeared.

The author writes from an experience which is probably unequalled. His treatment of the subject ranges from electrodiagnosis to the facilities for resettlement of the severely disabled person. Many of the concepts of re-education, the competitive games and the application of splintage spring from his imaginative mind. The training of sensory perception in a hand devoid of fine sensibility due to a peripheral nerve lesion is quite new and it is hoped that further research will be made in this direction.

The special hand unit he has created within the justly famed Rehabilitation Service of the Royal Air Force is a challenge to all interested in this work. The organization of a civilian department differs in character and discipline from Chessington, but the medical problems are the same. The stimulation of Wing Commander Wynn Parry's enthusiasm will continue to exert its influence upon us all.

January, 1966   R. Guy Pulvertaft

Preface to the Fourth Edition

Since the last edition of this book was published, I have left the Royal Air Force and taken up the post of Director of Rehabilitation and Consultant Rheumatologist at the Royal National Orthopaedic Hospital, London and Stanmore.

It has been my privilege to work with Mr Donal Brooks, Director of the Hand and Peripheral Nerve Unit, and I take this opportunity of paying tribute to his skill, wisdom and encouragement and to his kindness in accepting a physician into his team. As I have been working closely with a surgical team, it has seemed reasonable to describe the standard reconstructive procedures used at the Royal National Orthopaedic Hospital. A critic of the previous volume felt the intrusion of surgical descriptions inappropriate but, as the book is read by physiotherapists and occupational therapists, some account of current surgical thinking would seem helpful.

The Rheumatology Unit at Stanmore was developed by Derrick Brewerton who contributed the chapter on the rheumatoid hand in the previous edition and who is now at the Westminster Hospital. As I inherited his post as Director of the Medical Rheumatology Unit and have worked closely with the surgeons at Stanmore and Great Portland Street—in particular, Mr Brooks, Mr Lorden Trickey and Mr Michael Sullivan—it seemed appropriate that the chapter on the rheumatoid hand should come from the Royal National Orthopaedic Hospital and so I have undertaken to reflect current practice there by writing this chapter myself, while at the same time thanking Dr Brewerton for his brilliant contribution in past editions.

The sections on brachial plexus lesions, sensory re-education and reconstructive surgery have been entirely rewritten. A new extended section on pain has been added, and it is heartening to be able to report significant advances over the last few years in the treatment of many distressingly painful conditions of peripheral nerves. Other chapters have been updated as appropriate.

One of the inspiring features of working as a physician in a surgical team is the constant stimulus of new ideas, criticism and encouragement that typify the orthopaedic approach. My thanks are due in particular to Ian Bayley, FRCS, lecturer in surgery, Dr. Antonio Landi, Stephen Copeland, FRCS, and the occupational therapists, physiotherapists, social workers and nurses who work so hard to make rehabilitation a success—with special mention to Frances Perry, MAOT, Barbara Bannard, Senior MAOT, Alison Monteith, MAOT, and Susan Emerson, MAOT, head occupational therapist, Stanmore; Sarah Dobbs, MCSP, Vicky Frampton, MCSP, and Janet Lavery, MSCP, Joan Rix, social worker, Sister Moira Nurse, Dr Peter Smith and Mrs Elizabeth Hope, the indefatigable librarians at the Royal National Orthopaedic Hospital, William Seton, Senior Rehabilitation Officer, Royal National Orthopaedic Hospital, Stanmore, and Mr T. G. Evans, Mr John Heritage and Mr Michael Wardlow, orthotists, who have provided the brachial plexus splints.

My thanks also go to Gillian Clarke whose hard work will undoubtedly materially contribute to the success of this edition.

Finally, it is not possible adequately to thank Mrs Helen Ellis, secretary to the Rehabilitation and Rheumatology Unit, without whose untiring efforts none of this work would have been possible.

London, 1981   C. B. Wynn Parry

Preface to the First Edition

Cookery books tend to be the most irritating of all reference books. Sooner or later the phrase 'cook in the usual way' brings dismay to the learner. It is precisely 'the usual way' that, simple as it must be to the author, is a mystery to the reader.

It may be thought that there are already enough books dealing with the hand; none to our knowledge, however, has concerned itself with detailed conservative treatment, or the niceties of after-care. When the surgeon states that physiotherapy or occupational therapy should be given, following a surgical operation on the hand, it may not be clear which procedures are of help and for how long they should be maintained.

This book then is an attempt to provide details of 'the usual way' in the rehabilitation of hand disabilities.

We have been singularly fortunate in working in the closest co-operation with, and enjoying the confidence of, the Royal Air Force Plastic Surgery Centre, under its Director, Air Commodore G. H. Morley, OBE, FRCS, LRCP, and the Royal Air Force Orthopaedic Service, under its Director, Air Commodore L. M. Crooks, OBE, MB, MCh, FRCS. We owe an especial debt of gratitude to them for their encouragement and help, for permission to publish details of their cases, and for reading the manuscript and offering helpful advice and criticism. Mr R. G. Pulvertaft, FRCS, read the manuscript most carefully and offered numerous criticisms of extreme value; we are most grateful to him for his invaluable help. We wish to thank Lieutenant-Colonel P. R. Wheatley, DSO, MB, BS, FRCS, LRCP, for much valuable criticism of the manuscript and for permission to report his cases.

We should also like to thank Mr H. Osmond Clarke, CBE, FRCS, for his encouragement and help, Dr H. D. Darcus, BM, BCh, for his help in criticizing the chapter on anatomy and for providing the grip dynamometer, Wing Commander D. M. Keir, MB, ChB, FRCS(Ed), Mr D. Brooks, FRCS(I), Dr H. Glanville, DPhysMed, Dr F. B. Kiernander, MRCP, DPhysMed, Colonel A. MacMillan, MB, BS, FRCS, LRCP, Squadron Leader P. J. R. Nichols, DPhysMed, Dr V. Wilkinson, Mr R. G. T. Giddens and Mr A. A. Armour of the Government Training Centre and Industrial Rehabilitation Unit,

Waddon, for much helpful advice in the chapter on resettlement, and Mr R. Hannand, the Resettlement Officer, Kingston Labour Exchange, who has done so much to make the resettlement of the patients possible. We are very grateful also to Mr R. Carby for the drawings, Flight Lieutenant R. Jane, DPhysMed, for details of remedial games, and finally all the medical staff, physiotherapists, occupational therapists, remedial gymnasts and, not least, the long-suffering patients the the Royal Air Force Rehabilitation Unit, Chessington.

Our thanks are due to Mrs M. I. Lindow for her devoted secretarial assistance. Finally, we wish to thank also the Director General Medical Services, Royal Air Force, for permission to publish this book.

London, 1958   C. B. Wynn Parry

Preface to the Second Edition

The second edition of this book, like the first, reflects the methods and experience of the Royal Air Force rehabilitation units.

Since the last edition, Mrs Baker has left to be Superintendent Physiotherapist at University College Hospital, Ibadan, Nigeria, and Miss Natalie Smythe has become Chief Occupational Therapist to the Hong Kong Society for Rehabilitation. Their places have been taken by Miss Barbara Sutcliffe and Miss Doris Millar who have been responsible for the sections on physiotherapy and occupational therapy respectively.

This book has been extensively rewritten, in particular, the sections on functional anatomy of the intrinsic muscles, treatment of hemiplegia, physiotherapy techniques and the manufacture of splints. New sections have been added on sensory re-education, prostheses for amputations, conduction velocity measurements in localizing peripheral nerve lesions, lively stretch splints and games for re-education of hand function.

It is a pleasure to acknowledge again the help, encouragement and inspiration of Air Vice-Marshall G. Morley, RAF Senior Consultant in Plastic Surgery.

I have taken careful note of the constructive criticisms in the reviews of the first edition and hope that some of the defects have been corrected.

I have been constantly stimulated and encouraged by the members of the British Club for Surgery of the Hand, who are kind enough to allow a physician to be one of their number; to them this book is affectionately dedicated.

London, 1966

C. B. Wynn Parry

Preface to the Third Edition

In preparing the third edition of this book, the opportunity has been taken to make extensive revisions.

The chapter on functional anatomy has been brought up to date, the lively splints are all new, more space has been devoted to reconstructive surgery and the chapter on the spastic upper limb has been entirely rewritten and expanded.

The chapter on electrodiagnosis has been almost entirely rewritten, and an additional chapter on problems of upper limb amputation has been provided by Ian Fletcher whose experience is unrivalled in this field. Derrick Brewerton, assisted by A. W. F. Lettin, has largely rewritten his chapter on the rheumatoid hand, taking into account the new concept of the place of surgery in its management.

The separate chapter on techniques of treatment has been discarded—only specialized techniques relevant to the problem of the hand have been described and these have been included in the appropriate chapters.

Since the last edition Miss Maureen Salter has succeeded Miss Barbara Sutcliffe as Superintendent Physiotherapist at the Joint Services Medical Rehabilitation Unit, Royal Air Force, Chessington, and has contributed much of the material on physiotherapy.

This book is the result of a team working together over many years—only by close co-operation and mutual constructive criticism between surgeons, physicians and the remedial professions can the best results be obtained. It is a pleasure to acknowledge my incalculable debt to the skill, devotion and good humour of the therapists at the Service Rehabilitation Units at Chessington and Headley Court, and to my medical and surgical colleagues for their expertise and encouragement to us all. I wish to thank Wing Commander A. Honey for his invaluable help with recordings and documentations, and Miss Boreham for typing the manuscript.

Finally, my thanks are due to the Director General Medical Services, Royal Air Force, for permission to publish this new edition.

London, 1973   C. B. Wynn Parry

Contents

Functional Anatomy of the Hand 1

INTRODUCTION

The importance of a normally functioning hand needs no emphasis, whether in earning a living, practising a hobby or allowing independence in daily activities.

The hand is capable of the strongest grasp and the most delicate touch; its rich and complex sensory innervation allows the finest judgement of texture, volume and temperature. The value of a strong and well co-ordinated hand in such activities as writing, painting and manipulating tools is obvious. Less obvious perhaps is the extent to which the hand is a reflection of personality and a vital organ of expression. One has only to consider the manual signs and attitudes of an oriental dancer, the benediction of a priest, the gestures of a conductor or a Gallic raconteur, to realize how much more is the hand than a prehensile and sensory tool.

Injury, disease or surgical interference, therefore, do much more than interfere with grip or touch; they attack the personality itself. In disabilities of the hand more than in any other region of the body, the finest surgery and after-care are essential. Careless or inexperienced surgery, insufficient or non-existent rehabilitation are alike inexcusable. Only those who have not worked with patients whose hands are seriously disabled do not realise how deep the disaster may penetrate, and how much psychological trauma, often not manifest, can be caused.

All types of disease affect the hand – infections, arthritides, neoplasms and degenerations – but, unfortunately, the hand is also subject to injury to an alarming degree. Rank and Wakefield quoted USA statistics as 2 050 000 disabling work injuries in 1964 – 125 000 to hands and 350 000 to thumb and fingers. In some industries hand injuries account for more than 90 per cent of disabling accidents reported (Rank and Hueston, 1973).

Many industrial accidents are avoidable, and more stringent safety precautions and work studies will in time decrease their incidence. People will, however, continue to put their hands through window panes, knives will slip, hands will be burnt or crushed, and fingers lost.

It may not be widely appreciated how much can be done for the seriously disabled hand by intensive and long-continued conservative treatment, and to what extent rehabilitation can reinforce the dexterity and ingenuity of surgery.

It is accepted, of course, that the patient should be encouraged to use his hand as much as possible after tendon or peripheral nerve surgery. It is less well known that with full-time rehabilitation for many months, involving much attention to detail in departments of physiotherapy and occupational therapy, the majority of patients with neurotmesis of median and ulnar nerves may obtain a hand with function near normal.

Patients with severe crush injuries resulting in stiff and contracted fingers can regain a considerable degree of function with intensive serial stretches and specialized oil massage. Although this takes time, and may well involve the patient in several hours of treatment a day, the end-result may make the difference between returning to a skilled occupation, or taking a less skilled job, with all its financial, social and psychological implications to the patient, his family and the community as a whole.

During the last 20 years we have had an opportunity of studying and attempting to devise correct techniques of rehabilitation in a variety of hand disorders. We have come to the firm conclusion that only by intensive, if necessary, full-time treatment, the utmost attention to detail, and careful and realistic planning for future occupation can the best results be obtained.

The experience gained at the Royal Air Force Medical Rehabilitation Units and the Royal National Orthopaedic Hospitals, which has led us to realize the importance of detailed rehabilitation, is the apology for this book.

The treatment of hand injuries involves the development of muscle power, increase in joint range and redevelopment of co-ordination. As intelligent treatment depends on a sound knowledge of functional anatomy, this chapter is concerned with the anatomy of the hand and its function. In investigating the action of the hand muscles, electromyography, nerve stimulation and studies of the effects of nerve section in patients with nerve injuries have been studied. The fingers are referred to as index, middle, ring and little.

JOINTS OF THE HAND

Metacarpophalangeal joints

The joints between the head of the metacarpal and the base of the proximal phalanx allow flexion, extension, abduction, adduction and a certain amount of rotation. The heads of the metacarpals of the index and middle fingers have special features that deserve emphasis. On the radial side the condyle is larger than on the ulnar side and the ulnar condyle slopes proximally so that an extensor tendon is more liable to subluxate ulnarwards than radially, as happens when the metacarpophalangeal joint becomes swollen in rheumatoid disease. The capsule of the joint has a special development in its volar part, known as the volar plate. Distally it is cartilaginous and is inserted into the palmar surface of the base of the proximal phalanx. Proximally it is lax, thin and attached to the palmar aspect of the neck of the metacarpal. Laterally the volar plate is inserted into the transverse ligament which connects the metacarpophalangeal joints anteriorly. Dubousset (1971) has made the ingenious suggestion that the volar plates are really a differentiation of the transverse intermetacarpal ligament, which is itself the thickened distal portion of the deep palmar aponeurosis. Anteriorly the volar plate is closely adherent to the fibrous flexor sheath.

The volar plate is responsible for strengthening the capsule and provides a stabilizing force for the joint and, indeed, is really part of the joint – broadening the articular surface of the phalanx. The articular surface of the base of the phalanx, the volar plate and the collateral ligaments, with which it is continuous, act as a sort of cradle for the head of the metacarpal and increase its stability. The collateral ligaments are strong fibrous reinforcements to the capsule which maintain lateral stability of the metacarpophalangeal joints. They originate from the tuberosities on the heads of the metacarpals and run obliquely to be attached to the base of the lateral tuberosities on the base of the proximal phalanx (*Figure 1.1*).

The radial ligament runs obliquely, while the ulnar ligament is more vertical. This assists the element of rotation at the metacarpophalangeal joint in a radial direction with increasing flexion. Both run dorsal to the axis of the joint and become taut in flexion of the proximal phalanx and relaxed in full extension. Thus, lateral movements of the metacarpophalangeal joints are virtually impossible in flexion, but free in metacarpophalangeal extension. Abduction is greatest for the index finger – usually more than 50 degrees – and least for the middle and ring fingers.

In metacarpophalangeal extension, stability of the metacarpophalangeal joints is provided by the interossei. The accessory collateral ligaments or metacarpoglenoid fibres take origin also from the tuberosities on the metacarpal heads and insert in a fan-like manner into the volar plate and into the fibrous flexor sheath.

They lie volar to the axis of the joint and are therefore taut in extension and lax in flexion, and help to stabilize the flexor tendons in flexion.

There is a continuity between all the structures surrounding the metacarpophalangeal joint, for the extensor hood, extensor tendons, collateral ligaments, volar plate, and fibrous flexor sheath and capsule of the joint are all intimately interwoven. This continuity plays a valuable role in the stability of the joint. Also, each metacarpophalangeal joint is connected by the transverse metacarpal ligament and this, with the interconnection of the extensor tendons over the dorsum of the wrist and that of the flexors in the forearm, makes for co-ordinated action of all the fingers together.

Interphalangeal joints

The shape of these joints allows only flexion and extension. There are strong collateral ligaments with both lateral fibres and oblique fibres inserting into the volar plate, which is similar to that in the metacarpophalangeal joint and has a strong attachment to the fibrous flexor sheath.

The whole mechanism of the flexor tendon, its sheath and fibrocartilage to which it is attached at the metacarpophalangeal and interphalangeal joints, all move smoothly together – thus the slightest adherence due to scar from trauma, infection, burns, rheumatoid inflammation or prolonged immobilization, will be disastrous for effective hand function.

At the proximal interphalangeal joint is a specialized ligament – the retinacular ligament of Landsmeer. This has two main divisions: oblique fibres running anterior to the axis of the joint, and transverse fibres being directed anteroposteriorly.

Valentin (1962) has shown that the oblique fibres extend the distal phalanx passively but the transverse fibres keep the lateral tendons of the extensor digitorum communis taut and prevent dorsal dislocation during extension. These ligaments

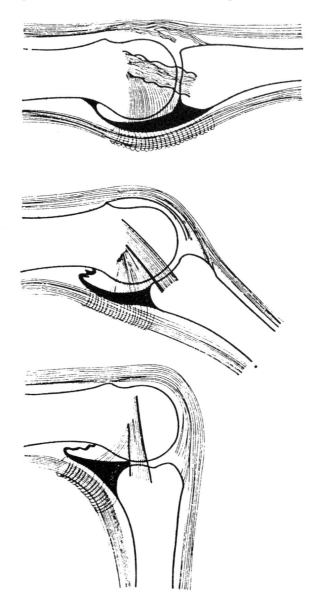

Figure 1.1   Lateral view of the metacarpophalangeal joint, showing the two parts of the collateral ligament—metacarpophalangeal and metacarpoglenoid fibres—with the joint extended and flexed. The volar plate or the glenoid fibrocartilage can be seen moving as one unit during flexion, due to the elasticity of its proximal part which is inserted on the palmar surface of the metacarpal head. (From Dubousset, 1971, by courtesy of Expansion Scientifique Francaise)

connect the proximal interphalangeal and distal interphalangeal joints and ensure that movement at one is reproduced by movement at the other joint (*Figure 1.2*). The tongue of the head of the proximal phalanx fits into the groove of the base of the middle phalanx, giving stability against rotatory and shearing stress. This is enhanced by the fact that the transverse dimension of the joint is double that of the vertical dimension.

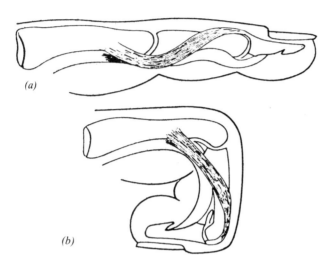

Figure 1.2   *The retinacular ligaments. (From Stack, 1962, by courtesy of the author and the Editors of* Journal of Bone and Joint Surgery)

The flexor digitorum sublimis is inserted several millimetres distal to the volar plate giving added leverage and power, whilst the flexor digitorum profundus inserts closer to the joint and movement is therefore less.

Thumb

The aponeurosis of the adductor pollicis and abductor pollicis brevis represents the lateral bands. Range of movement varies at the metacarpophalangeal joint between 5 and 100 degrees, depending on how flat or round is the head of the metacarpal. The major factor for lateral stability is the broad transverse diameter of the condyle. The sesamoids lie in the lateral margins of the volar plate – the radial sesamoid accepting the insertion of flexor pollicis brevis, and the ulnar sesamoid, the oblique head of the adductor pollicis. The arrangement provides a 'dumb bell' grip, forming a pulley groove over which the flexor tendons run.

The cartilaginous deep surface of the sesamoids is continuous with the intra-articular surface of the volar plate whose insertion is thin centrally and thick laterally, and it has been shown that the tensile strength of the ligament structure is three times that of the metacarpophalangeal joint of the fingers.

FLEXORS OF THE WRIST

In flexion and extension of the wrist, movement between the two rows of carpal bones exceeds that between the radius and the proximal row of carpal bones. Ulnar deviation involves movement mainly at the radiocarpal joint; radial deviation involves movement between the carpal bones themselves.

Flexor carpi radialis

The common flexor origin is on the medial epicondyle from which this muscle originates, and the insertion is on the palmar surface of the bases of the second and third metacarpals. Its antagonists are the extensor carpi radialis longus, which inserts into the dorsal surface of the base of the second metacarpal, and the extensor carpi radialis brevis, which inserts into the dorsal surface of the base of the third metacarpal. The function of the flexor carpi radialis is to flex the wrist and, with its antagonists, to deviate the wrist radially. The nerve supply is from the median nerve.

Flexor carpi ulnaris

The origin is the common flexor origin from the aponeurosis on the upper two-thirds of the posterior border of the ulna. The insertion is the pisiform bone and the base of the fifth metacarpal. The nerve supply is from the ulnar nerve. The function of the flexor carpi ulnaris is to flex the wrist and, with the extensor carpi ulnaris, to deviate the wrist in an ulnar direction.

Palmaris longus

When present, the palmaris longus muscle arises from the common flexor origin and is inserted into the flexor retinaculum and palmar fascia. It is supplied by the median nerve. Its action is to flex the wrist and tighten the palmar fascia, thus helping to cup the palm.

Clinical testing

To test the wrist flexors the patient is asked to flex the wrist slightly against the examiner's resistance applied at the level of the metacarpophalangeal joint of the thumb.

The tendon of flexor carpi ulnaris can be seen and felt on the ulnar border of the palmar surface of the wrist and that of flexor carpi radialis can be seen and felt about 2.5 cm from the radial border of the wrist just to the radial side of the palmaris longus tendon.

The palmaris longus tendon is seen and felt on wrist flexion but is best tested by asking the patient, with his wrist flexed, to touch the tip of his little finger with his thumb, when the tendon stands out boldly; it is not always present.

The wrist flexors are active in almost all activities of the hand. It is not possible to grade the power of each muscle accurately on the Medical Research Council (MRC) scale,* as they work in a group.

Clinically, the presence or absence of muscle action should be recorded and the power of wrist flexion, ulnar deviation and radial deviation assessed as a whole.

LONG FLEXORS OF THE FINGERS

Flexor digitorum profundus

The flexor digitorum profundus arises from the upper three-quarters of the anterior and inner surface of the ulna, and from the interosseous membrane joining the radius and ulna. It becomes tendinous about halfway down the forearm, lower than sublimis, and the four tendons (except indicis) pass below the flexor retinaculum at the wrist deep to the tendons of flexor digitorum sublimis.

Flexor digitorum sublimis

The flexor digitorum sublimis arises from the common flexor origin, from the coronoid processes of the ulna, the ulnar collateral ligament and a thin oblique line on the outer border of the radius between the bicipital tuberosity and the insertion of pronator teres. It becomes tendinous about halfway down the forearm and passes beneath the flexor retinaculum superficial to the tendons of flexor digitorum profundus. The tendons destined for the index and little fingers lie deep to those for the middle and ring fingers at the wrist. The tendons of both sublimis and profundus pass through the palm beneath the palmar fascia. Here they are enclosed by the synovial sheaths, that of the little finger flexors being continuous with the synovial sheath in the flexor tunnel, and enter the flexor tunnels in the fingers. The sides and roof of these tunnels are formed by the fibrous flexor sheaths which arise from ridges along the outer sides of the proximal and middle phalanges. Opposite the proximal interphalangeal joints the sheath arises from the fibrocartilaginous anterior ligament, which is grooved for the passage of the flexor tendons. The tunnel stretches from the metacarpophalangeal joint to the insertion of the flexor profundus tendon.

At the proximal phalanx the flexor sublimis tendon splits into two, allowing the tendon of flexor profundus to pass through. The sublimis tendon is then reunited to be inserted, after splitting again, into the base of the middle phalanx.

The profundus tendons, after splitting the sublimis tendons opposite the proximal phalanges, pass to their insertion into the palmar surface of the base of the distal phalanx. The alternating support thus given makes for better leverage.

The two tendons lie in a synovial sheath which is indivisible from the fibrous flexor sheath.

*MRC scale: 0, no contraction; 1, flicker; 2, definite contraction; 3, contraction against gravity; 4, contraction against gravity and resistance; 5, normal power.

The vincula are synovial threads carrying blood vessels to the flexor tendons. The vincula brevia are found in the angle between the insertion of the tendons and the phalanges. The flexor sublimis has two vincula longa which arise from the tendon at the site of its splitting and are attached to the fibrous flexor sheath at its lateral borders. The flexor profundus has one vinculum longum which arises from the tendon where it splits the sublimis and is attached to the roof of the synovial sheath.

The flexor tunnel is only just big enough to accommodate the various structures it contains. The slightest scarring after tendon suture will not allow true tendon play, and a stiff finger may result. Surgery of the flexor tendons in the sheath thus presents one of the most difficult problems in hand surgery.

Clinical testing

To test the flexor sublimis the hand is laid flat on the desk, palm upwards. Flexion of the other three fingers is prevented by the examiner holding the fingers down in extension, and the patient is asked to flex the free finger. Profundus action is then impossible, and independent sublimis action can be tested.

Similarly, the flexor profundus is tested by asking the patient to bend the terminal joint without bending the metacarpophalangeal or proximal interphalangeal joint, the middle phalanx being supported.

Nerve supply of the finger flexors

The flexor digitorum sublimis is supplied by the median nerve, the flexor digitorum profundus by the anterior interosseus branch of the median (tendons to index and middle fingers) and the ulnar nerve (tendons to ring and little fingers).

The main function of the flexor digitorum profundus is flexion at the terminal interphalangeal joint, but as it crosses the wrist, metacarpophalangeal joints and proximal interphalangeal joints, it will flex these joints as well, although it will only flex the metacarpophalangeal joints when the wrist and metacarpophalangeal joints are hyperextended. Sacrifice of the flexor digitorum sublimis in severe tendon injuries thus does not seriously impair flexor function of the hand.

The main function of the flexor digitorum sublimis is to flex the proximal interphalangeal joint, but it will also be able to flex the metacarpophalangeal joints, and the wrist, albeit weakly.

MOVEMENTS OF THE THUMB

The main function of the thumb is to hold objects between it and the fingers. The saddle-shaped joint between the first metacarpal and the trapezium allows movement in several planes.

Abduction is the movement of the thumb away from the palm at right angles to it. Adduction is the opposite movement, bringing the thumb down onto the index finger.

There are two types of abduction: palmar and radial. In palmar abduction the thumb is brought away from the index finger at right angles to it. In radial abduction the thumb is brought away from the index finger at an angle of 45 degrees, being at a diagonal, and outside the plane of the palm (*Figure 1.3*).

Flexion is the movement of the thumb across the palm and in the plane of the palm.

Extension is the opposite movement, bringing the thumb alongside the index finger.

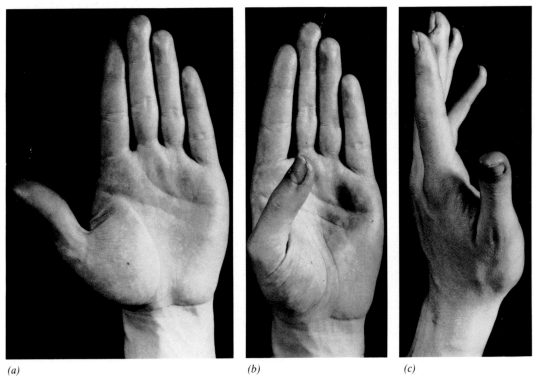

(a) *(b)* *(c)*

Figure 1.3   Extension: palmar and radial abduction of the thumb

Opposition of the thumb to one of the fingers is a complex movement comprising palmar abduction, flexion, rotation of the metacarpal towards the finger and adduction. Of these four components, palmar abduction is the most important.

In opposition, the thumb is held abducted at right angles to the palm, the metacarpophalangeal joint is stabilized by combined action of the long and short extensors, long abductor, and the flexors and adductors of the carpometacarpal and metacarpophalangeal joints, and the terminal joint stabilized in a variable degree of flexion by combined action of the long flexor and long extensor.

The extensor expansion of the long and short extensors of the thumb fuse with the fibrous flexor sheath. Opposition is carried out mainly by the abductor pollicis brevis which is instrumental in opposing the thumb to the index and middle fingers, the superficial head of the flexor brevis continuing the movement to the ring and little fingers. The opponens helps to rotate and flex the metacarpophalangeal joint.

The important part played by the abductor brevis and the superficial head of the flexor can be shown by seeing and palpating these two muscles as the thumb is opposed in turn to each of the fingers. This has been confirmed in two patients in whom the ulnar nerve supplied the opponens, the median supplying the short abductor and superficial head of brevis. Stimulation of the median nerve at the elbow produced significantly more opposition than stimulation of the ulnar nerve.

The importance of having the terminal joint of the thumb stabilized for power in opposition is reflected in the fact that all the short thenar muscles have an insertion into the extensor expansion of the thumb, so that their action of opposing inevitably results in stabilization of the terminal joint.

EXTRINSIC MUSCLES INVOLVED IN THUMB MOVEMENT

Extensor pollicis longus

The extensor pollicis longus arises from the radial border of the posterior surface of the ulna below the origin of abductor pollicis longus and above that of extensor indicis, from the interosseus membrane. It is inserted into the base of the radial aspect of the terminal phalanx of the thumb.

It is supplied by the posterior interosseus branch of the radial nerve. Its antagonists are the flexor pollicis longus and the muscles which oppose the thumb – opponens, abductor pollicis brevis and the superficial head of flexor pollicis brevis.

Its action is to extend the terminal joint of the thumb, and by virtue of its ulnar-sided pull it brings the thumb round in lateral (or external) rotation to lie flat against the fingers. It is also active in wrist extension, radial abduction of the thumb and adduction of the thumb, particularly when adductor pollicis is paralysed.

To test the muscle the patient is asked to extend the terminal joint of the thumb. The proximal phalanx must be supported by the examiner and the thumb held in adduction, otherwise the short abductor and flexor will also be active owing to their insertion into the extensor expansion.

Extensor pollicis brevis

The extensor pollicis brevis arises from the ulnar border of the posterior surface of the radius below the origin of pronator teres, and the interosseus membrane. Its tendon passes across the wrist together with that of abductor pollicis longus and is inserted into the posterior surface of the base of the proximal phalanx of the thumb.

It is supplied by the posterior interosseus branch of the radial. It is active in all movements connected with gripping as it stabilizes the metacarpophalangeal joint of the thumb. Its action is to extend and stabilize the metacarpophalangeal joint of the thumb.

To test this muscle the patient is asked to extend the thumb against resistance while keeping the terminal joint flexed. The tendon stands out well as the anterior boundary of the anatomical snuffbox.

Flexor pollicis longus

The flexor pollicis longus has an extensive origin from the anterior surface of the radius from the oblique line to just above the origin of pronator quadratus. The muscle becomes tendinous in the lower quarter of the forearm and passes under the flexor retinaculum. It is enclosed in a fibrous flexor sheath distal to the metacarpophalangeal joint, similar to those of the fingers, and inserts into the flexor aspect at the base of the terminal phalanx of the thumb. It is supplied by the anterior interosseus branch of the median nerve.

The flexor pollicis longus flexes the terminal joint of the thumb. It has also a slight action of wrist flexion and assists in adduction when the adductor is paralysed. Its antagonist is extensor pollicis longus.

To test the muscle the patient is asked to bend the terminal phalanx against the examiner's resistance with the thumb adducted and the proximal phalanx supported.

Abductor pollicis longus

The abductor pollicis longus arises from the middle third of the posterior aspect of the radius, the interosseus membrane and a thin line on the radial side of the posterior aspect of the ulna beneath the insertion of anconeus. It becomes tendinous near the wrist, often inserting by two tendons into the radial side of the thumb metacarpal. It may have two other insertions, into the trapezium or into the abductor pollicis brevis. It is supplied by the posterior interosseus branch of the radial nerve.

The main action of this muscle is to abduct the thumb in a radial direction; that is, at an angle of approximately 45 degrees with the index finger. It is also active in wrist abduction. It is active when objects are gripped hard between thumb and fingers. Its antagonists are adductor pollicis and flexor pollicis brevis. As its main action is to stabilize the thumb when the extensors are active, rather than to produce pure radial abduction, activity in the abductor pollicis longus always produces contraction in extensor carpi ulnaris.

The muscle is tested by asking the patient to bring his thumb away at an angle of 45 degrees in a radial direction.

INTRINSIC MUSCLES

Abductor pollicis brevis

The abductor pollicis brevis arises from the flexor retinaculum, the scaphoid tubercle and the ridge of the trapezium. It may occasionally also arise from the tendon of abductor pollicis longus. It is inserted into the radial side of the base of the proximal phalanx of the thumb and into the extensor expansion. It is supplied by the median nerve.

Its action is to abduct the thumb in the plane of the palm at right angles from the index finger, its main function being as a stabilizer.

Electromyography shows that it is highly active also throughout opposition of the thumb to all four fingers. It has a slight flexor action on the metacarpal and extends the terminal joint of the thumb. The muscle strongly contracts in the activities of holding a pen, painting and playing the piano.

The muscle is tested by asking the patient to lay the hand flat on the table, palm upwards, and to bring the thumb up at right angles to the index finger. Its antagonist is the adductor pollicis.

Flexor pollicis brevis

THE SUPERFICIAL HEAD

This arises from the flexor retinaculum and the ridge of the trapezium. It is inserted into the radial side of the base of the first phalanx and into the extensor expansion, and it has a sesamoid bone in its tendon. This superficial head is supplied by the median nerve. Its antagonist is the extensor pollicis brevis.

The superficial head of the short flexor flexes the first metacarpal, thus bringing the thumb across the palm in the plane of the palm. By virtue of its insertion into the extensor expansion it can extend the terminal phalanx weakly.

To test the muscle the patient is asked to bring the thumb across the palm with the terminal joint extended.

THE DEEP HEAD

This muscle is best considered as the first palmar interosseus. Its origin, insertion, action and nerve supply are similar in all respects to the interossei.

The origin is from the ulnar side of the base of the metacarpal of the thumb, and it is inserted into the ulnar side of the base of the proximal phalanx. It is supplied by the ulnar nerve, and its action is to bring the radially abducted thumb to the index finger. Further movement of the thumb across the palm is carried out by the deep head of the flexor brevis.

To test the muscle the patient is asked to bring the radially abducted thumb towards the index finger without flexing the terminal joint of the thumb. Alternatively, with the palm of the hand down on the table, the patient is asked to lift the thumb off the table and then bring it towards the index finger, as in testing the interossei.

Opponens pollicis

The opponens pollicis arises from the flexor retinaculum and the ridge on the trapezium. It is inserted into the whole length of the radial border and radial half of the lateral aspect of the metacarpal of the thumb. It is supplied by the median nerve and its antagonist is the extensor pollicis brevis and the long abductor and long extensor. Its action is to rotate the metacarpal towards the palmar surface of the fingers.

To test the muscle the proximal phalanx should be brought into abduction at a right angle to the index finger. Without bending the terminal joint of the thumb, the patient is asked to bring the thumb across to the tips of each finger in turn. It is essential to support the thumb in abduction for the opponens cannot work effectively until the thumb is abducted. If this is not done it is impossible to distinguish opponens paralysis from short abductor paralysis. This is important clinically because there may be an anomalous nerve supply – the ulnar nerve supplying the opponens, or the nerve to the short abductor only may be involved.

Adductor pollicis

The adductor pollicis has two heads: the oblique head arises from the palmar surfaces of the capitate, trapezoid, bases of the second and third metacarpals, and the palmar ligaments; the transverse head arises from the distal two-thirds of the palmar surface of the third metacarpal. The two heads are inserted into the ulnar side of the base of the proximal phalanx of the thumb. There is a sesamoid bone in this tendon. The muscle is supplied by the ulnar nerve. Its action is to bring the thumb down to the index finger from abduction and its antagonist is the abductor brevis. It is the muscle that enables objects to be firmly held between thumb and fingers.

To test the muscle the patient is asked to supinate the forearm and hold the forearm with the radial border pointing to the ground. He is then required to bring the abducted thumb up at right angles to the thumb against resistance without bending the terminal joint or hyperextending the metacarpophalangeal joint as both the long flexor and long extensor of the thumb can act as adductors.

MUSCLES OF THE HYPOTHENAR EMINENCE

It is logical to discuss the muscles of the hypothenar eminence next, as their main function is to assist in elevating the fifth metacarpal and opposing the little finger to the thumb.

Abductor digiti minimi

The abductor digiti minimi arises from the pisiform, pisohamate ligament and also from the tendon of flexor carpi ulnaris whose insertion is the same as the origin of the short abductor. The insertion is into the base of the lateral border of the proximal phalanx of the little finger, into the extensor expansion and occasionally into the capsule of the metacarpophalangeal joint. The nerve supply is from the deep branch of the ulnar. The main action is to abduct the little finger from the ring finger, but it is very active in opposition of the thumb to the little finger when it stabilizes the metacarpophalangeal joint. It is also a weak extensor of the little finger. The flexor carpi ulnaris always contracts to stabilize the ulnar border of the wrist when the abductor digiti minimi contracts.

To test the muscle the patient places the hand palm downwards on the desk, and is asked to raise the little finger upwards off the desk and move it sidewards away from the ring finger. This obviates the extensor digiti minimi and extensor digitorum communis deceiving the examiner by abducting because they are fully occupied in maintaining the little finger extended off the desk. The antagonist to the abductor digiti minimi is the third palmar interosseus.

Flexor digiti minimi

The flexor digiti minimi arises from the hook of the hamate and the flexor retinaculum, and is inserted with the abductor digiti minimi.

Opponens digiti minimi

The opponens digiti minimi arises from the hamate and flexor retinaculum, and is inserted into the whole length of the ulnar border of the fifth metacarpal.

Both muscles are supplied by the deep branch of the ulnar nerve and their action is to flex and rotate the proximal phalanx of the fifth finger towards the thumb in opposition.

Their antagonists are the extensors of the proximal phalanx of the little finger.

When the thumb is opposed to the little finger the fifth metacarpal is elevated by the flexor and opponens digiti minimi and rotated towards the thumb by the same muscles. The rotation is possible by virtue of the saddle–shaped joint between the fifth metacarpal and the hamate. The metacarpophalangeal joint is stabilized by those muscles and further by the short abductor and, most important of all, the fourth lumbrical.

EXTENSORS OF THE WRIST

Extensor carpi radialis longus

The extensor carpi radialis longus arises from the lower third of the lateral epicondylar ridge and the lateral intermuscular septum. It inserts into the dorsal aspect of the base of the second metacarpal. It is supplied by the radial nerve.

Extensor carpi radialis brevis

The extensor carpi radialis brevis arises from the common extensor origin and inserts into the base of the third metacarpal. It is supplied by the posterior interosseus branch of the radial nerve.

The action of these muscles is to extend the wrist and, acting synergically with the flexor carpi radialis, to deviate the wrist radially.

Their antagonist is the flexor carpi radialis, which has insertions on both the second and third metacarpals to balance them.

Extensor carpi ulnaris

The extensor carpi ulnaris arises from both the common extensor origin and the aponeurosis shared by flexor carpi ulnaris and flexor digitorum profundus. It is inserted into the dorsal aspect of the base of the fifth metacarpal. The nerve supply is from the posterior interosseus branch of the radial nerve.

It is an extensor of the wrist, and working synergically with its antagonist – the flexor carpi ulnaris – it produces ulnar deviation of the wrist.

The wrist extensors always contract strongly to stabilize the wrist and provide greater leverage when the fingers are flexed. The power of grip is poor when the wrist is fully flexed.

To test these muscles the patient is asked to extend the wrist with the metacarpophalangeal joints flexed. If the muscles are weak, the wrist must be supported in extension. The tendons can be seen and felt at the wrist.

EXTENSOR MECHANISM OF THE FINGERS

Extensor digitorum communis

The extensor digitorum communis arises from the common extensor origin and divides into tendons, one for each finger, in the lower third of the forearm. The tendons form the extensor expansion on the dorsal surface of the phalanges.

Intertendinous bands join the extensor tendons to the middle, ring and little fingers, while the index is usually free. Often, the common extensor to the little finger arises from that of the ring finger.

Opposite the metacarpophalangeal joint the extensor tendon becomes the dorsal ligament of the joint by virtue of fasciculi connecting it to the lateral ligaments. Over the dorsal surface of the phalanges it forms an aponeurosis – the so-called extensor expansion.

Extensor expansion

Landsmeer (1949) and Stack (1962) showed that the extensor expansion is a plexus of tendons rather than a sheet of tissue. The extensor digitorum longus tendon divides into three. The central tendon is attached to the base of the middle phalanx, being stabilized over the centre of the metacarpophalangeal joint by fibrous slips from the volar side of the tendon and by sagittal bands inserting into the deep transverse metacarpal ligaments; the lateral two tendons diverge from it but rejoin to insert into the distal phalanx. Into this basic tendon a number of other tendons are inserted. The dorsal interossei have one of their insertions into the extensor tendon along its length over the proximal phalanx, becoming continuous with that of the other side, forming the extensor hood. These transverse fibres are inseparable from the joint capsule and are attached to the transverse capitular ligament, thus providing a fixed point volarly, but are mobile on the dorsum so that the extensor tendon and this 'hood' can slip distally in flexion and proximally in extension. When the hood is pulled proximally by the long extensor, the interossei are most effective as extensors of the interphalangeal joints.

At the head of the proximal phalanx a lumbrical joins the extensor tendon on the radial side, while on the ulnar side a palmar interosseus is inserted. Each of these tendons divides into two parts – the superficial spiral fibres insert into the base of the

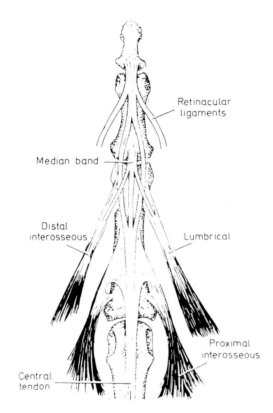

Figure 1.4   Extensor expansion assembly (after H. G. Stack)

middle phalanx, while the deep fibres insert into the lateral band of the tendon. Into the tendon over the middle phalanx, distal to the site where the lateral bands have rejoined, the retinacular ligaments of Landsmeer are inserted on each side (*Figure 1.4*).

Extensor indicis proprius

The extensor indicis proprius arises from the radial border of the posterior surface of the ulna below the origin of extensor pollicis longus and is inserted to one side of the extensor communis tendon to the index finger, in the extensor expansion.

Extensor digiti minimi

The extensor digiti minimi arises from the common extensor origin and is inserted into the extensor expansion of the little finger.

Both muscles are supplied by the posterior interosseus branch of the radial nerve. As the index and little fingers have two extensors, some abduction is possible in these fingers when the interossei are paralysed (see Chapter 3).

The main function of the long extensors of the fingers is to extend the metacarpophalangeal joints, and by virtue of their attachment at these joints they have normally little or no extensor action on the middle and distal phalanges. When the metacarpophalangeal joints are stabilized, however, they can exert some extensor action on these joints. When the capsule of the metacarpophalangeal joint is loose, as is sometimes seen, then the extensor digitorum can extend the interphalangeal joints as well as the metacarpophalangeal joints. Normally, however, the interphalangeal joints can be extended while the metacarpophalangeal joints remain fully flexed. When the metacarpophalangeal joints are fully flexed it is almost impossible to abduct the fingers owing to the tightening of their collateral ligaments.

THE INTRINSIC COMPLEX

Interossei

These are divided into dorsal and palmar interossei; there are four dorsal and three palmar interossei – unless one regards the deep branch of flexor pollicis brevis as a palmar interosseus muscle. This is logical, for the deep branch of the flexor pollicis brevis is concerned with approximating the thumb to the index finger and is supplied by the same nerve as the interossei, whereas the superficial head is usually supplied by the median nerve.

The dorsal interossei have two origins – the superficial belly from adjacent metacarpals, and the deep belly from the metacarpal on which it acts. In general the superficial belly inserts into the tubercle of the proximal phalanx, while the deep belly inserts into the wing tendon.

Zancolli (1968) showed that the insertions of the interossei have individual characteristics which are important. The first dorsal interosseus is a bulky and powerful muscle which is prominent when the thumb is approximated to the index in the plane of the fingers. It has two tendons of insertion – a dorsal tendon inserts into the lateral tubercle of the proximal phalanx which acts as a strong abductor, and a volar tendon which is inserted into the capsule and the collateral ligament of the metacarpophalangeal joint whose main action is flexion of the proximal joint.

Clearly in cases of permanent ulnar palsy when reconstructive surgery is required, the exact insertion of the tendon transfer (such as extensor indicis) is important – if inserted into the dorsal tendon it will abduct the index, if into the volar tendon it will flex the metacarpophalangeal joint.

In addition, the first dorsal interosseus has a middle fleshy portion which is inserted into the transverse fibres of the extensor hood. Zancolli showed that the function of this part of the muscle is to stabilize the long extensor in pinch grip between the tip of the index finger and the thumb. As the muscle does not reach the distal expansion, it qualifies for classification as a proximal interosseus (Stack, 1963). The second dorsal interosseus has, in addition, an insertion into the distal wing of the extensor expansion and thus extends the interphalangeal joints. By virtue of its insertion into the tubercle of the proximal phalanx and the extensor hood, it – like the first dorsal interosseus – is vitally concerned in stabilizing pinch grip between the middle finger and thumb.

Both the first and second dorsal interossei have strong rotatory actions at the metacarpophalangeal joints, allowing screwing and unscrewing movements which are characteristic of these digits.

The angle of approximation of the proximal interossei becomes greater as the metacarpophalangeal joint flexes, and thus rotation is greater and abduction less as the metacarpophalangeal joint is flexed further – precisely the action required on strong unscrewing and screwing.

The third and fourth dorsal interossei insert primarily into the distal wing of the extensor mechanism and thus are strong interphalangeal extensors. They also have an insertion into the volar glenoid ligament and the collateral ligaments of the metacarpophalangeal joints. The palmar (volar) interossei take origin by a single belly from the metacarpal on which they act and all insert into the extensor apparatus. They thus act as interphalangeal extensors as well as adductors of the fingers.

Lumbricals

There is considerable variation in the anatomy of these muscles. The usual situation is that the first and second lumbricals arise from the radial side of the tendons of flexor digitorum profundus to index and middle fingers, whilst the third takes origin from the adjacent sides of the tendons of flexor digitorum profundus to the middle and ring fingers, and the fourth from adjacent sides of flexor digitorum profundus to the ring and little fingers.

The ulnar head of the third lumbrical and the radial head of the fourth lumbrical arise also from the fascial sheath over the deep flexor tendon. Among the many variations from this conventional plan are that all lumbricals may arise from a single head only on the radial side of the corresponding deep flexor tendon, the fourth lumbrical may have two heads, or even all the lumbricals may have two heads each, suggesting that originally there were two lumbricals for each finger. The lumbricals pass volar to the transverse metacarpal ligament and are thus separated from the interossei.

INTRINSIC FUNCTION

A long series of brilliant experiments by Long and Brown (1964) and their colleagues in Cleveland, using electromyography with wire electrodes in all the muscles driving the middle finger, co-ordinated with cinephotography of hand positions and strain gauge dynamometry, has greatly enlarged our understanding of the activity of the intrinsic muscles.

In free movements – that is, without resistance – extension of all joints of the hand is achieved by extensor digitorum communis and the lumbricals. The lumbrical pulls the tendon of flexor digitorum profundus distally, relieving the interphalangeal joints of the passive force towards flexion caused by the viscoelastic properties of the profundus. Clawing of the hand (flexion of the interphalangeal joints and extension of the metacarpophalangeal joints) is exclusively achieved by the extrinsic muscles – extensor digitorum communis and flexor digitorum profundus.

Full flexion of all the joints is also achieved entirely by the extrinsics – flexor digitorum profundus, flexor digitorum sublimis and extensor digitorum communis. The intrinsics are most active in reaching and maintaining the position of metacarpophalangeal flexion and interphalangeal extension. In resisted movement the lumbricals are active in rotation movements of the index finger, as interphalangeal extensors, in stabilizing pinch grip and in extension of the interphalangeal joints against resistance – for example, in flicking objects. In pinch and precision grips the interossei act as abductors and rotators – that is, in anti-clockwise rotation the right first dorsal interosseus abducts and rotates and the first lumbrical stabilizes the interphalangeal joints in extension. In clockwise rotation the first volar interosseus rotates and adducts the index finger.

In pinch and opposition grips the interossei are active as metacarpophalangeal flexors, as are the lumbricals to some extent, as stabilizers of the interphalangeal joints. However, the main function of the lumbricals may well be to act as a source of information as to the position of the metacarpophalangeal and interphalangeal joints in relation to each other, to the state of tension in the various muscles acting on the particular digit and on the rate of change of position of the joints. The necessity for some such system can readily be appreciated when considering the technique of playing the piano. The pianist needs to know instantaneously and automatically the speed at which all movements are occurring at the metacarpophalangeal joints, for it is the state of tension in the metacarpophalangeal and interphalangeal joints which determines touch and dynamics.

It was shown by Rabischong (1962) that the lumbricals contain more annulospiral endings per unit length than any other muscle in the body. Their anatomical situation linking the main extrinsic flexor with the extensor mechanism is peculiarly suitable for them to act as indicators of degree and rates of change in the position and muscle tension of the digit they serve.

The long flexors and extensors acting alone cannot control the two-joint mechanism of metacapophalangeal and interphalangeal joints. A third muscle force is required to allow any of these joints to assume positions independent to each other. Thus it is possible to have a whole range of movements from full metacarpophalangeal and interphalangeal extension to full flexion of these joints, with all combinations of reciprocal static and dynamic movements between the two extremes. Thus the terminal interphalangeal joint can be hyperextended, the proximal interphalangeal joint flexed and the metacarpophalangeal joint of the index finger flexed as in writing, or the interphalangeal joints flexed and metacarpophalangeal joints extended as in a strong hook grip.

Precision activities rely also on interdependence of proximal and distal interphalangeal movements. When the proximal joint is fully flexed passively, extension of the distal joint is limited and weak, and, as the middle phalanx extends, so too does the distal phalanx. This interdependence is based on the double insertion of the intrinsic and extrinsic muscles on the middle and distal phalanges.

POSITION OF FUNCTION

When the hand has to be immobilized for any reason – in plaster after fractures, in splints during the acute stages of poliomyelitis or rheumatoid arthritis, in bandages and splints after operation – there is an optimum position of the hand in which, if stiffness does develop, it will function better than in any other.

The wrist should be in 20 degrees' dorsiflexion, the metacarpophalangeal joints in some 45 degrees' flexion (at 135 degrees), the proximal interphalangeal joints in 30 degrees' (at 150 degrees), and the distal interphalangeal joints in 20 degrees' flexion (at 160 degrees). The thumb should be in half palmar abduction and half opposition, the interphalangeal joint in a few degrees of flexion.

The elbow should be in 90 degrees' flexion and the mid-prone position and the shoulder in 45 degrees' abduction, 30 degrees' flexion and in neutral rotation.

ANOMALOUS INNERVATION

The innervation of the intrinsic muscles of the hand varies from the classical description more frequently than is generally realized. Seddon (1954) found that variations occurred in 20 per cent of 226 cases of peripheral nerve injuries studied. Every gradation is found from complete ulnar nerve supply to complete median innervation of the intrinsic muscles. The commonest variation is in the supply of flexor pollicis brevis. In one-third of cases the ulnar supplies both heads, in one-third the median, and in one-third there is a double innervation. The median nerve can supply the third lumbrical, and in some 10 per cent of cases we have seen, the ulnar nerve has supplied the opponens. Occasionally, the nerve supplying abductor pollicis brevis or the opponens, or both, takes a very tortuous course beneath the skin on emerging from under the flexor retinaculum. It is thus exposed to trauma and explains the puzzling phenomenon of isolated short abductor or abductor and opponens palsy sometimes seen.

It is extremely rare for anomalies to involve the radial nerve, though radial supply of the dorsal interossei has been described.

To test for the presence of anomalous innervation the median and ulnar nerves are stimulated at the elbow and wrist, and contraction looked for in the hand muscles. It is necessary to stimulate at the elbow as well as the wrist, for the nerve supply to the interossei may occasionally travel to the elbow in the median nerve and then cross over to the ulnar in the forearm.

SENSATION

The hand is a most important sensory organ, and its skin, particularly on the palmar surface, is richly supplied with all types of sensory receptor. As Napier (1956) wittily pointed out, the hand is an organ of touch which can feel round corners and see in the dark. The nail must also be considered a sense organ for it can judge textures and shapes when skin sensation is absent. In our experience the nerve supply to the palm of the hand is remarkably constant. In some 5 per cent of patients with peripheral nerve injuries, the median or ulnar nerve supplied the whole of the ring finger. Otherwise, anomalous sensory innervation was rare although wider variations are described. One patient was seen in whom the ulnar nerve supplied the little finger, the ring finger and the ulnar half of the middle finger. In this patient the ulnar nerve supplied all the hand muscles except abductor pollicis brevis.

The median nerve divides into lateral and median branches after piercing the flexor retinaculum. The lateral branch supplies the short muscles of the thumb and then gives off three digital branches, two to the thumb and one to the radial side of the index finger. The medial branch divides into two digital branches, one supplying the ulnar side of the middle finger and the radial side of the ring finger. This branch anastomoses with the ulnar nerve. The digital nerves also communicate with the radial nerve on the dorsal surfaces of the proximal phalanx. The ulnar nerve divides into superficial terminal and deep terminal branches beneath the flexor retinaculum. The deep terminal branch is a motor nerve to the third and fourth lumbricals, interossei, adductor pollicis and deep head of the flexor pollicis brevis. The superficial terminal branch divides into two branches, one supplying the ulnar border of the little finger and the other the radial side of the little finger and the ulnar side of the ring finger, and also supplies the hypothenar muscles.

The palmar cutaneous branch of the median arises in the lower part of the forearm and supplies the skin of the thenar eminence where it anastomoses with the radial nerve and the skin of the palm.

The palmar cutaneous branch of the ulnar nerve arises about the middle of the forearm and supplies the skin of the palm communicating with the median nerve.

On the dorsal aspect of the hand the terminal phalanx of the thumb, the middle and distal phalanges of the index and middle fingers, and the radial half of the middle and distal phalanges of the ring finger is supplied by the median nerve.

The ulnar nerve supplies via its palmar digital branches the dorsal surface of the ulnar side of the middle and distal phalanges of the ring finger and the dorsal surface of the distal phalanx of the little finger. By its dorsal branch and via these digital branches the ulnar nerve supplies the fifth metacarpal and proximal and middle phalanges of the little finger and the ulnar half of the proximal phalanx and metacarpal of the ring finger. It communicates with the radial nerve.

The rest of the back of the hand is supplied by the median and radial and occasionally the ulnar nerves; the exact supply is very variable. In some people the radial nerve only supplies autonomously skin over the first dorsal interosseus space – severance of the radial nerve often results in no loss of sensation in the hand at all, but many people have a volar innervation on the pulp of the thumb from the radial nerve. In the majority of 30 patients whose median nerves Fetrow (1970) blocked with local anaesthetic, there was 10 mm radial innervation on both radial and ulnar borders of the thumb. The sensory distribution in the hand is shown in *Figure 1.5*.

Physiology of sensation

Earlier workers described two types of sensation – crude or protopathic and fine or epicritic. Return of sensation after peripheral nerve injuries was supposed to be in two stages – protopathic first and later epicritic. This theory no longer holds its ground; the intensification of sensation in the early stages of nerve regeneration, or so-called protopathic sensation, is now believed to be due to lack of insulation of the growing nerve fibres which disappears as they acquire their myelin sheaths.

There are four primary modes of sensation – touch, pain, cold and warmth. 'The relation of light touch to painless pressure remains obscure' (Walshe, 1942). As Walshe pointed out, pressure may derive from the activity of both cutaneous and deep sensory mechanisms; it is a concept rather than a primary sensation.

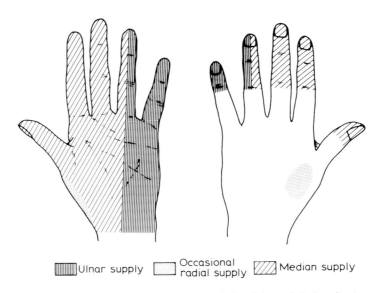

Ulnar supply   Occasional radial supply   Median supply

Figure 1.5   Sensory supply of the hand as deduced from clinical studies in peripheral nerve injuries

Similarly, two-point discrimination is a judgement, not a primary sensation, and to some extent depends on the patient's intelligence.

In a peripheral nerve injury, testing for sensation reveals two areas of sensory disturbance: an outer area where sensation is diminished but not absent (due to adjacent nerves overlapping), and an inner area where it is completely lost. Normal skin does not respond to temperatures within −5°C (5°F) of the skin temperature. Thermal hypoaesthesia consists in widening of the indifferent range and diminished intensity of thermal sensation (Walshe, 1942).

Trotter (quoted by Walshe, 1942) pointed out that there is transitory hyperalgesia for some hours after nerve section, then for 10 days it disappears, only to reappear for 6 weeks and then disappear entirely.

Clinically, all modalities of sensation should be tested – pain, touch, joint sensation, temperature, stereognosis and two-point discrimination. The patient should first be asked to indicate the affected area, and to say if feeling is completely absent, diminished, excessive or altered.

LOCALIZATION

A most important parameter of sensation is the ability to localize correctly with the eyes shut.

In recovered peripheral nerve injuries there is almost invariably a degree of cross-reinnervation, which leads to incorrect localization of stimulus. This may seriously hamper function although much can be done to overcome this by re-education.

The examiner touches the blindfold patient in various places, which should include finger tip, palmar, lateral and dorsal surfaces of proximal, middle and distal phalanges, thenar and hypothenar eminences and middle of the palm. The patient is asked to describe where he has been touched and, if he finds this difficult, to indicate where on the unaffected hand. A record is kept of the number of correct answers and the sites where inaccuracies were found.

STEREOGNOSIS

The more one's experience with the functional assessment of rehabilitation of nerve injuries increases, the less attention one is inclined to pay to academic tests of sensation. The function of sensation is to allow recognition of texture, weight, shape and size, and if activity is required, to relate this to power of grip. Thus, the only rational way of testing sensation is by function.

The authors have introduced a system of sensory re-education into the rehabilitation of peripheral nerve injuries which is fully described in Chapter 3.

A subject with normal sensory function should be able to recognize quickly when blindfold, textures of materials in common use, such as wool, felt, sandpaper, the nature and shape of everyday objects such as buttons, coins, safety pins, keys, corkscrews, and to gauge correctly the difference in weight between objects in each hand to a few grams. Tables have been compiled of average times taken in such tests, in normal people, and are presented in Chapter 3.

We feel that abnormalities of sensation are more realistically described and assessed in terms of slowness or inaccuracy in recognition of the nature of objects than in more academic tests, which are often difficult to perform accurately and require a high degree of co-operation, intelligence and patience on the part of the subject.

SWEAT TESTS

These may occasionally be useful when it is difficult to map out the area of sensory loss in a patient. The dye method involves applying quinazarin powder to the affected limb and heating the patient in a special hot chamber. When the dye changes colour to deep blue, sweating is present. Where sweating is absent no change in colour occurs. Alternatively, the skin resistance may be measured by electrical means. High values indicate absence of sweating, as the skin resistance is always higher in dry than in moist skin.

The sensory innervation and sweat distribution are by no means always coincident.

TEMPERATURE

Elaborate systems of temperature measurement are not called for. The surface of a clinical tuning fork is adequate for testing cold sensation and a test tube of warm water for heat.

PAIN

Pain is tested by applying a sharp needle perpendicularly and at a constant pressure over the skin to detect the dividing line between present and absent or altered sensation. The needle is dragged slowly and at a uniform pressure across the skin. The test should be repeated before the area of pain sensitivity is finally mapped out.

TOUCH

A von Frey's hair is the most accurate method of testing touch, though cotton wool used carefully and with a fine applied tip may be adequate.

JOINT SENSATION

Each joint is moved several times with constant pressure in all directions, the joints above and below being supported by the examiner. The patient is asked to say which joint is being moved and in which direction. This test should be explained carefully to the patient and demonstrated first on the unaffected hand. A record should be made of whether the patient detects fine or only gross movements, and in what proportion of tests he is correct in judging the direction.

Table 1.1   Two-point discrimination in the hand (measured in millimetres; figures in parentheses denote extremes)

Site	Thumb		Index		Middle		Ring		Little	
	Dorsal	Palmar	Dorsal	Palmar	Dorsal	Palmar	Dorsal	Palmar	Dorsal	Palmar
Terminal phalanx	2.5 (1–6)	2.75 (1.5–2.75)	3.5 (1.5–6)	2.25 (0.5–4)	2.75 (1–7)	2 (1.5–3)	4 (1–12)	2.5 (0.5–4)	3.5 (2–6)	2.5 (0.5–5)
Middle phalanx			3.5 (0.5–5)	3.3 (1–6)	3.1 (1–8)	3.25 (1–6)	3 (1–7)	5 (2.5–7)	4 (2–8)	2.5 (2–6)
Proximal phalanx	4.25 (1–9)	4.5 (2.5–7)	4.5 (1–12)	5 (3.5–8)	3 (1–7)	5 (2–8)	3.5 (0.5–10)	4.5 (2–6)	2.5 (0.5–4)	4.5 (2–8)
Thenar eminence:										
Base		3.75 (1–6)								
Middle		11 (10–13)								
Distal crease				6 (5.5–7)		6 (3.5–8)		8 (3–10)		4 (2–6)

Mid-palm: 9 (4–15)   Hypothenar eminence: middle, 7 (5–9); base, 3 (1–3.5)

TWO-POINT DISCRIMINATION

A compass can be used to measure the least distance between the two points at which the patient can feel two and not one prick. We prefer Mannerfelt's 'preprogrammed' apparatus (*Figure 1.6*). Comparable areas on the normal hand should be tested and measurements made, because this modality varies in different people and is said to vary in different occupations. *Table 1.1* shows the values for normal found by the author in 50 young male subjects; the values did not seem to bear any relation to occupation.

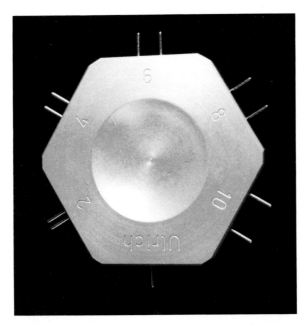

Figure 1.6 Mannerfelt apparatus for estimating two-point discrimination

The presence of accurate two-point discrimination is related directly to precision grip. Moberg, Swanson and Wynn Parry (1971) have stated that 6 mm two-point discrimination is required for winding up a watch, 6–8 mm for sewing, and for handling precision tools 12 mm. Periodic estimates of two-point discrimination at the finger tip, over the thenar and hypothenar eminences and over the proximal and middle phalanges depending on the peripheral nerve involved, are useful as a guide to anatomical reinnervation.

Functional recovery, however, is of more importance and this is tested best by assessing stereognosis.

It is our practice in examining sensation, first to ask the patient to map out the area of sensory loss and sensory abnormality with a finger. Then with his eyes shut, pain sensation is tested with a pin, and touch with the examiner's finger and the von Frey hair.

Finally, a base line is taken of the performance in the sensory function tests.

In testing for all types of sensation the patient must be asked to describe what he feels as accurately as he can, particular attention being paid to added sensation or altered response.

When testing for touch the patient must be asked to say if the sensation is that of touch, pressure, tinglings or a numb sort of feeling. Similarly, when testing for pain, inquiry should be made into the presence of excess pain or a feeling of pressure only.

JOINT RANGE

The range of movement of the metacarpophalangeal and interphalangeal joints is said to depend very much on the patient's occupation and age. It is always advisable to note the range of movement in the equivalent unaffected joints when examining joints with a limited range of movement.

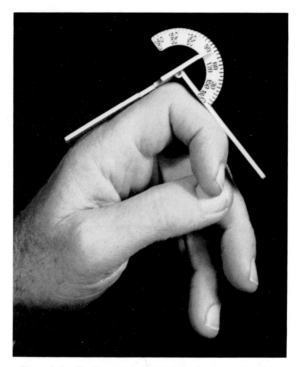

Figure 1.7   Goniometer for measuring finger movements

When testing joint range a small goniometer in the form of a protractor with moveable arrow indicators is used (*Figure 1.7*).

Tables 1.2 to *1.5* give the range of movement of flexion and extension in the joints of the finger and thumb found by the author in 100 normal young adult males. It is remarkable how little trade and laterality affect the range of movement.

Table 1.2 Average range of movement in normal proximal interphalangeal joints and normal metacarpophalangeal joints (by degrees)

Joints	Preferred hand			Non-preferred hand		
	Skilled	Sedentary	Heavy	Skilled	Sedentary	Heavy
Proximal interphalangeal						
Index	105	107	100	106	106	103
Middle	103	106	103	102	104	102
Ring	104	109	105	108	107	105
Little	100	105	100	101	102	100
Metacarpophalangeal						
Index	86	84	82	84	84	79
Middle	87	87	86	88	87	85
Ring	85	87	86	85	86	84
Little	87	87	89	89	86	88

Table 1.3 Limits of normal range of movement in proximal interphalangeal and metacarpophalangeal joints (by degrees)

Joints	Preferred hand			Non-preferred hand		
	Skilled	Sedentary	Heavy	Skilled	Sedentary	Heavy
Proximal interphalangeal						
Index	90–130	90–125	90–115	90–130	80–120	85–115
Middle	90–115	90–130	90–125	90–125	90–120	80–115
Ring	75–120	90–125	90–125	90–135	90–126	80–120
Little	70–120	85–150	85–120	85–125	90–130	90–115
Metacarpophalangeal						
Index	75–95	70–95	75–90	70–95	60–95	70–90
Middle	80–100	80–95	70–95	80–100	65–95	75–90
Ring	75–90	75–95	75–95	75–95	80–100	70–95
Little	75–95	65–95	70–95	75–100	75–105	80–100

Table 1.4 Average range, and limits (in parenthesis), of movement in normal distal interphalangeal joint (by degrees)

Fingers	Preferred hand			Non-preferred hand		
	Skilled	Sedentary	Heavy	Skilled	Sedentary	Heavy
Index	72 (55–90)	72 (55–90)	71 (60–90)	73 (45–85)	74 (60–90)	73 (60–95)
Middle	75 (60–100)	75 (65–95)	70 (65–90)	76 (45–90)	78 (65–95)	75 (50–95)
Ring	73 (55–95)	73 (55–90)	70 (60–85)	73 (45–90)	73 (60–95)	70 (50–90)
Little	76 (60–90)	73 (50–90)	77 (60–90)	79 (55–95)	79 (55–85)	76 (50–85)

Table 1.5   Average range, and limits (in parentheses), of movement in normal interphalangeal joint of thumb (by degrees)

Preferred hand			Non-preferred hand		
Skilled	*Sedentary*	*Heavy*	*Skilled*	*Sedentary*	*Heavy*
90	97	89	88	91	88
(65–115)	(65–135)	(70–120)	(70–110)	(65–110)	(65–105)

When measuring joint range the values from full extension to full flexion possible both actively and passively must be recorded; for example, the measurements given in *Table 1.5* might be recorded following tendon grafting.

Joint range
Index finger, left hand

Terminal interphalangeal joint	Active	10–30	=	20 degrees of flexion
	Passive	10–90		
Proximal interphalangeal joint	Active	30–60	=	30 degrees of flexion
	Passive	30–70		
Metacarpophalangeal joint	Active	10–90	=	80 degrees of flexion
	Passive	10–80		

Not, as one often sees recorded:

Terminal interphalangeal joint	20 degrees	(80 degrees passive)
Proximal interphalangeal joint	30 degrees	(80 degrees passive)
Metacarpophalangeal joint	80 degrees	(90 degrees passive)

When an increase in range is recorded the latter method does not allow one to judge if the flexion deformity is being overcome or if further flexion is occurring due to increased excursion of the tendon, or both.

When there is limitation of movement in the metacarpophalangeal or carpometacarpal joints of the thumb, the range of maximum palmar abduction should be measured in centimetres to get a value of the web stretch, and flexion and extension measured by the distance the thumb with the interphalangeal joint extended can flex and extend from the index finger. Opposition can be roughly measured by taking the angle the thumb pad makes with the horizontal; abduction and adduction can be measured passively by taking the distance between the proximal end of the nails of two adjacent fingers.

GRIP

Apart from the long flexors of the fingers and thumb, the intrinsics and wrist and finger extensors are of great importance as stabilizers in gripping.

During recovery in an ulnar or median nerve lesion, the value of grip increases markedly when the interossei begin to recover. Similarly, in a radial nerve palsy the power improves greatly as the wrist and metacarpophalangeal extensors recover.

Commonly, the grip is only 20 per cent of normal when the wrist and finger extensors are paralysed.

We use the Mannerfelt dynamometers, which have three bulbs of different sizes according to the size of the hand (*Figure 1.8*).

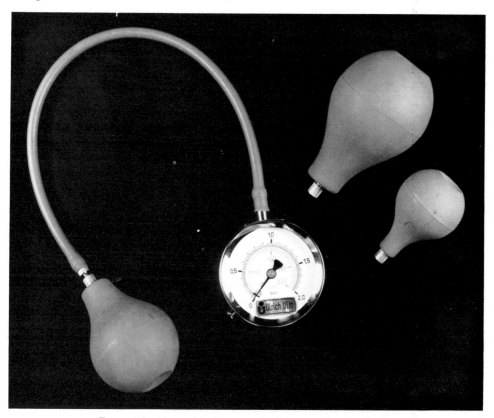

Figure 1.8   Mannerfelt dynamometer for measuring hand grip

Table 1.6   Average force in the power grip of 100 persons: 50 male and 50 female (in kg force)

			Skilled	*Sedentary*	*Manual*
Male	Major hand	47.6	47	47.2	48.5
	Minor hand	45	45.4	44.1	44.6
Female	Major hand	24.6	26.8	23.1	24.2
	Minor hand	22.4	24.4	21.1	22

The patient is asked to grip the bulb as hard as he can while the examiner supports the instrument round the stem. Three readings are taken at intervals of 15 seconds. The difference in the readings between the normal and the affected hand is recorded, thus allowing for changes in the pressure with use. Both hands should always be

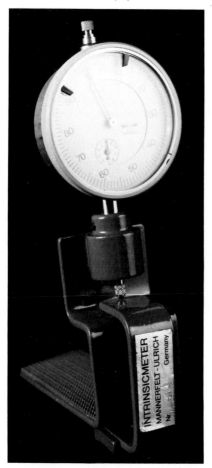

Figure 1.9   Mannerfelt dynamometer for measuring the power of the intrinsic muscles

tested, as the power of the unaffected hand invariably improves with treatment; it is the difference between the two hands which is of significance.

Pinch grip and the power of individual intrinsic muscles can be conveniently measured with the Mannerfelt strain gauge dynamometer (*Figure 1.9*). *Tables 1.6 to 1.10* show average values of grip. Wainerdi (1950) found values of 5.9–8.8 kg for women and 6.8–10 kg for men.

Table 1.7   Variation of the force of power grip according to age (in kg force)

	Age (years):	<20	20–30	30–40	40–50	50–60
Male	Major hand	45.2	48.5	49.2	49	45.9
	Minor hand	42.6	46.2	44.5	47.3	43.5
Female	Major hand	23.8	24.6	30.8	23.4	22.3
	Minor hand	22.8	22.7	28.0	21.5	18.2

Napier (1956) showed that grip can be broadly divided into two types – precision grip and power grip – and this classification has been universally accepted.

Power grip is exemplified by holding a hammer; the wrist is in 10–20 degrees' dorsiflexion and slight ulnar deviation, the thumb and fingers adducted at the metacarpophalangeal joints and the fingers flexed at the interphalangeal joints. In a precision grip, as in holding a paintbrush, the thumb is opposed to the index finger which is abducted and rotated and the fingers slightly flexed at all joints, and the wrist is held in very slight dorsiflexion. The pulp of the finger tip can adjust to the shape of whatever is being gripped. Very broadly speaking, the median nerve is most important for precision and the ulnar nerve for power.

In pinch grip, such as holding a key to open a lock, adduction of the thumb to the index finger using the adductor pollicis and the first dorsal interosseus and firm apposition of thumb tip to index tip, is required using the long flexors and extensors of

Table 1.8   Average force of the precision grip (in kg force)

			Skilled	Sedentary	Manual
Male	Major hand	7.9	7.3	8.4	8.5
	Minor hand	7.5	7.2	7.3	7.6
Female	Major hand	5.2	5.4	4.2	6.1
	Minor hand	4.9	4.6	4.0	5.6

Table 1.9   Average force in the pinch grip (lateral grip) (in kg force)

			Skilled	Sedentary	Manual
Male	Major hand	7.5	6.6	6.3	8.5
	Minor hand	7.1	6.4	6.1	7.7
Female	Major hand	4.9	4.4	4.1	6.0
	Minor hand	4.7	4.3	3.9	5.5

Table 1.10   Average of pinch with separate finger (in kg force)

		Index	Middle	Ring	Little
Male	Major hand	5.3	5.6	3.8	2.3
	Minor hand	4.8	5.7	3.6	2.2
Female	Major hand	3.6	3.8	2.5	1.7
	Minor hand	3.3	3.4	2.4	1.6

the thumb and the flexor digitorum profundus of the index finger. Pinch grip is often the only function left in rheumatoid disease when the metacarpophalangeal joints are disorganized and there is severe ulnar drift, and it is remarkable how wide a range of functional activities are still possible (*Figure 1.10*).

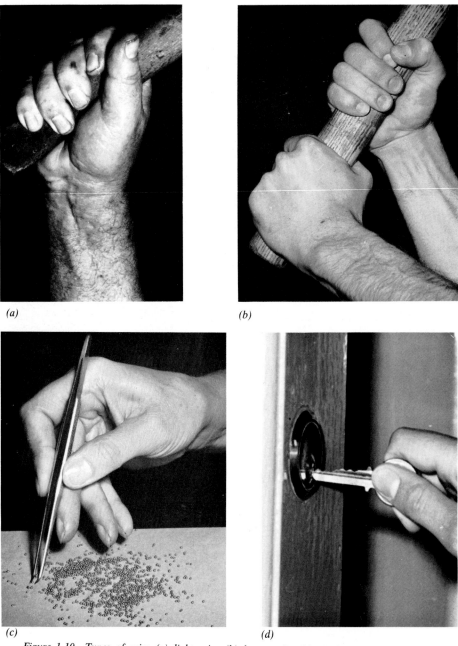

(a)   (b)

(c)   (d)

Figure 1.10   Types of grip: (a) light grip; (b) heavy grip; (c) pinch grip; (d) key grip

Swanson noted (Moberg, Swanson and Wynn Parry, 1971) that the various pinch patterns are used with different frequencies:

Prehensive movement	*Pulp*	*Lateral*	*Tip*
Picking up	50%	33%	17%
Holding	88%	10%	2%

and emphasized that, if one is lost, the other can be used well to perform the task. There is one other type of grip used when prolonged power grip is required: the hook grip, using flexion of the proximal interphalangeal joints by the action of flexor digitorum sublimis, as in carrying a heavy suitcase.

Apart fom the various types of grip, the fingers are used in free movements, such as typing, playing musical instruments, picking up objects, flicking, brushing, buttoning and unbuttoning. All these activities depend primarily on movement and stability at the metacarpophalangeal joints and their integrity is vital to hand function. Thus the correct positioning of these joints, when immobilization of the hand is necessary for any reason, is of paramount importance and when the hand becomes stiff it is mobility of the metacarpophalangeal joints that must be restored.

With fixed metacarpophalangeal joints and mobile interphalangeal joints only a hook grip is possible. With mobile metacarpophalangeal joints and stiff interphalangeal joints most hand functions are possible. This explains the specialized anatomy of the metacarpophalangeal joints, their more varied range of motion and the complexity of the ligamentous arrangement as compared with the interphalangeal joints.

For very powerful activities the hand is used to grasp the object and the power is provided by the shoulder, elbow and wrist in diminishing proportions. The shoulder depressors, pectorals and deltoid are the most important at the shoulder. To maintain stability at the elbow a strong triceps and brachialis are required. At the wrist, the flexor carpi ulnaris is probably the most important, being marginally stronger than the flexor carpi radialis, and should be the last muscle to be considered for tendon transfer.

Tables 1.6 to *1.10* indicate the force of various types of grip (Moberg, Swanson and Wynn Parry, 1971).

SUMMARY OF NERVE SUPPLY TO MUSCLES

Ulnar nerve in the hand
Hypothenar group – abductor, flexor and opponens digiti minimi
Third and fourth lumbricals
All interossei
Adductor pollicis
Half flexor pollicis brevis (deep head)
(All have root supply C8, T1)

Median nerve in the hand
Thenar group – opponens pollicis, abductor pollicis brevis, half flexor pollicis brevis (superficial head)
First and second lumbricals
(All have root supply C8, T1)

Radial nerve
Triceps (C6, 7)
Brachioradialis (C5, 6)
Extensor carpi radialis longus (C6, 7)

Posterior interosseus nerve
Supinator (C5, 6)
Extensor carpi radialis brevis (C6, 7)
Extensor carpi ulnaris (C7, 8)
Extensor digitorum communis (C7, 8)
Extensor digiti minimi, extensor indicis
Extensor pollicis longus (C7, 8)
Extensor pollicis brevis (C7, 8)
Abductor pollicis longus (C7, 8)

ROOT SUPPLY OF SENSATION

Based on a study by Inouye and Buchthal (1978) in which spinal nerve potentials were recorded at the level of the fifth to eighth cervical roots, potentials were evoked by stimulation of the fingers, radial nerve at the wrist, musculocutaneous nerve at the elbow and the axillary nerve over the deltoid. Considerable individual variation was found.

	Usual supply	*Variation*
Over deltoid	C5	C6
Elbow	C6	–
Dorsal side of hand	C7	C6–8
Thumb	C6	C7
Index finger	C7	C6–8
Middle finger	C7	C8
Little finger	C7	C8

REFERENCES AND BIBLIOGRAPHY

Backhouse, K. M. and Catton, W. T. (1954). Experimental study of functions of the lumbrical muscles in the human hand. *Journal of Anatomy* **88**, 133–141
Bunnell, S. (1970). *Surgery of the Hand*, 5th edn. Ed. by J. H. Boyes. Philadelphia, Pa: Lippincott
Dubousset, J. (1971). Functional anatomy of the capsulo-ligamentous apparatus of the joints of the fingers. In *Traumatismes Osteoarticulaires de la Main*, pp. 3–26. Paris: Expansion Scientifique
Duchenne, G. B. (1949). *Physiology of Motion*. Translated and edited by E. B. Kaplan. Philadelphia, Pa: Lippincott
Fetrow, K. (1970). Practical and important variations in sensory nerve supply to the hand. *The Hand* **2**, 178–184

Inouye, I. and Buchthal, F. (1978). Segmental sensory innervation determined by potentials recorded from cervical spinal nerves. *Brain* **100**, 731–748

Kaplan, E. B. (1965). *Functional and Surgical Anatomy of the Hand*, 2nd edn. Philadelphia, Pa: Lippincott

Landsmeer, J. M. F. (1949). The anatomy of the dorsal aponeurosis of the human finger and its functional sigificance. *Anatomical Record* **104**, 31–44

Long, C. (1960). An electromyographic study of the extrinsic intrinsic kinesiology of the hand. *Archives of Physical Medicine and Rehabilitation* **41**, 175–181

Long, C. and Brown, M. E. (1964). Electromyographic kinesiology of the hand. Muscles moving the long finger. *Journal of Bone and Joint Surgery* **46A**, 1683–1706

Mackenzie, W. C. (1930). *The Action of Muscles,* p. 103. London: Lewis

Moberg, E., Swanson, A. and Wynn Parry, C. B. (1971). Report to International Federation of Societies for Surgery of the Hand

Napier, J. R. (1956). The prehensile movements of the human hand. *Journal of Bone and Joint Surgery* **38B**, 902–913

Rabischong, P. (1962). L'innervation proprioceptive des muscles lombricaux de la main chez l'homme. *Revue Chirurgie Orthopedique et Reparatrice de l'Appareil Moteur* **48**, 234–245

Rank, B. K. and Hueston, J. T. (1973). *Surgery of Repair as Applied to Hand Injuries*, 4th edn. Edinburgh: Livingstone

Seddon, H. J. (Ed.) (1954). *Peripheral Nerve Injuries*. Medical Research Council Report Series No. 282. London: HMSO

Stack, H. G. (1962). Muscle function in the fingers. *Journal of Bone and Joint Surgery* **44B**, 890–892

Stack, H. G. (1963). A study of muscle function in the fingers. *Annals of the Royal College of Surgeons of England* **33**, 307–322

Valentin, P. (1962). Contribution à l'etude anatomique physiologique et clinique de l'apparell extenseur des doigts. Thesis, Paris

Wainerdi, H. R. (1950). Simple ergometers for measuring the strength of the hand grip. *Journal of the American Medical Association* **144**, 619–620

Walshe, F. M. R. (1942). The anatomy and physiology of cutaneous sensibility. *Brain* **65**, 48–112

Wood-Jones, F. (1942). *The Principles of Anatomy as Seen in the Hand*. Baltimore, Md: Williams & Wilkins

Zancolli, E. (1968). *Structural and Dynamic Bases of Hand Surgery*. Philadelphia, Pa: Lippincott. (2nd edn, 1979)

Injuries to Tendons 2

In this chapter the management of the hand after surgery for tendon lesions is described in detail. The conventional division of flexor tendon lesions into those at the wrist and those in 'no man's land' has been adopted and lesions of the extensor tendons divided into those at the wrist and over the dorsum of the hand, and those in the fingers. Our material comprises 440 flexor tendon lesions of the fingers, 80 lesions of flexor pollicis longus and 79 severe lesions of the extensors.

FLEXOR TENDONS

The anatomy of the flexor tendons was described in detail in Chapter 1, but it will be recalled here that there is a very small space between the metacarpophalangeal joint and the proximal interphalangeal joint in which the sublimis and profundus tendons glide. In the palm there is more room for the tendons to move and greater elasticity of the surrounding tissues, so injuries of the tendons at this site are less likely to result in adherence. At the wrist there is plenty of space surrounding the tendons, and damage here is less likely to cause adherence than in the palm. Owing to the confined space in which the tendons move in the finger itself, injuries to the finger tendons are far more disabling and present much greater problems than in the palm or at the wrist.

INJURIES OF THE FLEXOR TENDONS AT THE WRIST

Causative factors

The commonest cause of tendon injuries at the wrist is a fall on glass or on sharp objects such as stones, metal and the edges of tins. Accidents with knives are fairly common, as are the results of plunging the hand through a window pane. Patients who sustain injuries to the flexor tendons through window panes usually damage one or other of the nerves and almost invariably the ulnar or radial artery.

Frequency

The commonest tendons to be affected in order of frequency are the palmaris longus, the flexor carpi radialis, flexor carpi ulnaris, sublimis and profundus tendons of the fingers. The ulnar artery is often involved with the tendon injury. When the nerves are affected the tendons involved depend on which nerve is severed. In our series of nerve injuries at the wrist, the tendons involved most often with an ulnar nerve lesion were the flexor carpi ulnaris, the flexor profundus and flexor sublimis to the ring and little fingers; the ulnar artery was involved almost as commonly. When the median nerve was affected, the tendons involved most frequently were the flexor pollicis longus, the flexor of the index finger, the flexor carpi radialis and the palmaris longus. When both median and ulnar nerves are affected, it is usual for most structures in front of the wrist joint to be severed. It is unusual to have a nerve injury at the wrist without tendon involvement, but it is quite common to have tendon injuries without nerve involvement.

Treatment

Simple lesions of the tendons at the wrist present no problems and normally do not require formal rehabilitation.

If the tendons have been cut above the carpal tunnel, primary suture is always successful provided the wound is clean, has been caused by a sharp implement and is seen within 8 hours. If, however, the injury has been associated with crushing, or is dirty, or a skilled surgeon is not available, skin suture only should be performed and secondary tendon suture undertaken 3 weeks later.

If all flexor tendons have been cut within the carpal tunnel, most surgeons excise the sublimis and suture only the profundus to avoid adherence of tendons to each other or to the skin, causing a flexion deformity at the proximal interphalangeal joints.

Following multiple tendon suture, mobilization is usually allowed 3 weeks after surgery, and some 10 days' active exercises under the supervision of a physiotherapist is all that is required.

Severe lacerating wounds at the wrist, involving all tendons and nerves, often result in adherence of the tendons to each other and to the skin. In these circumstances, intensive rehabilitation is essential if any sort of reasonable function is to be obtained. Oil massage is given gently at first, progressing to stronger and deeper massage with circular, transverse and longitudinal movements to break down the adhesions.

Following 10 minutes of such massage, slow, gentle, passive stretch is put on the tendons whilst supporting the metacarpophalangeal joints and trying gradually to extend the proximal interphalangeal joints. This is done at first with the metacarpophalangeal joints in full flexion. As the deformity resolves, increasing extension of the metacarpophalangeal joints can be allowed during this manoeuvre. After the slow gentle stretch a plaster splint is applied to the palmar surface of the forearm, palm and fingers, and bandaged on, being maintained in this position between each treatment session; four to six such sessions are given daily. It is known that such techniques produce cell multiplication and permanent lengthening. A plaster splint is worn at night, which gives some three-quarters full correction. A full correcting splint would be too painful to be worn in the night. In the early stages of recovery plasters may need to be changed once or even twice a day, later every other day and then twice a week. The plasters are used to maintain the movement gained by physiotherapy – they are not *corrective* in the sense of causing continuous stretch. We strongly oppose the type of dorsal splint which produces active stretch with pulleys, elastics or springs, as these tend to produce more deformity than they are attempting to correct. This treatment should not be painful – the secret is slow, gentle correction, to obtain only a degree or two at a time. This, however, is cumulative and over a period of several weeks even very severe deformities can be corrected. The surgical team for whom we work feel that such conservative measures are superior to tenolysis and dissection of fibrous tissue which is always a much more formidable prospect than would appear from clinical examination through the intact skin. Following these physiotherapy sessions, active exercises, games and occupational therapy are prescribed – all to encourage general flexion and function of the hand.

Case 2.1   Figure 2.1 illustrates such a patient who cut all flexor tendons and both median and ulnar nerves at the wrist, with secondary infection and a frozen hand. Intensive oil massage, slow stretches and serial plasters were required, as well as occupational therapy, games and exercises, and the patient made an excellent tendon and neurological recovery.

INJURIES OF THE FLEXOR TENDONS IN THE PALM AND FINGER

In the mid-palm, suture of the flexor tendons gives good results, particularly if the sublimis is excised and the lumbrical wrapped round the sutured profundus so that adherence does not occur. No more formal rehabilitation is usually necessary than for simple lesions at the wrist (when tendons are involved in severe crush or blast injuries the management is entirely different and is discussed on page 37). The management of lesions in the distal part of the palm and in the fibrous flexor sheath, however, present complex problems, the solution of which is still a matter of much debate and controversy. It is usually claimed that suture of both tendons in the fibrous flexor sheath is not feasible, for there is so little room within the sheath that the slightest additional tissue in the form of scarring leads to adherence and a stiff finger, and flexion will occur only at the proximal interphalangeal joint. This area has been termed 'no man's land' and it has been common practice to excise both tendons and to put in a free graft. In the opinion of most authorities this is the treatment of choice unless the surgeon is especially skilled and all the conditions are ideal for primary suture in the flexor tendon sheath.

However, the results of flexor tendon grafts, even in the best hands, still give rise to concern, for the proportion of excellent results remains unsatisfactory and one cannot expect full finger flexion with the tip of the finger flexing to the distal palmar crease in more than 75 per cent of patients. For this reason a number of experienced surgeons undertake suture of the tendon in the fibrous flexor sheath, provided that the wound is clean, seen early within the first 6 hours and that the surgeon is skilled. This is discussed further on pages 51–53. 'No man's land' has been renamed 'châsse gardée'

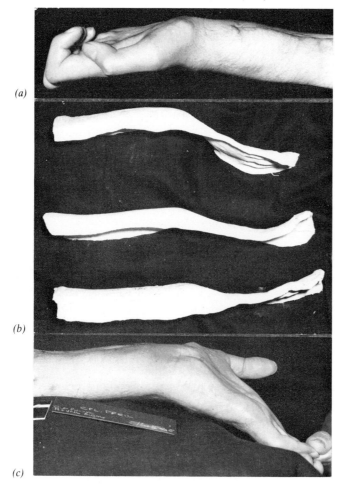

(a)

(b)

(c)

Figure 2.1 Tendon adherence. (a) Lacerating wound extending from mid-forearm to mid-palm with infection, and division of median and ulnar nerves and all flexor tendons. Severe fibrosis developed 5 months after injury. The patient presented for rehabilitation with a frozen hand. There was no active or passive movement at wrist, metacarpophalangeal or interphalangeal joints. (b) Serial plasters used in correction of deformity. (c) Passive correction obtained after 3 months' intensive treatment. (Case 2.1)

(Verdan and Crawford, 1971), indicating that surgery in this area should be reserved for the expert, who may elect to perform primary suture rather than grafting in special circumstances.

Flexor tendon grafts

Grafting can be either secondary, usually 3–4 weeks after injury, which is the commonest technique used, or primary.

Harrison (1969) compared 60 grafts in 57 patients in whom he performed the conventional secondary grafting, 30 with primary grafts and 30 with delayed primary grafts (5–8 days after injury). Secondary grafts were better than primary grafts because at the secondary operation the degree of fibrosis could be seen and excision effected. Harrison prefers delayed primary grafts in which 83 per cent had good results, compared with 75 per cent with secondary grafts and 66 per cent with primary grafts, and return to work was quicker. However, secondary graft is always indicated when there has been skin loss, fracture, crushing or infection. The advantages of early grafting are that the gliding mechanism is intact and withdrawal of divided tendon atraumatic in the absence of fibrous adhesions, and the exact length of tendon replacement can be measured accurately.

Pathology

Skoog and Persson (1954) carried out some interesting experiments on rabbits in order to study the early healing of sutured tendons. They found that the scar tissue which forms between the cut ends of a tendon arises from the peritenon and paratenon, whereas the tendon itself does not appear to make any contribution. It appeared that the paratenon was the most important structure in healing. When a tendon was cut and enclosed in a thin sheath of stainless steel, no significant regeneration occurred during the first 3 weeks. In the case of grafts, the graft was replaced partly by new connective tissue which grew along its entire surface. The endotenon played no active part and the peritenon had no specific role, but in its presence the action of the surrounding tissues was less violent, resulting in somewhat less firm adherence between the graft and its surroundings. Skoog and Persson point out that tissues with a tendency to lay down connective tissue are unhealthy neighbours for a recently operated tendon because of their liability to lay down organized adherence to the peritenon.

Surgical treatment – flexor tendon grafting

The incision is made along the mid-lateral line from the pulp to the base of the finger, and a flap raised to expose the digital theca. This is removed except over the head of the metacarpal and opposite the proximal and middle phalanges where it is preserved as pulleys for the graft. The donor tendon is usually the palmaris longus or, if absent, the plantaris or a toe extensor. The palmaris longus is drawn out through a superior incision in the upper part of the forearm, after being freed by an incision at the wrist. The graft is threaded through the pulleys, the proximal end is sutured, the profundus tendon sutured at the level of the lumbrical muscle belly and the distal end to the tendon stump or terminal phalanx (Campbell Reid, 1966) (*Figure 2.2*).

The length of time for which a finger is immobilized after flexor tendon grafting varies from surgeon to surgeon, but an average time is 17–21 days, during which time the finger is kept completely at rest. Some surgeons take the finger out of plaster at the tenth day and allow active exercises, but most keep the finger completely immobile for up to 3 weeks. It has been shown that there is no advantage in early movement and indeed a tendon does not gain its vascular supply before the third week, and there is therefore a definite danger in starting movements before then. Often there will be some local oedema in the finger and it is important to remove this as early as possible to prevent fibrosis. This means that the hand may need to be kept in elevation at night and indeed during the day, in between sessions of exercise and physiotherapy. For this purpose a special sling has been devised at our Unit which allows the hand to be put in any position of elevation (see Appendix A, *Figure 2.17*).

The skin may be scaly and it is often helpful for the physiotherapist to give some light oil massage to the skin.

For the first 2 weeks the only active exercises allowed are those in which the physiotherapist supports the finger at the metacarpophalangeal, the proximal interphalangeal and the terminal interphalangeal joints and encourages the patient to flex at each joint in turn. Resistance can be given after 5 weeks to the other fingers and such facilitation encourages the graft to work more strongly. It is unwise to give resistance to the affected finger before the sixth week. Thereafter resistance can gradually be increased, first with the physiotherapist preventing the movement and then giving active resistance.

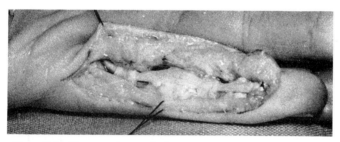

Figure 2.2   Flexor tendon graft; finger at operation. (From Morley, 1956, by courtesy of the author and the Editor of British Journal of Plastic Surgery)

There is usually some degree of adherence of the graft, either in the finger or in the palm, and more often than not it is necessary to give some light massage to loosen these adhesions. This can be given twice a day and may become gradually more vigorous after the sixth week. Friction is best given when the graft is put under tension and is more effective than trying to relieve adherence in the relaxed position. In the early stages oil massage is advisable; later, lanolin can be given as this can produce a deeper effect. At the start of formal rehabilitation some 2–3 weeks after grafting, there is usually a flicker of movement at the terminal interphalangeal joint and up to 10 degrees at the proximal interphalangeal joint. The finger is usually held in about 30 degrees' flexion at the proximal interphalangeal joint, and 10–20 degrees' flexion at the terminal interphalangeal joint. There is no doubt that if the finger is put in marked flexion during the stage of immobilization after grafting, it is extremely difficult to gain reasonable function. Flexion of more than 30 degrees at the proximal interphalangeal joint is likely to lead to a permanent flexion deformity.

Some surgeons are in the habit of bandaging the finger right down in full flexion in the palm, and in our experience such cases do extremely badly. We have never seen in our Unit a patient whose hand was so splinted regain anything like reasonable function.

As well as active exercises between the third and sixth weeks, specific hand games can be played in the physiotherapy department. Games involving string, such as cat's cradles and knotting, making houses with cards, games with matches and simple ball games are all useful, as is any activity involving picking up objects. Occupational therapy is most important, for here the patient is using his hand for functional and absorbing activities.

The following techniques are used in the various stages after grafting in the occupational therapy department at our centres.

Occupational therapy

Occupational therapy activities should be selected to suit the patient; for example, the traditional crafts such as weaving and basketry may well be rejected by young servicemen.

Men prefer using tools and lathes and like to see something useful as a result of their labours. When possible we try to provide activity which will help in the upkeep of the unit. Thus the Gestetner duplicating machine is most useful for providing copies of forms for the administrative work of the centre and the handle of the machine can be padded to provide light repetitive grip in the early stages of activity after tendon surgery. Printing presses have been devised with adaptations which can be quickly and easily adjusted for most hand movements; various grip attachments provide large handle grip, span grip, disc attachments, narrow tubular grips and bilateral grips. Handles can be covered with material enabling the patient with sensory impairment to feel more easily; for example, rough surfaces such as a roller can be covered with cotton string and provide a better sense of grip than a smooth shiny metal handle. Work can be varied in resistance from light to very heavy work. Type-setting using composing sticks and various-sized tweezers provides light resistance. For general office work, preparation of card and paper can be carried out on various guillotines with adaptations similar to those on the printing presses.

Brushmaking. Wire-twisting on a special machine provides hand movement with resistance, and brushes can be made for the hospital or centre.

Cardboard box manufacture. Gripping of small hand tools – small craft knives, stapling machines and rulers – is involved in making boxes, and these can often be produced in bulk for local manufacturers and the profit put back into the department. Polythene bag sealing provides light work and co-ordination to feed polythene into the machine. Movement is mainly at the metacarpophalangeal joints and opposition of the thumb for pinch grip. This activity can provide covers for books and documents as well as a variety of sizes of bag.

Ornamental brick-making. This provides work in the later stages of treatment where resistance is necessary, but it can be graded from light to very hard, depending on the moulds used and the weight of cement in the box 'shaper'. Bricks can be sold for garden reconstruction.

Painting and decorating. A 'do-it-yourself' room is much appreciated where patients can paint walls; various grips are provided for each stage, i.e. for cleaning down the walls, filling and preparing surfaces and scraping.

Cement mixing. This gives really heavy work required in the later stages of tendon rehabilitation. Once more, depending on the nature of the disability, the grips can be specifically constructed to achieve accurate tendon movement. Shovel handles can be altered, different working methods used and the weight of shovels varied. Flagstones and garden seats can be made for the hospital.

Gardening. Provided the patient enjoys gardening, a wide variety of hand movements can be employed: watering, using a trowel and planting out in the greenhouse, in the early stages, as well as digging, fencing and mowing in the later stages.

Wrought iron. This is a useful activity in the later stages of treatment; metal strips are cut to a specific length, shaped round a jig and assembled prior to welding. Applications can be decorative or functional and this activity is very popular.

Carpentry. Carpentry offers a wide range of hand movement: gripping with a saw, rotation with screwdrivers, cylinder grip with a hammer and controlled finger movements with a chisel.

Games. Whenever possible, rehabilitation should be made as enjoyable as possible and so a wide variety of games are provided, all using specific hand movements. These include blow football, using rubber bulb syringes for grip, flip football, using a leather bag on the hand, which encourages extensor movements of the fingers, draughts of varied weights, car race game, beat the clock, rod football in which the handles of the rod carry small wooden figures and can be of varying shape to suit the stage of disability, and magnetic jigsaw puzzles providing light pinch grip (the board can be put upon the wall so that the patient with oedema can work in elevation). All the activities in the occupational therapy department are discussed and illustrated in Chapter 6.

One of the problems in rehabilitation of flexor tendon grafts is that on attempting to flex the interphalangeal joints, the joints are paradoxically extended – this is most common in the middle finger if the graft is too long – for then the shift of the flexor digitorum profundus will exert traction on the lumbrical insertion and extend the interphalangeal joint. It is also seen when there has been too long a delay between the original injury and the flexor tendon grafting, for the patient gets in the habit of flexing the finger by the intrinsic muscles working at the metacarpophalangeal joint only.

To try to overcome this the metacarpophalangeal joint is held in extension and the patient concentrates on moving the interphalangeal joints only. Once resistance is given the splinting effect often returns and it has been found useful at this stage to provide a form of lively splint, such as the Capener (1949) splint (see Appendix B of this chapter, *Figure 2.18*). A double finger stall can often be helpful in overcoming this splinting effect; indeed, double finger stalls are valuable whenever patients find difficulty in flexing the interphalangeal joints and can be introduced at the sixth or seventh week if recovery is slow (*Figure 2.3*). However, conservative treatment may be unsuccessful and, in this event, Parkes (1970) has shown that division of the lumbrical tendon will cure the disability of 'the lumbrical plus finger'.

Course

In an uncomplicated flexor tendon graft there should, by the sixth week, be 30 degrees' movement at the proximal interphalangeal joint and 10–15 degrees'

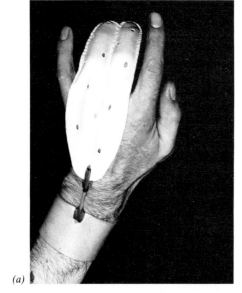 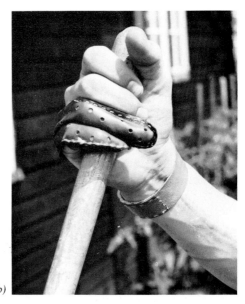

(a)   (b)

Figure 2.3   (a) Double finger stall used in rehabilitation following flexor tendon graft to encourage the use of the grafted finger in the early stages. (b) Double finger stall used in rehabilitation following flexor tendon graft of the little finger.

movement at the terminal interphalangeal joint. By the eighth week there should be at least 45 degrees at the proximal interphalangeal joint and some 20–30 degrees at the terminal interphalangeal joint. It may be some months before full flexion is obtained, and of course in many cases full flexion in which the interphalangeal joints can be brought down to the distal palmar crease never returns, but a reasonable result demands an extension deformity at the proximal interphalangeal joint of no more than 30 degrees and the ability of the finger to touch the palm.

Individual work is of great importance in the re-education of flexor tendon grafts. Occupational therapy and gymnasium activities are vital but there is never any substitute for the physiotherapist giving individual attention at each interphalangeal joint and progressing treatment, particularly by proprioceptive neuromuscular facilitation techniques.

A patient with a simple uncomplicated flexor tendon graft should be fit to return to work 8 weeks after surgery. This implies 5–6 weeks of active rehabilitation. There is no doubt that in adults the best results are obtained if intensive treatment is given daily for at least half a day and if possible for a full day, for by this means the quickest result will be obtained and the maximum amount of movement will be regained. The results of flexor tendon grafts cannot be assessed for at least a year after surgery, for movement continues to increase and power to improve as time goes on, particularly if the patient uses the hand.

Case 2.2 This patient slipped off a chair, put his right hand through a pane of glass and divided the flexor digitorum profundus of the little finger. A secondary graft using the palmaris longus was carried out 1 month later and rehabilitation started 3 weeks after this. On admission to the rehabilitation centre no movement was seen at the terminal or proximal interphalangeal joint. There was 25 degrees' movement at the metacarpophalangeal joint, which was held in 60 degrees of flexion. Five weeks later there was a flicker at the terminal joint, and 20 degrees at the proximal joint. Grip, however, was excellent. At this stage hard work was started in the workshop on engine servicing. He was discharged 13 weeks after grafting, with 40 degrees' movement at the proximal interphalangeal joint and 20 degrees at the terminal joint. When reviewed 11 months after graft he had full flexion and a fully function hand (*Figure 2.4*). This case illustrates the continuing improvement that occurs with time and use in tendon grafts and that the final result must not be judged in less than a year.

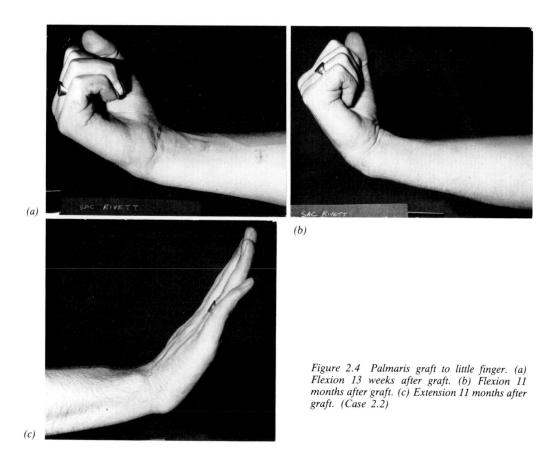

(a)

(b)

(c)

Figure 2.4   Palmaris graft to little finger. (a) Flexion 13 weeks after graft. (b) Flexion 11 months after graft. (c) Extension 11 months after graft. (Case 2.2)

Manual workers usually obtain better results than clerical or sedentary workers. For this reason patients who are in sedentary trades and who do not make demands on their hand, require a more intensive and a longer period of rehabilitation than those who use their hand at work, for their rehabilitation can be work itself, from the eighth week onwards.

It is wiser not to let people return to really heavy manual work for 8–10 weeks after surgery, in case they put too much strain on the graft.

In our experience lesions of the little finger take longer to recover, perhaps because there is no tendon on the ulnar side to help in mass flexion movements.

Results

MEASUREMENTS

When examining the hand in the clinic, the following measurements should be made and recorded.

(1) Range of passive movement at each affected joint.
(2) Range of active movement at each joint.
(3) The distance from the tip of the finger to the distal palmar crease. If there is only a little flexion at the joints, this is not easy to perform and the best measurement is then the perpendicular from the tip of the finger to the palm of the hand.
(4) Power of grip, using a small dynamometer.
(5) Active extension should be looked for and recorded at both interphalangeal and metacarpophalangeal joints.

When testing the range of active movement, the joint should be stabilized and the patient asked to bend the joint as much as possible. Resistance is given to the equivalent joints of the normal fingers for three or four pulls and the joint range measured with a small goniometer. The range should be recorded as extension to flexion, that is, 0 to 80, *not* 80 degrees of movement, for there is almost always a flexion deformity in the early stages after tendon grafts and it is important to record this. Accurate measurements of joint range are essential, for it is only by this means that deterioration in the condition can be assessed. The examiner should be aware of the ability of the extensor to trick the flexor action by its relaxation after contraction. If the joint is palpated carefully, trick action can always be detected because the opposite movement to that desired is always produced first.

The active range should be measured with the metacarpophalangeal joints extended and flexed.

In the thumb it is important to test the range of function in both flexion and extension of the carpometacarpal joint; in full extension the interphalangeal joint may go into flexion and it is important to record this.

An important function of the flexor pollicis longus is the power of pinch between the thumb and fingers, and this should always be tested by asking the patient to pinch between the thumb and index finger and assessing the amount of resistance to this pinch.

ASSESSMENT OF RESULTS

There is a certain amount of controversy about the assessment of good and bad results. Many reports of series of flexor grafts do not specify exactly what is meant by good and bad results. Flynn's (1953) good result is 90 degrees' movement at each interphalangeal joint, and the finger within 1.25 cm of the distal crease in flexion. A fair result is 45 degrees' movement at each interphalangeal joint and with the finger within 3.8 cm of the distal crease in flexion, while a poor result is one in which there is less than 45 degrees' movement at the interphalangeal joints and more than 3.8 cm from the distal crease in flexion. Morley (1956), on the other hand, suggests, as an excellent result, full extension, flexion to within 0.6 cm of the mid-palmar crease; good, full extension, flexion to within 2.5 cm of the mid-palmar crease; fair, full extension, flexion to within 5.0 cm of the mid-palmar crease; and poor, less than that defined for a fair result.

Much of the success in a tendon graft depends on what the patient is going to do with his hands, but it would seem wise to record all the information available so that long-term assessment can be made. In this series Morley's criteria are used; in addition, the range has been recorded in the equivalent joints of the other hand.

FACTORS AFFECTING THE RESULTS OF FINGER GRAFTING

An analysis of the tendon grafts treated at the Joint Services Medical Rehabilitation Unit showed that they fell into the following three main groups.

Group 1. Those that made a rapid recovery and achieved 50 degrees at the proximal interphalangeal joint and 45 degrees or more at the distal joint by the end of the third month after operation. In this group there were no complications either during or after operation, and the preoperative condition of the finger was good; furthermore, the patient was keen to get the hand better as quickly as possible.

Group 2. In this group, fairly good function of the hand was regained, but less movement at the joints was obtained. The average range of movement on discharge was 30 degrees at the proximal joint and 25 degrees at the distal joint.

Group 3. In this group there was a very poor range of movement at the interphalangeal joints, although power of grip and general function were usually fairly good.

On referring to the operative findings it was found in the second and third groups that there were definite complicating factors. In group 2, the commonest complication was adherence of the scar, either in the palm or finger, or both. Other complicating factors included a poor preoperative state of the finger in that the joints were stiff and the circulation was poor. There was destruction of the lumbrical muscles in some cases. Moderate scarring was present due to the injuries being ruptures rather than clean cuts, and injury to digital nerves as well as tendons at the time of injury.

All the severe complications were found in group 3. These included gross adherence, infection, scar contraction, destruction of the fibrous flexor sheath, haematoma formation, gross oedema, crush injuries, excessive scarring and fibrosis, or a long history of previous operations and even previous grafts.

The general progress of each group was quite distinct.

In group 1 (the uncomplicated cases) the most movement occurred in the first 8 weeks after operation. There was usually a flicker of movement of both interphalangeal joints by the twenty-seventh day after operation. By the seventh week after operation there was some 50 degrees' movement in the proximal interphalangeal joint and 35 degrees or more at the terminal interphalangeal joint. The finger flexed down to the palm well, and the power of grip was excellent, usually being up to only 0.9 kg less than the normal hand. These patients were fit to return to work between the eighth and twelfth weeks, depending on their jobs, and when reviewed at 6 months or a year later, still showed signs of increasing movement in the joints and improvement of function. By one year almost all patients had a full range of movement at all joints and could make a complete fist.

In group 2 movement started about the same time after operation as in the above cases but by the sixth week after operation there was never more than 30 degrees' movement in the proximal joint and 10–15 degrees at the terminal joint. From the sixth to the ninth week very little progress was noted. From the tenth week onwards gradual progress continued, however, and most patients in this group were fit to return to work between 14 and 16 weeks after operation. A gradual increase in function was noted on subsequent review, even 1 year after operation when there was an average of 25 degrees more movement in the interphalangeal joints.

In group 3 no movement at either interphalangeal joint was seen for the first 6 weeks after operation. None of the patients in this group every achieved more than 30 degrees' movement at the proximal interphalangeal joint or more than 10 degrees' movement at the terminal interphalangeal joint and, of course, they were not able to bring the finger down into the palm. Despite this, general function was often good and for this reason intensive treatment was justified.

On review 1 year after operation a few patients showed an increase of 15 degrees or so in range over and above their range on discharge, but most showed none. One or two patients whose work did not involve much use of the hand showed a slight decrease in range.

These patients require a much longer period under treatment than either of the first two groups because there is so much more to be done. A grossly scarred palm, for example, requires intensive oil massage several times a day. Many of the patients, moreover, need stretching and plaster splints. Those patients with gross oedema in the early stages must have their hand in elevation until the oedema has subsided, so that not only are they unable to start intensive work earlier, but they inevitably develop considerable fibrosis, particularly if the oedema is disregarded.

The preoperative condition of the finger is important and a first-class result was never obtained in a finger that had not a full range of passive movement and that had more than minimal scarring before operation.

Complications

The complications of flexor tendon grafts can be summarized as follows.
(1) Abnormalities of the circulation, particularly where digital arteries have been severed.
(2) Involvement of the digital nerves.
(3) Marked fibrosis – some patients have a capacity for forming fibrous tissue very easily and this may hinder movement of the graft.
(4) Injuries in which there has been a tearing or wrenching strain or rupture of the tendon rather than clean division, thus damaging the sheath throughout its length.
(5) Crush injuries, when fibrosis inevitably develops.
(6) Infection which is liable to lead to fibrosis and therefore to limitation of movement.

(7) Cases where suture or grafting has been undertaken at more than 2 months after injury.
(8) Patients in whom immobilization has been prolonged for more than 4 weeks and particularly where the finger has been held in marked flexion.
(9) Patients in whom there have been multiple injuries – although multiple tendon grafting can give good results, rehabilitation is more difficult and takes longer.

Motivation is of extreme importance; if the patient wants to get better and is prepared to work hard he will obviously get a much better result than the patient who expects the physiotherapist to do all the work for him.

The quality of surgery is obviously of extreme importance; the more experienced the surgeon and the more skilled he is, the better the result. This is a field in which surgery is best left to the expert and is not the province of the orthopaedic surgeon who makes an occasional foray into the hand.

Should tenolysis be necessary it is important to establish active rehabilitation straight after surgery – which means the next day if possible, and certainly well before the stitches come out.

Although there are many causes of stiffness and lack of movement after flexor tendon grafts, the management of the problems these present is basically the same – that is, restoration of gliding motion of the tendon by reducing the adherence, and encouraging movements at the stiff joints and power of the tendon. The principles are the same whether the cause of stiffness is excessive fibrosis, severe infection, stretching of the tendon sheaths in a tearing injury, or involvement of the digital nerves giving lack of proprioceptive feedback.

ADHERENCE OF THE GRAFT

If the graft has become adherent, it is important to try to relieve this by intensive lanolin massage, four times a day, followed by intensive active work against resistance. Clearly this cannot be done until at least 6 weeks after the graft. Intensive treatment of this sort can often mobilize an adherent tendon, and even quite surprisingly stiff fingers can become mobile in a matter of 3–4 weeks. If adherence has caused oedema, it is important to eradicate it as soon as possible for, if allowed to persist, more fibrous tissue will be formed and an even stiffer finger will result. The best way to relieve oedema is by elevating the hand and applying ice. Heat, particularly in the form of wax baths is contraindicated where there is oedema, for this causes more swelling. Ice treatment is of great value – crushed ice is applied in towelling to the part affected with the arm elevated, for increasing periods starting with 5 minutes and increasing to 10 or 15 minutes after a few days' treatment. This is followed by massage and active exercises. The limb is elevated between treatment sessions and kept in elevation above the head at night.

STIFF INTERPHALANGEAL JOINTS

If there is a permanently stiff interphalangeal joint in flexion, serial plasters may be required to try to obtain extension, although if the patient has no more than a 30 degree extension lag this is acceptable for function.

If the flexion deformity is 45 degrees or more, the finger will usually get in the way – the extent to which this interferes with function can be found out by trial at the patient's work, or a mock-up of his work in the occupational therapy department. Often extension can be improved by intensive oil massage, slow gentle stretches given by the physiotherapist with the finger fully supported, and then the application of a plaster of Paris splint to the palmar surface of the finger. Some workers have found that putting the finger actually into a plaster cylinder for a few days may be a more effective way – although one is loath to immobilize a finger for more than a few hours at a time, as one is concerned to obtain power in the graft as well as range of active movement.

These techniques can often successfully overcome very severe flexion deformities, but it is important that they be used in the relatively early stages. If a finger has been stiff in flexion for more than 3 months, it is extremely unlikely that conservative treatment will overcome the deformity, and it may then be necessary to carry out some form of surgery on the interphalangeal joints, such as the Curtis (1971) procedure (page 241). If this is unsuccessful it may be necessary to amputate the finger.

DIGITAL NERVE INVOLVEMENT

It has been our experience that patients who have sustained severance of the digital nerves take longer to regain reasonable function than those in whom the digital nerve has been intact. Long-term assessment of a group of patients with digital nerve involvement did not show that they had any decrease in final range or function (Morley, 1956), but the experience of physiotherapists treating such patients is that they are more difficult to rehabilitate for they lack the sensory feedback that will tell them how strongly their muscle is contracting and in what position their joint is, under various circumstances.

It is therefore important to know if somebody has sustained a digital nerve lesion for they will need more intensive and individual work and may require a long period under full-time rehabilitation.

RUPTURE OF THE GRAFT

Occasionally, during rehabilitation, a snap may be heard and movement may immediately be lost, and it is often thought that this indicates tearing or snapping of the graft.

In fact, such a circumstance is extremely rare, and the majority of cases in which such a situation arises are due to snapping of an adhesion. Under these circumstances the finger should immediately be rested for 2 or 3 weeks and then graduated active exercises started without resistance for a further 2 weeks. In almost all cases good function will return, but if it is clear that there is no movement at all at such a stage then exploration and regrafting may be necessary. Usually, in such cases, after a week of immobilization it is permissible to ask the patient to try to get active movement and if the graft has not been snapped there will be a flicker of movement at one or both joints. This indicates that further immobilization will be successful.

Sometimes one sees a remarkable range of movement quite soon after flexor tendon grafting; for example, we have seen a number of patients in whom there has been 30 degrees' movement at the proximal interphalangeal joint and 20 degrees' movement at the terminal interphalangeal joint at 4 weeks after grafting. Such patients are likely to stretch the graft at a later stage, and indeed we are suspicious of a patient with much movement at an early stage – we prefer to see a small range of movement, gradually increasing as the weeks go by, than a rapid recovery of movement in the early stages, which usually means the graft has not got a secure bed and is thus more vulnerable.

In severe injuries, a good case has been made for a temporary replacement of the tendon mechanism by Silastic rods. The patient is encouraged to use his hand as much as possible for 10 weeks and then secondary tendon grafts can be performed (Helal, 1969).

Suture

Controversy rages and will rage for many years to come on the question of whether primary grafting, delayed primary grafting, secondary grafting, or primary or secondary suture of the flexor tendons in the tendon sheath is the treatment of choice. Much depends on the availability of a skilled surgeon and on good after-care, and it is very difficult to compare results from one surgeon to another.

McFarlane, Lamon and Jarvis (1968) reviewed 100 flexor tendon injuries in the finger – 64 grafts and 36 in which primary suture had been performed. If the ends of the tendons can be joined without excessive tension, suture is recommended as the treatment of choice, but this could be achieved in only 36 patients. Suture is contraindicated when there is much scarring, damage to the sheath or joint, multiple tendons and in older age groups. These authors emphasize that the same attention to detail is required in sutures as in grafts and that it is not an easier operation.

Bolton (1970) prefers suture to graft if the following conditions are satisfied: a clean incised wound, the injury is seen within the first few hours and an experienced hand surgeon is available. Only the flexor digitorum profundus is sutured, the flexor sublimis digitorum being excised. One slip is left stretching from its insertion to just proximal to the proximal interphalangeal joint and tacked to the side of the fibrous sheath to prevent hyperextension. The fibrous flexor sheath is excised for 0.6 cm on either side to allow gliding. If the lesion is distal to the proximal interphalangeal joint, he will repair the tendon by primary suture even if it is a late case, provided that the division is distal to the attachment of the vinculum when the proximal part will not retract. If the lesion is proximal to the vinculum and the patient must have flexion at the joint (as in a musician), a plantaris graft is put from the terminal phalanx to the flexor digitorum profundus near its attachment to the lumbrical. If the movement is not essential, arthrodesis of the terminal interphalangeal joint gives excellent results.

Winston (1972) reviewed the results of treatment of flexor tendon injuries in 131 patients, primary suture being carried out in 105 patients; 83 of these had good results – that is, the finger tip within 2.5 cm of the distal palmar crease in full flexion. He recommends primary suture as the method of choice, provided that the wound is tidy and seen within 8 hours of injury. If both tendons are divided between the distal palmar crease and the insertion of flexor sublimis digitorum, suture of flexor digitorum profundus only is advised, while primary suture is indicated when flexor digitorum profundus is divided distal to the insertion of flexor sublimis digitorum. Verdan and Crawford (1971) reported 36 patients in whom primary repair had been effected of either both tendons (14), or at the profundus only (11) with sublimis excision; 93 per cent had flexion to within 2.5 cm of the distal palmar crease, and they prefer primary suture to grafting, saving the patient's time and money.

Madsen (1970) treated 53 patients – 43 with lesions in the fingers and 10 in the thumb – by delayed primary suture 1–3 days after injury, immobilizing for 3 weeks after surgery; 79 per cent had good results in which the finger touched the palm and lacked only 20 degrees' full extension at the proximal interphalangeal joint; good results were obtained in 60 per cent of the grafts to the thumb.

Jaffé and Weckesser (1966) reported on 30 profundus grafts with the sublimis intact and showed that 30 degrees' movement at the terminal interphalangeal joint could be obtained but it was not clear if proximal movement, which is by far the most important, had been lost. Generally speaking, surgeons are very loath to jeopardize a good range at the proximal interphalangeal joint by surgery at the terminal interphalangeal joint.

Kleinert and his colleagues (1973) perform primary repair of both tendons provided the injury was not caused by a human bite, has not been infected and there is no skin loss. They apply dynamic splinting using a dorsal plaster splint with the wrist in flexion and the fingers in the neutral position.

Dynamic rubber band traction is applied to the finger nail, holding the finger in flexion but permitting full active extension. During finger extension, the flexor muscle relaxes by synergistic reaction. On attempted flexion the rubber band immediately flexes the finger, removes tension on the tendon juncture and lessens the likelihood of rupture as the flexor muscles contract. The splint and sutures are removed at 3 weeks. Active exercises start earlier – at 10 days.

Kleinert and colleagues believe that this technique prevents flexion contractures – they emphasize the importance of rehabilitation. We believe that this technique is probably most useful when there is no possibility of providing intensive rehabilitation after tendon surgery. We insist on readmission at 3 weeks for 2–3 weeks' full-time rehabilitation and therefore have not used the dynamic splinting technique. Kleinert *et al.* sacrifice the sublimis if there is a crush injury or extensive damage.

In 360 cases they had 75 per cent good or excellent results. *Excellent* was flexion within 1 cm of the distal palmar crease and less than 15 degrees' loss of extension; *good* was flexion within 1 cm of the distal palmar crease and less than 30 degrees' loss of extension; *fair* was 2–3 cm flexion and less than 50 degrees' extension.

Our experience over the last 15 years, during which time a number of patients have been referred to us in whom suture rather than grafting has been carried out, suggests that the results are equally good.

The rehabilitation after tendon suture is similar to that after grafting. In the last 20 years we have had personal experience of rehabilitating 440 patients with flexor tendon grafts and sutures in the fingers. The majority have been grafts but in recent years there have been more sutures performed and we have figures for 50 primary sutures of profundus in the sheath. The average time between operation and surgery has been 3 weeks for both grafts and sutures, and the average stay at the rehabilitation centre 5 weeks. The range of movement was 53 degrees at the proximal and 25 degrees at the terminal interphalangeal joints on discharge both in the patients treated by grafting and in those treated by suture. However, one is comparing patients in whom the ideal situation exists in the case of sutures, for if there are complicating factors the case is most likely to be treated by secondary grafting, so it should not be concluded from these figures that suture is the treatment of choice. However, we feel that if ideal conditions exist – a clean incised wound, the patient seen within a few hours and an experienced hand surgeon available – primary suture is the treatment of choice, for the end-result is as good as in grafting but the patient will be back at work much sooner.

In cases where there were complications such as infection, fibrosis, digital nerve involvement and multiple tendon grafts, the average stay at the rehabilitation centre was 8 weeks before function was judged to be adequate for the patient's job. The average range in this series was found to be 22 degrees at the terminal and 50 degrees at the proximal interphalangeal joints. In some patients only a flicker was obtained at the terminal interphalangeal joint but a good range at the proximal joint (45 degrees or more). The finger almost touched the palm, grip was strong and function good.

Ruptures

In ruptures of the tendon, for example at rugby, the range of movement is more limited after grafting. This is due to the damage done by tearing and the profuse fibrosis that follows along the whole length of the tendon sheath. In the best results movements were 45 degrees at the terminal and 55 degrees at the proximal interphalangeal joint but several had virtually no movement at the terminal and 30 degrees only at the proximal interphalangeal joint, while in one the terminal interphalangeal joint had to be arthrodesed. However, all had acceptable function, only 1 of 12 having to change his trade due to stiffness of the finger.

Lesions distal to the insertion of sublimis

Primary repair is preferred. If the tendon is lacerated distal to the vincula, retraction is limited and secondary repair is possible. Grafting is difficult and may prejudice good sublimis action. The choice, if tendon suture is impossible, lies between arthrodesis and tenodesis – the latter is preferred, as loss of passive movement can be a problem.

Case histories

Case 2.3 Lack of postoperative rehabilitation. An 18-year-old civilian apprentice engineer cut the flexor digitorum profundus to the right index and little fingers in an accident at work. Four months later a palmaris longus graft was carried out to the right index finger and 6 months later to the right little finger. No formal rehabilitation was given. Eighteen months later a tenolysis on both tendons was carried out for lack of movement. He was referred to the Medical Rehabilitation Unit (MRU) 2 weeks later. Movements before and after 5 weeks of intensive treatment are shown in *Table 2.1*.

Table 2.1   Movements (degrees) before and after intensive treatment (Case 2.3)

Finger	Terminal interphalangeal	Proximal interphalangeal	Metacarpo-phalangeal	Finger to palm
Before treatment				
Index	30–31	55–75	0–65	5 cm
Little	0–5	0–45	0–65	4.5 cm
After intensive treatment				
Index	20–35	20–85	Full	–
Little	10–35	0–75	Full	–

Grip was 70 per cent normal

He was assessed in the workshops and found fully fit for his job. This case illustrates two points: the danger of not providing rehabilitation after tendon grafting and the good results that can be obtained with intensive treatment despite a long delay after grafting, given a co-operative and well motivated patient.

Case 2.4 Delay in surgery.   A 24-year-old fireman cut his right middle finger on a broken beer glass, dividing the flexor digitorum sublimis and flexor digitorum profundus but not the digital nerves. Skin suture was performed. Four months later he sought advice as the finger was getting in his way, and palmaris longus grafting was performed; 26 days later he was admitted to the MRU, when there was 10 degrees' movement at the terminal interphalangeal joint (0–10) and 30 degrees at the proximal interphalangeal joint (0–30) with, as expected, a poor grip.

Routine rehabilitation was given and 8 weeks later movements were 0–80 at the metacarpophalangeal joint, 0–80 at the proximal interphalangeal joint and the finger could touch the palm 1.9 cm from the mid-palmar crease. He was assessed and found fully fit for duty. On review 6 months after discharge he had almost normal flexion.

This case illustrates the excellent results that can be obtained despite a long delay between injury and grafting. In one of our patients the delay between injury and grafting was 8 years – 10 degrees at the terminal interphalangeal joint and 30 degrees at the proximal interphalangeal joint only resulted, but grip was full and function excellent.

Case 2.5 Blast injuries.   A 25-year-old surface worker sustained deep wounds of the palmar surface of his hand when a varnish bottle he was holding exploded. Skin suture was effected the same day. It was not clear, owing to gross oedema and pain, what structures had suffered and he was transferred to the MRU 20 days after injury with deep scarring in the palm, some residual oedema and lack of activity in the flexor digitorum profundus of the index finger. Electromyographic studies showed absent sensory potentials on the index finger. Intensive oil massage, slow stretches, active work in physiotherapy, and gymnastics and workshop activities were given.

Two months after injury he returned to hospital where very dense scarring was dissected out. The medial digital nerves to the thumb and both digital nerves to the index finger were sutured, the flexor digitorum sublimis to index excised and flexor digitorum profundus sutured with silk. Twenty-one days later he returned to the MRU with 20 degrees' movement (30–50) of the terminal interphalangeal joint, and 15 degrees' movement (30–65) at the proximal interphalangeal joint.

Two months later the scar in the palm was supple and non-adherent. The terminal interphalangeal joint had an active range of 45 degrees (15–60), and the proximal 50 degrees (40–90). Grip was 3.2 kg on the affected side and 5.4 kg on the normal side. Sensation was returning. He was tested on his job and found fit for all but heavy lifting, and returned to duty. This case illustrates the value of intensive treatment in conditions where gross scarring follows blast injuries.

Case 2.6 Dissolution of graft and regrafting.   Rupture of the flexor tendons of the left ring finger occurred in this patient whilst playing rugger. A palmaris graft was performed 1 month later. It was noted at operation that both tendons were firmly adherent in the palm. Both tendons were excised. The patient came to the MRU 22 days later when it was observed that he had 20 degrees' movement in the terminal interphalangeal joint, 30 degrees at the proximal interphalangeal joint, and the grip was half that of normal. A fortnight later the tendon snapped while the patient was doing a free exercise, and 2 weeks later a new graft was inserted using the second toe extensor. Rehabilitation recommenced a month later when there was a 15 degrees' movement at the terminal interphalangeal joint (0–15) and 10 degrees at the proximal interphalangeal joint (10–20). After treatment for 1 month (i.e. 8 weeks after the second operation) movement at the terminal interphalangeal joint was 0–60, at the proximal interphalangeal joint 0–85, and at the metacarpophalangeal joint 0–90. The finger came to within 1.9 cm of the mid-palmar crease. The patient returned to work as a mechanic at this stage, with excellent hand function (*Figure 2.5*).

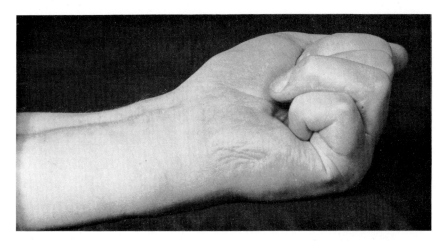

Figure 2.5   Maximum flexion of the ring finger on discharge, 7 weeks after regrafting. (Case 2.6)

Case 2.7 Infection.   A 42-year-old supplier put his right hand through a window, severing extensor tendons to the right middle and ring fingers, which were repaired by primary suture, and severing flexors to the ring and little fingers at the level of the proximal interphalangeal joints and the digital nerves and arteries to these fingers. Three weeks later he was readmitted to hospital with gross infection of the affected fingers.

He was admitted to the MRU for mobilization prior to tendon grafting. This required 2 months' intensive oil massage, stretching, active exercise and games for there was gross scarring in the palm, oedema of the fingers and only 20 degrees' passive range in the interphalangeal joints, from 30 to 50 degrees. Subsequently the right ring finger was grafted using palmaris longus, but the little finger was left owing to the gross scarring and stiffness of the interphalangeal joints. Twenty days later he was readmitted to the MRU with 27–35 degrees' active range at the proximal interphalangeal joint and 27–31 degrees at the terminal interphalangeal joint. The little finger was stuck at 40 degrees at the terminal and 45 degrees at the proximal interphalangeal joint. Seven weeks later, after intensive treatment which included the use of a double finger stall, movements of the ring finger were 20–60 at the terminal and 10–80 at the proximal interphalangeal joint. The finger was able to be flexed to within 3.5 cm of the palm, and grip was 60 per cent of normal. He was found fully fit for duty and the stiff little finger was not in the way.

Case 2.8 Adherence of graft.   This patient divided both flexor tendons of the left index finger and the digital nerve at the radial aspect on a circular saw. Two months later a palmaris graft was inserted and the digital nerve sutured. He started rehabilitation 5 weeks later. At this time there was no active movement at the terminal joint and a passive range of 10 degrees from 10 degrees of full extension. At the proximal joint there was 10 degrees' active movement from 30 degrees. There was some adherence of the graft in the palm. Ten days later intensive oil massage was started four times a day to the adherent scar in the palm and hard work began 2 weeks later. Eleven weeks after grafting function was excellent and he was able to return to full duty as an infantryman.

Case 2.9 Development of hyperextension deformity.   This patient sustained a tear of the flexor tendons of the right index finger and an open wound which became infected. One year later the tendons were seen at operation to be adherent and there was much capsular thickening. Sublimis was excised, a graft inserted, the lateral ligaments resected and the capsule thinned. On admission to the MRU 17 days after operation the terminal interphalangeal joint was held at 30 degrees and the proximal interphalangeal joint at 45 degrees. Nine days later there was 5 degrees' movement at the terminal interphalangeal joint and 20 degrees at the proximal interphalangeal joint.

Four weeks later the proximal interphalangeal joint began to go into hyperextension (*Figure 2.6a*) and a plaster splint was made which the patient wore when not actively engaged in treatment (*Figure 2.6b*). The hyperextension persisted, although it diminished under treatment, and prevented proper initiation of flexion by the graft as so much

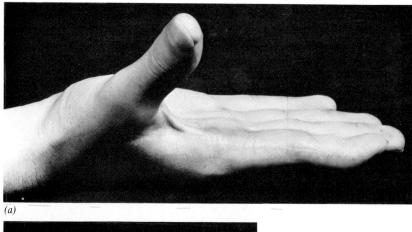

(a)

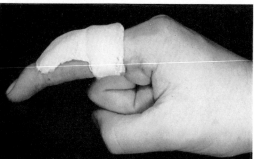

(b)

Figure 2.6 (a) Hyperextension
of proximal interphalangeal
joint of the index finger. (b)
Plaster splint used in treatment.
(c) Maximal voluntary flexion
possible. (Case 2.9)

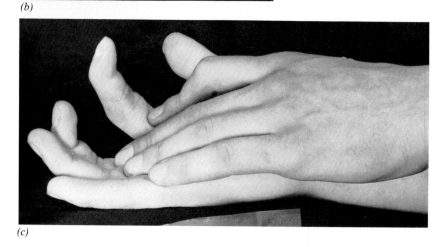

(c)

'slack' had to be taken up before flexion could start (*Figure 2.6c*). Grip, however, was good, and the patient returned to duty after 3 months' rehabilitation.

In another case of hyperextension of the proximal interphalangeal joint, Mr R. Furlong opened the joint and scarified the flexor aspect of it. This prevented the joint from hyperextending and an excellent result was obtained.

Case 2.10 Surgery contraindicated.   This patient cut his left index finger with a chisel, dividing the flexor digitorum profundus. No surgery was attempted and he spent 2 weeks at the rehabilitation centre to gain maximum power and function. He was assessed in the Britannia Simulator, and throughout a series of preflight taxiing and take-off checks, as well emergencies during flight, he had no disability. Both the captain and the monitoring flight engineer was fully satisfied with his performance.

Case 2.11 Late surgery. This patient sustained rupture of the flexor digitorum profundus of the left ring finger, falling off a chair. One year later, as he was inconvenienced by lack of range of movement, a graft using a toe extensor was put in. He was transferred for rehabilitation 4 weeks later. The scar was thickened and the finger was held at 30 degrees' flexion in the terminal interphalangeal joint and 25 degrees at the proximal interphalangeal joint. He required serial plaster stretches and a Capener splint to encourage flexion. On discharge 5 weeks later he had a flexion deformity of 30 degrees at the proximal joint but could make a full fist, and was fit for his trade as a carpenter.

Case 2.12 Multiple grafts. This patient cut all flexor tendons to all fingers of the right hand on a glass window, at the level of the proximal interphalangeal joint. Secondary grafting using plantaris was performed 5 weeks later to the index finger; 4 months later the middle and ring fingers were grafted using palmaris longus. Intensive rehabilitation was given after both operations, and 2 months after the second operation movements were as shown in *Table 2.2*.

The index finger lacked the thenar eminence by 0.5 cm, the middle finger by 1 cm and the ring finger by 1.75 cm. He was assessed and found fully fit for his trade as a wireless mechanic (*Figure 2.7*).

Table 2.2 Movements (degrees) after intensive rehabilitation following operation (Case 2.12)

Finger	Terminal interphalangeal	Proximal interphalangeal
Index	10–35	0–75
Middle	20–15	0–75
Ring	0	0–75

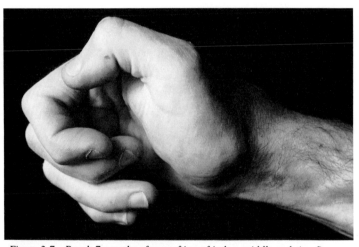

Figure 2.7   Result 7 months after grafting of index, middle and ring fingers. (Case 2.12)

Case 2.13. This patient fell into a hole in Malaya, lacerating the middle and ring fingers, and severing the tendons of the flexor digitorum sublimis and flexor digitorum profundus. Secondary grafting of the flexor digitorum profundus with palmaris tendons, excising the sublimis, was carried out 1 month later and he was transferred to the MRU 3 weeks after this. After 8 weeks' intensive treatment he achieved at the middle finger 0–90 at the proximal joint, 0–10 at the terminal joint; ring finger 0–95 at the proximal joint and no movement at the terminal joint. Function was excellent and he returned to work as a gunner.

Case 2.14. This patient cut all the flexor tendons and digital nerves to the right hand at the level of the metacarpophalangeal joints on a panga knife in a fight with terrorists. He was admitted to the MRU for preoperative mobilization of his metacarpophalangeal and interphalangeal joints. Two months after injury grafts were put in to the index and middle fingers. Three weeks later intensive rehabilitation started. At this stage there was 10 degrees' active movement at the proximal interphalangeal joints and a flicker at the terminal interphalangeal joints. Seven weeks later movements were 0–75 degrees at the proximal joint, index; 10–75 degrees at the proximal joint, middle; 0–15 degrees at each interphalangeal joint. The ring finger was then grafted and rehabilitation recommenced 3 weeks later. Six months after injury he returned to work with movements of 0–90 degrees at the proximal joint, index; 20–90 degrees at the proximal joint, middle; 20–40 degrees at the proximal joint, ring; and 0–30 degrees at each terminal joint. The workshop supervisor reported him as fully fit for his trade as an air wireless fitter, and he has subsquently improved steadily. On review 6 years later he had retained movement and increased power.

Case 2.15.   This young man lacerated his right index, middle and ring fingers at the level of the proximal interphalangeal joints, dividing all the flexor tendons.

He underwent three operations over the following 18 months, including repair, tenolysis and Silastic rod implants, but no flexion was possible at any ot the joints.

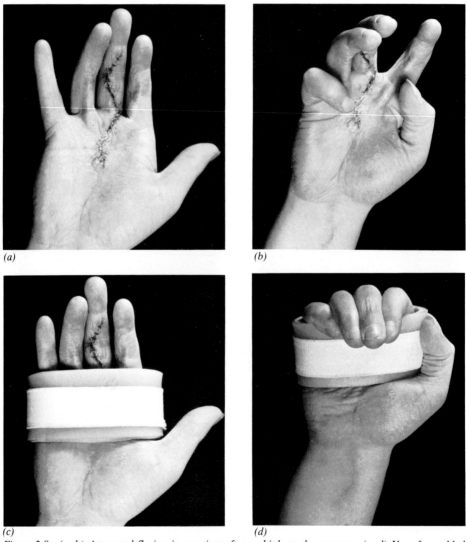

(a)

(b)

(c)

(d)

Figure 2.8   (a, b) Attempted flexion in a patient after multiple tendon surgery. (c, d) Use of a padded wood board to facilitate flexion at the interphalangeal joints. (Case 2.15)

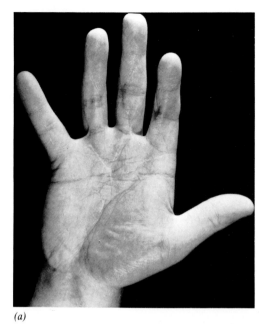
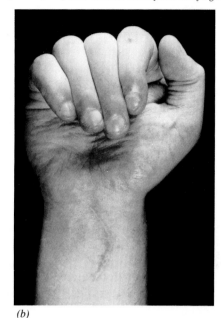

(a)   *(b)*

Figure 2.9 Final result of Figure 2.8. (Case 2.15)

Two years after the original injury, the index finger was grafted, using palmaris, removing the sublimis. The ring finger was grafted using a toe extensor. Three months later the right middle finger was tenolysed. Intensive rehabilitation followed for 3 months. A padded bar of wood was helpful in concentrating the patient's tendon effort at the proximal interphalangeal joint (*Figures 2.8* and *2.9*).

This case shows that with first class surgery and intensive rehabilitation an excellent result can be obtained despite failed tendon surgery previously and a lapse of nearly 2 years.

Case 2.16. This patient severed both tendons to the index and middle fingers at the level of the proximal interphalangeal joints in January 1975. Tendon suture failed and in February 1976 Silastic rods were put in to prepare a bed for the subsequent tendon graft which was carried out in May.

In July he came to the rehabilitation centre when the fingers were swollen, tender and stiff. Movements recorded on admission and in subsequent weeks are shown in *Table 2.3*.

Table 2.3 Movements (degrees) on admission and over the subsequent 4 months (Case 2.16)

Joint and finger	8 July	22 July	28 July	9 Sep.	3 Oct.	4 Nov.
Metacarpophalangeal						
Index	55–90	40–100	25–95	0–110	0–115	0–110
Middle	45–90	20–93	10–90	−10–110	0–110	0–110
Proximal interphalangeal						
Index	65–80	50–71	40–65	25–73	25–90	20–90
Middle	70–75	69–77	50–70	58–80	50–90	45–87
Terminal interphalangeal						
Index	Nil	22–26	10–20	0–15	0–20	1–17
Middle	60–63	43–50	40–47	30–45	20–30	17–37

Serial plasters were of great value in this case, where further surgery would have been undertaken only with great reluctance. *Figure 2.10* shows the serial plasters used and the end-result.

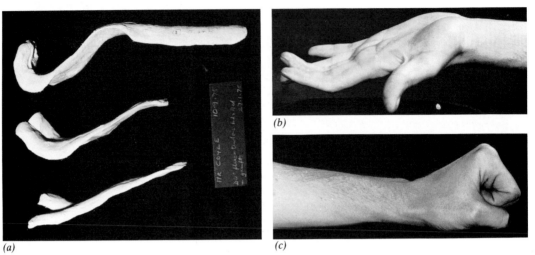

(a)   *(c)*

Figure 2.10   (a) Serial plasters. (b) Active extension obtained 2 months later. (c) Full flexion. (Case 2.16)

Multiple disorders

There are various circumstances under which tendons may be damaged incidentally to a severe hand lesion. These include crush injuries, blast injuries, Dupuytren's contracture, multiple fractures or fracture dislocations. Tendons may either be divided or, more commonly, bound down by massive fibrosis or adhere to callus. Each severe hand injury of this sort presents its own problem but the general principles are the same: attempts to mobilize the tendons and skin by frequent sessions of oil massage, the use of stretch plasters, polyethylene foam (Plastazote) wedges to increase the excursions of the thumb web and interdigital spaces, intensive active exercises and functional activities in the occupational therapy workshop.

The more severe the lesion the more important it is to institute full-time intensive treatment. Massive scarring causing a 'frozen hand' is not amenable to surgery, other than skin cover when appropriate. Even very severe stiffness can be remarkably improved by conservative measures.

INJURIES OF THE FLEXOR TENDONS IN THE THUMB

Flexor tendon injuries to the thumb can be treated either by suture or by graft. Complications such as infection, excess scarring and adherence occur as in lesions of the fingers and, in such circumstances, the usual management is required, including oil massage and stretches. However, results of flexor tendon injury to the thumb are usually good whether there are complicating factors or not – the main criterion for good thumb function is a strong pinch in opposition to the finger tips and this does not require more than 30 degrees' active flexion at the interphalangeal joint. Power is relatively easy to restore by physiotherapy and occupational therapy as already described. The average range of movement obtained at the interphalangeal joint after 3 weeks' rehabilitation in uncomplicated cases was 60 and 35 degrees in cases where infection or scarring were complicating factors.

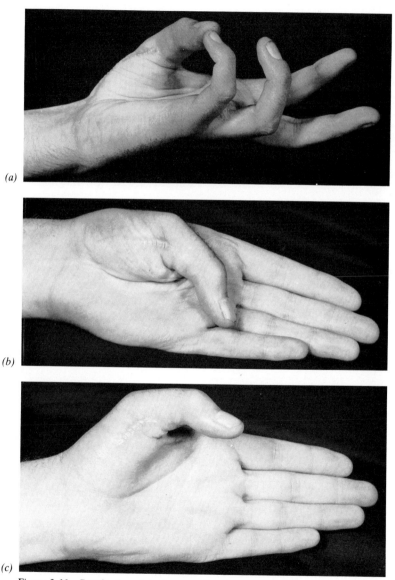

(a)

(b)

(c)

Figure 2.11   Result of graft to flexor pollicis longus 12 weeks after operation. (a) Opposition to minimus. (b) Flexion; in this position with a poorly functioning graft the interphalangeal joint falls easily into extension. (c) Flexion with carpometacarpal joint extended. (Case 2.17)

Case 2.17   This patient cut his flexor pollicis longus and digital nerves. A palmaris graft was carried out after 4 months and the nerves were sutured. Rehabilitation started 6 weeks later when it was noted that the tendon graft was adherent to the scar in the thumb. Active range was 8 degrees at the interphalangeal joint. After intensive treatment he was discharged 3 weeks later with 48 degrees at the interphalangeal joint and a grip of 4.5 kg compared with 6.4 kg on the normal side. He returned to his job as an air frame fitter 2 months after grafting (*Figures 2.11* and *2.12*).

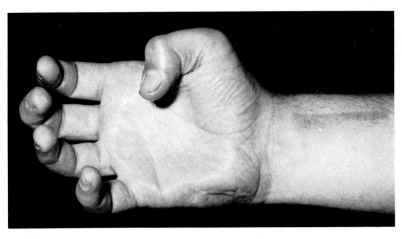

Figure 2.12   Result of palmaris graft for severed flexor pollicis longus 5 months after grafting. (Case 2.17)

EXTENSOR TENDONS

Repair of extensor tendons at the wrist or over the dorsum of the hand is relatively easy, for there is plenty of loose areolar tissue and adherence does not occur. After repair the wrist is put in full dorsiflexion so that the metacarpophalangeal joints need not be immobilized in full extension. Few problems are presented in rehabilitation unless there is adherence of the extensor mechanism in fractures, crush injuries, infection or burns. In such a situation the principles are the same as in complicated flexor tendon injuries – oil massage to overcome the adherence, and intensive active exercises with graded resistance, occupational therapy and games.

Rupture of the extensor pollicis longus at Lister's tubercle is not uncommon and is best treated by a transfer of the extensor indicis to extensor pollicis longus.

Extensor tendon injuries in the finger can offer considerable problems in rehabilitation, particularly if adherence occurs over the dorsal surface of the finger. Here it may be impossible to obtain active movement at the interphalangeal joints and the aim of treatment is to develop strong grip. It is less easy to provide specific physiotherapy for extensor tendons than it is for flexor tendons. Flexion and grip are easier and stronger movements to retrain. Proprioceptive neuromuscular facilitation techniques are of particular value in re-educating extensor function using flexion, abduction, external rotation patterns, and extension, abduction and internal rotation patterns to obtain a maximum extensor movement of shoulder, elbow, wrist, finger and thumb, by irradiation. Games such as jacks, cat's cradles with string, tiddly-winks, matches and pennies are all valuable in the physiotherapy department to

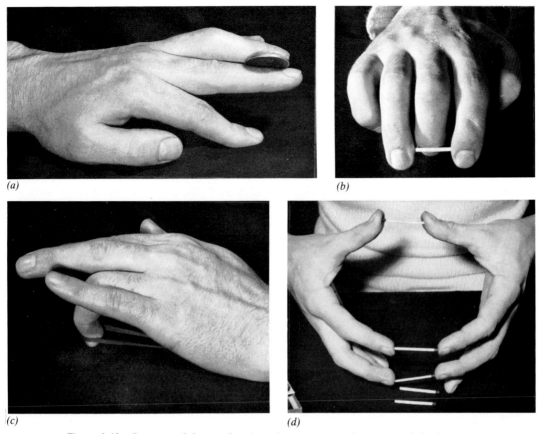

(a) *(b)*

(c) *(d)*

Figure 2.13 Games used for re-education after extensor tendon suture of the fingers

encourage the extensor tendons to contract (*Figure 2.13*). Electrical stimulation can be most valuable for extensor tendons to give the patient the idea of the movement but only as an assistance, never to replace the patient's active efforts. The patient should be encouraged to contract his muscles with the current; then intermittently the current is turned off and the patient tries to activate the tendon by himself. The stimulus is then reapplied. As the session progresses the patient may often find he is much more successful in initiating movement than at the beginning. In our experience electrical stimulation is of no value for the re-education of flexor tendon grafts or sutures, but has a definite place in the management of extensor tendon injuries.

Sometimes a spring wire splint is useful to assist extension or to provide resistance to extension.

GAMES SUITABLE FOR PATIENTS RECOVERING FROM TENDON SUTURE

(1) Flick light material such as cotton wool, progressing later to hard objects such as marbles.

(2) Balance a penny on the back of the terminal phalanx and attempt to transfer it to the back of each terminal phalanx in turn, one from another (*Figure 2.13a*).

(3) As power improves, the same game as in (2) is used, but with marbles.

(4) The patient is asked to hold a match across the back of the affected terminal phalanx, the two fingers on either side are pressed down on top of the match and an attempt made to break it. This shows up very well the extensor tendon action at the wrist (*Figure 2.13b*).

(5) A rubber band is placed around the wrist and another hitched to it which goes up to the volar surface of the finger and pulls over the back of the finger at different levels starting at the proximal phalanx and working to the tip where leverage is greatest, the patient attempting to extend the finger against the resistance of the rubber band. The rubber band can also be placed over all the fingers and the thumb at about the level of the proximal interphalangeal joints, and the patient separates the fingers and thumb against the resistance of the band. Following this each finger in turn is lifted in and out (*Figure 2.13c*).

(6) Rolling and unrolling a crepe bandage, and later a rubber bandage, as described for the flexor tendons is useful.

(7) Tiddly-winks is excellent for the later stages of re-education of extensor tendon action.

(8) Cat's cradle.

(9) Jacks.

(10) Picking up five matches between the finger tips of both hands (*Figure 2.13d*).

(11) Yo-yo.

(12) Pick-a-stick.

(13) Plasticine modelling.

(14) Card tricks and making card houses.

(15) Ball games.

DEFORMITIES

Swan neck

This deformity is one of hyperextension of the proximal interphalangeal joint and flexion of the terminal interphalangeal joint. It is caused by dorsal subluxation of the lateral extensor bands. This can occur in intrinsic contractures due to rheumatoid arthritis, cerebral palsy or Parkinson's disease, or when there is an instability of the proximal interphalangeal joint due to lesions of the volar glenoid ligament, paralysis of the flexor digitorum sublimis or mallet finger. Flexion takes place in two stages: at first the proximal interphalangeal joint extends further; then when the terminal interphalangeal joint is fully flexed the longitudinal bands are displaced in a volar direction and then the flexor digitorum sublimis becomes effective. Treatment is by correcting the cause – release of intrinsic contracture, or synovectomy – and then to stabilize the proximal interphalangeal joint either by tenodesis of the flexor digitorum sublimis or shortening the glenoid ligament.

Boutonnière

In this condition the deformity is the exact opposite of the swan neck. There is flexion of the proximal interphalangeal joint and hyperextension of the terminal interphalangeal joint. This is due to damage to the central slip of the extensor tendon over the proximal joint, and can be caused by trauma, burns, Dupuytren's contracture, rheumatoid disease or congenital disease. As flexion occurs at the proximal joint so the dorsal retinacular ligament is stretched, the lateral extensor slips subluxate volarwards, producing hyperextension of the terminal joint and also of the metacarpophalangeal joint. If the terminal joint can be flexed when the proximal joint is supported, the retinacular ligaments have not yet contracted and the proximal joint is splinted in extension to encourage terminal interphalangeal joint flexion with either a static splint or a dynamic Capener splint. If the ligaments have contracted the deformity will be severe and surgery is essential. The scar over the dorsum is resected and the lateral bands sutured together over the middle phalanx. Plaster is applied for 5 weeks.

Chronic heroin addicts suffer from a particularly unpleasant hand lesion as a result of too hasty an injection into a hand vein, causing rupture of the vessel and sloughing of the tissues. When the dorsum of the finger is used, the extensor mechanism is destroyed, causing a boutonnière deformity, the skin sloughs and the proximal interphalangeal joints become septic.

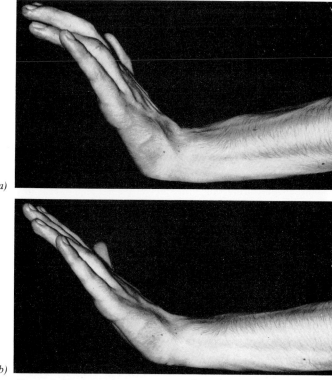

(a)

(b)

Figure 2.14 Division of extensor tendon to ring finger. (a) One month after suture, at start of rehabilitation. (b) Result after 20 days' treatment. (Case 2.20)

Case 2.18 This patient was involved in a road traffic accident, sustaining a fracture of the parietal bone, and a rupture of the extensor tendon of the left index finger over the proximal phalanx. Three weeks later a 0.6 cm gap was repaired in the tendon and some glass splinters were removed. She was put in plaster of Paris and started rehabilitation 15 days later. There was 22 degrees' active flexion of the proximal interphalangeal joint which lacked 10 degrees' extension. Nine days' intensive exercises gave her full passive range of movement and good power but she still had an extension lag at the proximal interphalangeal joint. She was supplied with a Capener splint and allowed to return to duty as a driver wearing the splint all day.

On review 6 weeks later she had overcome the lag fully.

Case 2.19 This patient cut the base of his thumb when he fell through a glass door and divided the extensor pollicis longus. At operation 2 months later the proximal ends could not be found, and the extensor pollicis brevis was therefore transferred to the distal end of the extensor pollicis longus. He was in plaster for 3 weeks and rehabilitation started on its removal. The scar was adherent and required intensive massage. Ten weeks after surgery he had an excellent result with normal grip, and he was fit to return to full duty in the infantry.

Case 2.20 This patient tried to walk through a glass door and cut the extensor tendon over the left ring finger, producing a boutonnière deformity. Three weeks later the scar was excised and the lateral slips of the extensor expansion approximated. Seventeen days later he was transferred to the MRU and after 1 month's intensive exercises, occupational therapy and games he returned to duty as a teleprinter operator, fully fit (*Figure 2.14*).

Case 2.21 This patient cut the back of his left index finger across the proximal interphalangeal joint and divided the extensor tendon. This was repaired at secondary operation 5 weeks later, as the wound was infected. Two months later he attended for intensive rehabilitation because he had a lag and poor grip. A Capener splint proved very useful in encouraging flexion and, after 3 weeks' intensive exercises, games and carpentry, he obtained full function (*Figure 2.15*).

Case 2.22 This patient was involved in a road traffic accident, lacerating the dorsum of his hand on the windscreen. Skin grafting was required and also suture of the cut extensor tendons; gross adherence of the tendons presented a problem for rehabilitation, and flexion of the metacarpophalangeal joints was virtually nil (*Figure 2.16a*).

Intensive oil massage and active exercises and games gave a good result within 4 weeks and he returned to his work as a supplier. *Figure 2.16b* and *c* shows the result at follow-up 4 months after the injury.

Case 2.23 An 18-year-old armament mechanic put his right hand through a window and severed the extensor pollicis longus over the proximal phalanx. Three weeks later secondary suture with wire was carried out and he was transferred to the MRU 3 weeks after this. Full extension was present but power was poor. After 2 weeks' intensive treatment, including racket games and workshop activities, he was discharged back to full duty, power being the same as measured by a dynamometer on the two hands and work assessment, showing that he could manage a full day's work on his job.

Case 2.24 An 18-year-old radar mechanic injured his right hand when he fell on some glass, cutting the extensor pollicis longus of the right thumb and the extensor tendons to the middle and ring fingers of the right hand. Primary suture was carried out and he was referred to the MRU 3 weeks later. There was a marked stiffness of the metacarpophalangeal joints, measurements being: metacarpophalangeal joint of little finger lacked full extension by 10 degrees, and there was 60 degrees of active flexion; the ring finger lacked full extension by 10 degrees and there was 40 degrees of active flexion; the middle finger lacked full extension by 20 degrees, and there was 45 degrees of active flexion; the right thumb had 10 degrees' movement only, the metacarpophalangeal joint being held at 20 degrees. Two weeks later his grip still measured 0.5 kg only, and 3.2 kg on the right. He was given routine active exercises in physiotherapy, racket games in the gymnasium and intensive functional activities on electronic apparatus in the workshops, related to his trade. Three weeks after starting treatment it was clear that his motivation towards the service was poor and, despite intensive treatment and the exhortations of the therapists, he failed his workshop tests and was regarded as being a danger if he returned to work. In such situations it is pointless to continue attempts to return the patient to his former work; he was invalided and resettled into light work.

CONCLUSION

It will be seen that the results of treatment in tendon lesions depend on a variety of factors – whether the lesion is in the 'châsse gardée', if it involves infection, digital nerve involvement, associated fracture or crushing, a long period between injury and

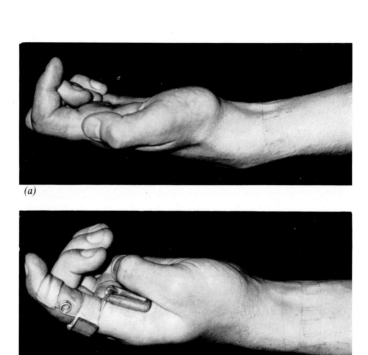

(a)

(b)

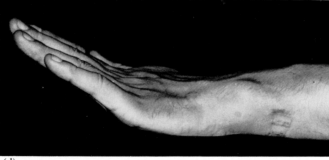

(c)

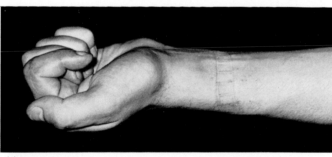

(d)

Figure 2.15   Division of extensor tendon of index. Primary suture. (a) At start of rehabilitation, 2 months after suture at proximal interphalangeal joint. (b) Use of Capener splint. (c) Flexion and (d) extension on discharge 3 weeks later. (Case 2.21)

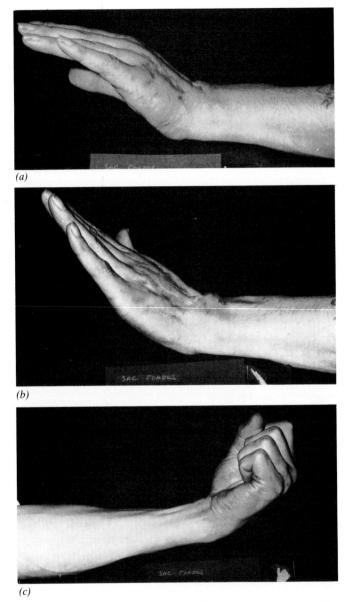

*Figure 2.16   Laceration of extensor tendons over dorsum of wrist with
skin loss. Adherence of tendons to grafted skin and underlying tissues.
(a) Attempted extension 49 days after accident. (b) Final result 6
months later—extension. (c) Final result—flexion. (Case 2.22)*

treatment or poor motivation. But our experience leads us to believe that the two
over-riding factors are skilled surgery and proper rehabilitation. Only a surgeon
versed in the techniques of hand surgery with a wide experience and critical outlook
can obtain the best results, and it is the writer's opinion that the occasional surgeon
who does not make a special study of the hand cannot hope to be as successful as the
dedicated hand specialist. Rehabilitation can help a first class surgeon to achieve a

first class end-result. Often rehabilitation can offer much better function after indifferent surgery than no rehabilitation at all. Certainly the more complications that exist the more important is intensive full-time skilled rehabilitation, using all the resources of modern physiotherapy and occupational therapy, in order to gain function. Physiotherapy and occupational therapy can offer the surgeon a means of obtaining the maximum range of passive movement and muscle power preoperatively in order to facilitate postoperative recovery, and can provide the means to regain function after surgery quicker and to a higher standard than if the patient is left to his own devices.

Such treatment, however, must be realistic, active, dynamic, related to the patient's interests and work, and supervised in detail from day to day.

The operation is only one event – albeit the most important one – in a chain of circumstances, starting with the preparation of the hand for surgery in the best state and continuing until the patient has adequate function for all the varied activities to which he wishes to put his hand.

At the Royal National Orthopaedic Hospital it is the custom after tendon surgery to readmit the patient 3 weeks later for 2–3 weeks of intensive rehabilitation.

APPENDIX A: CHESSINGTON ARM SLING (*Figure 2.17*)

This sling is valuable in any condition where the arm needs rest, and in particular when the hand is oedematous, as the height of the hand can be adjusted by buckles and the weight is taken on the opposite shoulder.

Materials required

A piece of strong canvas 119 x 18 cm; 114 cm of 2.5 cm webbing, either cotton or nylon; old aluminium black splint for gutter, maximum width being 15 cm; two 2.5 cm roller buckles with prong; linen thread; and felt for lining gutter.

Method (*Figure 2.17c*)

(1) Taking the length of canvas, mark one end '1' and the other end '2'. Make a hem across end 1, by turning it in for 2.5 cm and then machine stitching.
(2) Fold end 1 inwards towards centre for a distance of 45 cm (for gutter pocket) and mark a cross on the canvas on both sides. Open out again and mark a line where the canvas became a fold across the end.
(3) Using the 2.5 cm webbing, cut two lengths approximately 10 cm long. Mid-way along each length fix a buckle through the webbing, and fold over to make two buckle holders, one for each side of the gutter pocket.
(4) Place the buckle holders just inside the fold line on the canvas so that they can be stitched into the side seam in one movement. (If they are not inserted now, it can be done at the very end, when the pocket is turned the right way out, but this means extra stitching.)

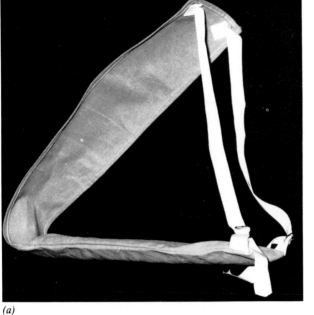

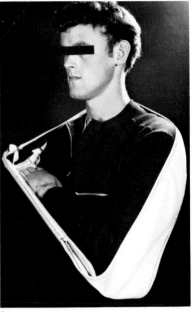

(a)   (b)

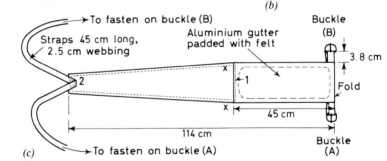

Figure 2.17   The Chessington sling

(5) Now with end 2 of the original canvas, cut off 30 cm on each edge and gradually taper off until just beyond the original 'X' marks on the canvas is reached. Turn in both the long edges, also the narrow one across end 2, and machine to just beyond the crosses.

(6) Replace end 1 exactly back to the 'X' marks, and stitch down the sides to make a pocket for the gutter, at the same time incorporating the two buckle holders. Turn inside out.

(7) Take the 91 cm length of webbing, fold in half to make a 'V' and stitch on to edge 2.

(8) Cut the aluminium gutter to 43 cm rounding off the ends. File all edges.

(9) Pad with felt and place inside gutter.

(10) Place sling under patient's forearm, bend up elbow, pass end 2 across and upwards over the back of the patient's injured arm to reach the top of the uninjured shoulder. Carry the end over to the front, and fasten the two straps to the buckles as illustrated. Adjust the buckles so that the arm is in the required position of elevation.

APPENDIX B: SPRING WIRE FINGER SPLINTS (*Figure 2.18*)

Spring wire splints can be quite easily made in the occupational therapy department, provided the occupational therapist has a basic understanding of soldering techniques and has the necessary equipment.

Uses of spring wire splints

(1) To correct flexion (or extension) weaknesses or deformities of the interphalangeal joints.
(2) To prove increased resistance for the long flexors or extensors.

Materials required

Two coiled springs, reversed for right and left side of the finger, either type A or type B (*Figure 2.18e*) made from spring steel wire, s.w.g. 19 (this is an average strength and must be increased or decreased according to resistance desired).

Two pieces of spring steel wire, s.w.g. 17, 3.8 cm in length (this requires to be two gauges thicker than the wire used for the flat springs).

One piece of tin (an old syrup tin or cocoa tin will do), 13 cm².
Tinman's shears.
Flux for soldering.
Soldering iron.
Watchmaker's pliers.
One piece of gloving leather (for covering), 19 cm².

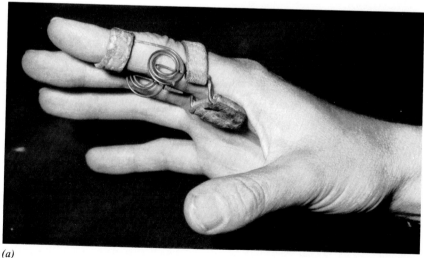

(a)

Figure 2.18 (a–m) Spring wire finger splints

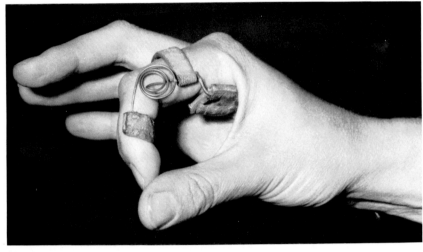

(b)

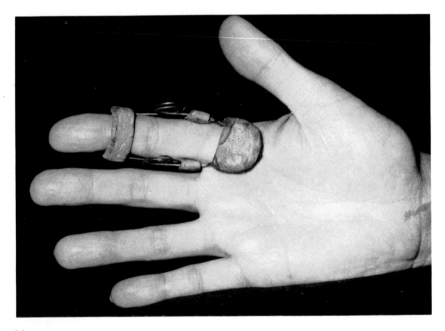

(c)

Figure 2.18 (cont)

Method of construction

It must first be decided which type of spring is to be used. Both can be made in the occupational therapy department, but type A takes longer to construct than type B, and requires practice. Type B can be constructed with a simple jig or can be easily made by hand.

TYPE A (FLAT SPRING)

Spring wire, s.w.g. 19, is bent to the shape shown in *Figure 2.18e* with the aid of watchmaker's pliers. A straight piece of wire about 15 cm long is the most satisfactory to work with, as it has been found that a short piece makes it difficult for the occupational therapist or technician to hold while putting in the 'twists'. The pliers are placed halfway along the wire then bent to form a semi-circle (*Figure 2.18f*).

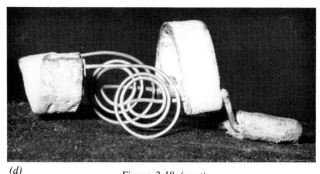

(d)

Figure 2.18 (cont)

From then on, it is a matter of squeezing the wire gently round into position, moving the pliers along only a small distance each time to avoid 'kinking', or a series of little straight lines instead of a smooth curve. It is a slow and tedious task because of the nature of spring wire, but with practice, the occupational therapist quickly develops a 'feel' for the necessary movement, and speeds up the working time. To try to turn the wire into a flat coil with only a few turns results in a faulty spring (*Figure 2.18g*).

It is important to keep each round as close to the next as possible, with only a little space between each so that it is not clumsy on the finger. A space equal in width to the size of the wire would be about right. After the original first turn is made, it will be noticed that the wire will fall to one side of it. For this reason, it is necessary to reverse the spring for the other side of the finger, and to let the wire fall into position on the original turn, on the other side.

TYPE B (ADJACENT COILS)

This is much quicker to make, and can be done on the jig designed for the purpose, or by hand, using the watchmaker's pliers. Any occupational therapy department with a technician should be able to construct the simple tool from the diagram, and make the coil in a few seconds. If made with the watchmaker's pliers, the same working techniques apply as in type A, except that only two coils are made, and they are of the same diameter and lie adjacent to each other, as in the ordinary 'coiled' type of spring.

Once the type of spring has been decided upon, proceed as follows: for example, using type A.

(1) Using the tinman's shears, cut out a semi-circle about the size of a 2-penny piece (2.5 cm diameter) or a little more, the width being the measurement of the finger from medial to lateral sides (*Figure 2.18h*).

Flat spring coils

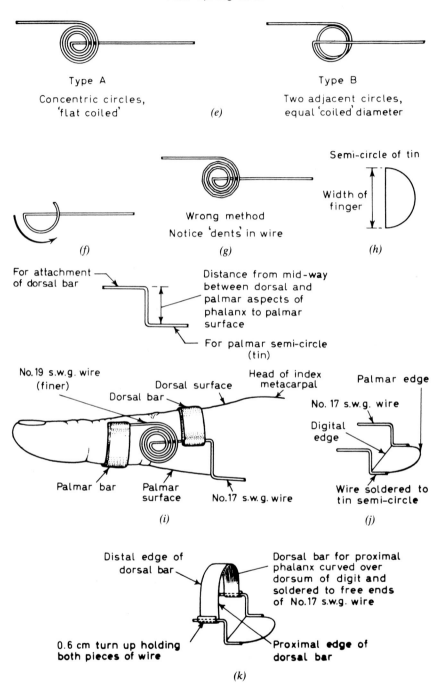

Type A
Concentric circles,
'flat coiled'

(e)

Type B
Two adjacent circles,
equal 'coiled' diameter

Semi-circle of tin

Width of
finger

(f)

Wrong method
Notice 'dents' in wire

(g)

(h)

For attachment
of dorsal bar

Distance from mid-way
between dorsal and
palmar aspects of
phalanx to palmar
surface

For palmar semi-circle
(tin)

No. 19 s.w.g. wire
(finer)

Dorsal surface

Dorsal bar

Head of index
metacarpal

Palmar edge

No. 17 s.w.g. wire

Digital
edge

Palmar bar   Palmar
surface

No. 17 s.w.g. wire

Wire soldered to
tin semi-circle

(i)

(j)

Distal edge of
dorsal bar

Dorsal bar for proximal
phalanx curved over
dorsum of digit and
soldered to free ends
of No. 17 s.w.g. wire

0.6 cm turn up holding
both pieces of wire

Proximal edge of
dorsal bar

(k)

Figure 2.18 (cont)

(2) Cut two strips of tin 0.9 cm in width: (*a*) one measuring three-eighths of the width across the dorsum of the patient's proximal phalanx (from midline on the medial aspect to midline on the lateral aspect of the digit) – allow 1.2 cm for turning over wire (0.6 cm at each end); (*b*) the other measuring three-eighths of the width across the palmar aspect of the middle phalanx (from midline on the lateral aspect to midline on the medial aspect) plus 1.2 cm for turning over wire (0.6 cm at each end).

(3) Bend the two pieces of spring wire No. 17 s.w.g. (the stronger wire) as shown in *Figure 2.18i*.

(4) Solder the two pieces of No. 17 s.w.g. wire on to the sides of the semi-circular palmar piece, keeping the distance between them the width of the proximal phalanx from medial to lateral sides. Trim off surplus tin (*Figure 2.18j*).

(5) Curve the dorsal bar for the proximal phalanx over the dorsum of the phalanx to obtain the correct shape, and then solder the free ends of the No. 17 s.w.g. wire to it (*Figure 2.18k*).

(6) The two coils are now soldered into place on either side of the dorsal bar, making sure that the fulcrum of the movement of the coil is opposite the proximal interphalangeal joint. The proximal portions of the wire will require to be cut from the length from the fulcrum to the proximal edge of the dorsal bar (*Figure 2.18i*).

(7) The palmar bar for the middle phalanx is next curved into shape, and soldered on to the free ends of the coils, one on each side. The bar should lie mid-way along the middle phalanx, and the surplus wire cut off.

(8) The splint should then be neatly covered with thin gloving leather, which can be stuck to the tin with any good adhesive and finally trimmed with scissors.

Precautions

(1) The bars across the phalanges must lie mid-way down each phalanx, and not infringe upon the joint and impede movement.

(2) The splint must not be too tight on the finger, nor be allowed to rub against the skin.

Variations

Instead of the semi-circular palmar piece, the proximal phalanx can be completely encircled, as in wearing a ring, and the coil springs attached in the same way on either side.

JIG TOOL FOR MAKING SPRING WIRE COILS (*Figure 2.18l* and *m*)

The jig consists of two parts, as follows. One (part A) is a 22.5 cm length of steel tubing, outside diameter 9.5 mm and 1.1 mm thick, the inside diameter being 4.5 mm. A vertical slot about 5 cm long is cut down one end. The other (part B) is a

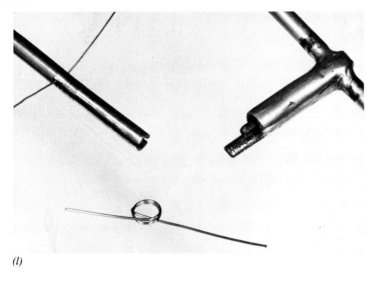

(l)

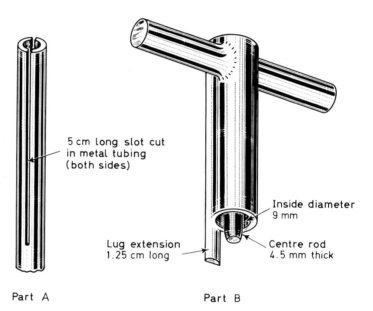

5 cm long slot cut
in metal tubing
(both sides)

Inside diameter
9 mm

Lug extension
1.25 cm long

Centre rod
4.5 mm thick

Part A   Part B

Figure 2.18 (cont)

3.8 cm length of steel tubing, of which the inside diameter is 9 mm, to fit over the outside diameter of part A. Down the centre of this tube is a rod 4.5 mm or just under, which protrudes 0.6 cm beyond the end of the hollow tube. This has to fit inside the rod part A. To the outside of the hollow tube a 1.2 cm lug is attached. A horizontal bar, at least 15 cm long, is fixed to part B at right angles (at the other end from the lug) to provide leverage when coiling the spring wire.

Method of use

Part A is mounted vertically in a vice, the slot uppermost. To begin, cut a length of No. 19 s.w.g. wire about 15 cm long, and place one-third of this through the base of the slot, the remaining two-thirds being necessary to make the coil. Part B is then fitted over part A, when the lug in part B will contact the wire in the slot. Holding the short end in one hand, the handle is then turned smoothly and firmly in order to counteract the springiness of the wire, and continued for two and one-half revolutions. Care must be taken to raise the handle slightly at each revolution in order that the coils lie one upon the other (this 'raising' is the thickness of the wire). Clockwise turning of the handle will produce a spring for one side of the finger, and an anti-clockwise turn for the other.

REFERENCES AND BIBLIOGRAPHY

Bolton, H. (1970). Primary tendon repair. *The Hand* **2,** 56–57

Bunnell, S. (1970). *Surgery of the Hand,* 5th edn. Ed. by J. H. Boyes. Philadelphia, Pa: Lippincott

Campbell Reid, D. (1966). Tendon injuries. In *Clinical Surgery,* Vol. 7: *The Hand,* pp. 114–128. Ed. by R. Guy Pulvertaft, Charles Rob and Rodney Smith. London: Butterworths

Capener, N. C. (1949). The use of orthopaedic appliances in the treatment of anterior poliomyelitis. *Postgraduate Medical Journal* **37B,** 59

Curtis, R. (1971). Capsulectomy of the interphalangeal joints. In *Traumatismes Osteoarticulaires de la Main.* Paris: Expansion Scientifique Francaise

Flynn, J. E. (1953). Problems with trauma to the hand. *Journal of Bone and Joint Surgery* **35A,** 132–140

Harrison, S. H. (1969). Delayed primary flexor tendon grafts. *The Hand* **1,** 106–107

Helal, B. (1969). Silastics in hand surgery. *The Hand* **1,** 120–121

Jaffé, S. and Weckesser, E. (1966). Profundus tendon grafting with sublimis intact. *Journal of Bone and Joint Surgery* **48,** 614

Kleinert, H. E., Kutz, J. E., Alasoy, E. and Stormo, A. (1973). Primary repair of flexor tendons. *Orthopedic Clinics of North America* **4,** 865–876

McFarlane, R. M., Lamon, R. and Jarvis, G. (1968). Flexor tendon injuries within the finger. A study of the results of tendon suture and tendon graft. *Journal of Trauma* **8,** 987–1003

Madsen, E. (1970). Delayed primary suture of flexor tendons cut in the digital sheath. *Journal of Bone and Joint Surgery* **52B,** 264–267

Mason, M. L. and Aiken, H. S. (1941). Rate of healing of tendons – experimental study of extensile strength. *Annals of Surgery* **113,** 424–459

Morley, G. H. (1956). Flexor tendon injuries. A review of results. *British Journal of Plastic Surgery* **8,** 300–311

Parkes, A. H. (1970). The lumbrical plus finger. *Journal of Bone and Joint Surgery* **53B,** 236–239

Pulvertaft, R. G. (1950). Repair of tendon injuries in the hand, with special reference to flexor tendons. *Postgraduate Medical Journal* **8,** 81

Rank, B. K. and Hueston, J. T. (1973). *Surgery of Repair as Applied to Hand Injuries,* 4th edn. Edinburgh: Churchill Livingstone

Skoog, T. and Persson, B. H. (1954). An experimental study of the early healing of tendons. *Plastic and Reconstructive Surgery* **13,** 384–399

Stack, H. (1969). Mallet finger. *The Hand* **1,** 83

Verdan, C. and Crawford, G. P. (1971). Flexor tendon suture in the digital canal. In *5th World Congress of Plastic and Reconstructive Surgery.* Sydney: Butterworths

Winston, M. E. (1972). The results of treatment of injuries to the flexor tendons. *The Hand* **4,** 45–52

Wood-Jones, F. (1942). *The Principles of Anatomy as Seen in the Hand,* p. 274. Baltimore: Williams & Wilkins

Peripheral Nerve Injuries   3

INTRODUCTION

All three nerves supplying the hand are liable to damage which may well result in very severe loss of function.

Damage to the median nerve is the most serious, for two reasons. First, because the majority of sensation in the hand is supplied by the median nerve and, second, because the muscles that supply the grip between thumb, index and middle finger are supplied for the most part by the median nerve. The ulnar nerve, on the other hand, supplies little sensation in the hand, and complete paralysis of the muscles supplied by the ulnar nerve is consistent with good function, provided that the patient does not require very fine co-ordinated activity.

An ulnar nerve lesion in a heavy labourer is little disability; of course, in a concert pianist it is disastrous. Permanent paralysis of muscles can often satisfactorily be replaced by tendon transfers; for example, sublimis transfer for opposition in median nerve palsies and Brand's many-tailed operation for correcting clawing of the hand in ulnar nerve palsy. Replacement of sensation, however, is a much greater problem. The most serious injuries, therefore, are those involving damage to both nerves and all the tendons of the wrist together with a great deal of soft tissue damage resulting in fibrosis, tendon adherence, contractures, stiff joints and, if untreated, a crippled hand for life.

In this chapter, the cause and significance of peripheral nerve injuries and detailed assessment of damage and appreciation of subsequent recovery are discussed. The results of various types of lesions, with and without complications, are presented in the light of the authors' experience, and the various treatments of physiotherapy, occupational therapy, remedial exercises, lively splintage and retraining are all fully described. This chapter is based on the personal study of 659 peripheral nerve injuries involving the hand: 286 lesions of the ulnar nerve, 180 of the median nerve, 118 of the radial nerve and 75 combined median and ulnar nerve lesions.

CAUSES

Peripheral nerve injuries can result from trauma or from pressure lesions.

Trauma

RADIAL NERVE

The following are the main causes of injury to the radial nerve in order of frequency: fractures of the humerus involving the nerve in the spiral groove; direct blows to the nerve in the upper arm; traction lesions; damage to the nerve by pressure in sleep – as in a Saturday night palsy – fractures of the radius and ulna; and direct blows to the forearm involving the posterior interosseus branch. The posterior interosseus nerve is also liable to pressure lesions, due to compression of the nerve in the forearm. Pressure lesions to all nerves in the upper limb are treated in a separate section (see page 80).

In the series of peripheral nerve injuries discussed by Seddon and Brooks (1954) in the Medical Research Council report, of 102 nerve injuries due to fractures, 44 were radial palsies following fractures of the humerus. Seventy per cent of the cases in the Medical Research Council series achieved spontaneous recovery. This accords with our experience. It is usually obvious from the X-ray or coexistence of severe soft tissue damage if the nerve is likely to have been severed and exploration is necessary.

MEDIAN NERVE

The most common cause of damage to the median nerve is by falling on glass or putting the hand through a glass window pane and severing the nerve at the wrist. Next in frequency are lacerations of the wrist due to a multitude of causes such as cuts by glass, knife wounds and falls on hard objects. Then come various lesions at the elbow – lacerations, fractures and ischaemic paralysis. Other causes are traction injuries involving the median nerve roots, and compression of the nerve in the carpal tunnel by the flexor retinaculum (see page 83).

A strange phenomenon is sometimes seen when the thenar muscles are spared following complete division of the median nerve at the wrist. We have seen eight such cases when the median nerve was reported by highly skilled hand surgeons to be completely divided and which was then sutured.

On admission to the rehabilitation unit, all the muscles normally supplied by the median nerve were functioning normally and only partial sensory loss was present. It is known that motor fibres can leave the median nerve in the forearm and cross to the ulnar nerve by a communicating branch, continuing distally in the ulnar nerve to the hand. A lesion at the wrist would therefore not affect the thenar muscles.

This can be demonstrated by stimulation of the median nerve at the elbow when thenar action will be seen, whilst at the wrist stimulation produces no activity. Conversely, stimulation of the ulnar nerve at the elbow will produce no activity in the thenar muscles, but stimulation at the wrist will do so. Similarly, but less commonly, the ulnar-supplied intrinsics in the hand may be spared after ulnar nerve lesions at the elbow, due to the presence of a communicating branch from the median nerve in the forearm.

ULNAR NERVE

The most common site of injury of the ulnar nerve is at the wrist, and by far the most common cause is, again, putting the hand through a glass window pane. The next most common are lacerations due to knives and glass. Lesions at the elbow are common – associated with fractures, dislocations or direct severance. Many years after fracture of one of the bones of the elbow joint, pressure on the ulnar nerve may be caused by gradual progressive deformity (cubitus valgus).

Arthritis of the joint is a rarer cause. Traction lesions may involve the nerve roots in the neck.

MEDIAN AND ULNAR NERVES

The most common cause of damage to both nerves at the wrist is by falls on glass or putting the hand through a glass window pane. One or more tendons are almost invariably severed also and frequently one of the arteries. The combination of division of both nerves and all tendons at the wrist is perhaps the most devastating injury that can befall the hand – the tendon complications and their management are considered in Chapter 2 (page 37).

Both can be damaged in severe fractures of the forearm bones and are vulnerable also at the elbow by direct violence, involvement in fractures or dislocations of the joint, or injuries from falls through windows. In the neck and axilla, gunshot wounds and traction lesions in traffic accidents are the most common causes of damage. The nerves can be involved in crush injuries, particularly in traffic accidents and industrial injuries at any level in the upper limb. Too tight plasters can cause direct nerve damage as well as through vascular damage indirectly such as Volkmann's ischaemic contracture.

Pressure lesions

An increasing number of conditions have been recognized whereby peripheral nerves can be compressed at some level in their course down the limb. These have been given the generic title of entrapment neuropathies. They can be due to pathological conditions such as ganglia, lipomata, malunited fractures; to anomalous anatomical structures; or to pressure of tight normal anatomical structures. The underlying pathology is local disturbance of the myelin at the site of pressure, which may produce a neurapraxia only or may be sufficiently severe to cause complete wallerian degeneration demanding exploration and release, and all stages of partial lesions between these two extremes.

CERVICAL SPINE

Prolapsed intervertebral discs, osteophytes in cervical spondylosis and rheumatoid disease of the cervical spine are the most common causes; rarer causes include infections of the vertebrae, primary and secondary bone tumours and Pancoast tumour. Pain and paraesthesiae in the root distribution are the most frequent symptoms – marked wasting and weakness in the hand muscles do occur but are rare in cervical spine disorders and all other causes of neuropathy must be excluded before attributing the neuropathy to cervical spondylosis which is extremely common over the age of 50. Clumsiness and difficulty in fine movements, reduced tendon reflexes and sensory changes are common but not actual wasting of the small muscles of the hand.

ROOT OF NECK

This is referred to as the thoracic inlet or outlet syndrome. Strictly speaking, it should be termed the thoracic inlet, but the term outlet is widely used, although in a postgraduate examination asking for a description of the thoracic outlet, a candidate who described the structures emerging from the thorax to the abdomen could not be marked down. Here pressure by cervical ribs, anomalous bands or scalenus anticus tendon can cause nerve pressure, particularly on the medial cord affecting the ulnar supplied muscles. Usually there are marked vascular symptoms and pain, which help to distinguish the syndrome from more distal pressure lesions at the elbow or in the axilla.

Lain (1969) described a partial lesion of the C5–6 roots in cadets required to perform the 'military brace', with strong retraction and depression of the shoulders and the chin down for 30 minutes or more several times a day. This occurred in 13 of 1000 cadets. The condition recovered completely with cessation of the abnormal posture. It was thought to be due to contraction of the scalene muscles, causing ischaemia of the C5–6 roots, due to an anomalous relationship between a muscle and the roots. One of our patients developed a complete C5 palsy after carrying a 13.5 kg rucksack on his back strapped round the shoulders for 10 minutes – complete recovery occurred in 5 weeks.

There are certain pressure lesions peculiar to each nerve in the arm and these will now be considered.

RADIAL NERVE

This can be compressed in the axilla against a chair, as in the well known Saturday night palsy, or by axillary crutches.

Recently a new cause of radial nerve compression has been described by Lotem (1971): a fibrous arch 2 cm distal to the insertion of the deltoid from the lateral head of the triceps can compress the radial nerve. Three cases were described of radial palsy following resisted action of the shoulder muscles, such as loading a truck, pushing a heavy load and exercising with heavy weights, and it was shown that the nerve was compressed by muscular contraction against the arch. A fibrous arch has also been demonstrated over the posterior interosseus nerve on its course through the supinator and intense muscular activity can cause compression, with the characteristic clinical picture of paralysis of finger and thumb extensors and sparing of the extensor carpi radialis longus.

POSTERIOR INTEROSSEUS NERVE

The two layers of the supinator muscle can compress the nerve against the aponeurosis of the extensor carpi radialis brevis. The nerve can also be compressed by lipomata, ganglia, fibromata and fibrosis after trauma.

ULNAR NERVE

This can be compressed in the axilla, causing the well known crutch palsy, and is seen in people who have had axillary crutches for many years. The introduction of elbow crutches should have banished this condition for ever.

The most common site of compression is at the elbow where the nerve is superficial as it runs along the medial epicondyle. The nerve passes through a tunnel, the roof of which is a fibrous band across the two heads of the flexor carpi ulnaris. Osborne (1970) has shown that this band tightens in elbow flexion and the capsular floor bulges up. Thus, in cubitus valgus or arthritis of the elbow joint, the floor of the tunnel can become elevated and compress the ulnar nerve against this band. In the early stages this causes a conduction block only, but in due course adhesions may form, binding the nerve down and producing wallerian degeneration. A sudden minor injury may trigger off a severe nerve lesion in a subclinical chronic compression syndrome and this has a bad prognosis in view of the long-standing nerve changes.

Osborne distinguishes another type, the acute-on-normal lesion, in which a minor injury such as sleeping on the elbow, compression at operation or a trivial blow, may compress a normal nerve in a tunnel narrowed by a tight band. These cases respond dramatically to operation and there is no need to perform a transplantation with the disturbance to the blood supply that this demands. Such views coincide well with Payan's (1970) work, in which he showed that ulnar transposition has surprisingly little effect clinically, and with our experience that once wasting, weakness and objective sensory loss are present, transposition is ineffective because permanent damage has been caused due to intraneural fibrosis – a complete barrier to reinnervation. The good results of surgery are probably due to division of the bands in Osborne's 'acute-on-normal' cases. It is strongly recommended that all patients with symptoms of ulnar neuritis be subjected to conduction studies as described in Chapter 4 (page 218) to ensure that there is evidence of a localized conduction block at the elbow.

Patients with the carpal tunnel syndrome can refer their symptoms to the little and ring fingers, and we routinely study both median and ulnar nerves at the upper arm, forearm and at the wrist in any patients with symptoms referred to either ulnar or median nerves. Moreover, 'ulnar neuritis' may be the first manifestation of a generalized polyneuropathy – detection of generalized slowing of conduction in the nerve with no localizing features must be followed up with measurement of conduction velocity in other nerves.

COMPRESSION AT THE WRIST AND IN THE PALM

Just as the median nerve is compressed in the carpal tunnel, so the ulnar nerve can be compressed as it passes through the canal of Guyon at the wrist. This canal is bordered on the medial side by the tendon of the flexor carpi ulnaris and the pisiform; the floor is the flexor retinaculum and the roof is the superficial part of the retinaculum. Beyond the tunnel the nerve divides into its superficial and deep branches, the deep branch passes through a tunnel bounded by the pisohamate ligament and the origin of the hypothenar muscles.

The deep branch makes a sharp turn round the hook of the hamate between the origins of the abductor digiti minimi, and the sensory fibres lie superficial to the motor branch in the canal. The nerve can be compressed proximal to or within the canal by ganglia, in which case both branches are affected giving weakness of abductor digiti minimi and sensory loss in the little finger as well as weakness of interossei, adductor pollicis and the medial two lumbricals. If the lesion is in the canal or at the hook of the hamate, only the motor branch is affected and this produces the classic deep branch syndrome, seen in people whose occupations demand pressure on the heel of the palm such as despatch riders pressing on their handlebars, lorry drivers 'crashing' their gears or workmen operating heavy tools whose handles press into the palm. Occasionally the deep branch is spared and only the superficial branch is affected, resulting in sensory loss only. Other causes of compression in this area are fractures of the carpus, tumours, osteoarthritis and aberrant muscles or nerves (Shea and McClain, 1969).

The site of compression and the distinction between lesions at the wrist and the elbow can be determined by conduction studies (page 220).

MEDIAN NERVE

Compression at elbow

The median nerve can occasionally be compressed by a musculofibrous band from the deep to the superficial head of the pronator teres. It almost always occurs in men and is aggravated by the use of the forearm muscles, particularly pronator teres. There is also a fibrous arch from the origins of the flexor digitorum sublimis, and the median nerve can be compressed by this, causing isolated weakness of the flexor digitorum sublimis and the flexor digitorum profundus.

Compression at wrist

The most common cause of entrapment neuropathy in the upper limb is the carpal tunnel syndrome. Compression of the median nerve within the carpal tunnel may be caused by an increase in the volume of the contents, decrease in the volume of the tunnel due to deformity of the bone trough (such as in osteoarthritis or after fractures), thickening of the transverse carpal ligament (probably due to thickening of the flexor retinaculum with age) and anomalous structures within the tunnel. Among common symptomatic causes of carpal tunnel syndrome are tenosynovitis, myxoede-ma, acromegaly, amyloid disease, neuroma of the median nerve, dislocation forward of the lunate and the result of a Colles' fracture set in a bad position (Robins, 1961). One of the earliest manifestations of rheumatoid arthritis is a carpal tunnel syndrome due to pressure of rheumatoid flexor tendon synovitis on the median nerve. This may precede articular manifestations. The most common cause is the idiopathic variety seen particularly in middle-age women with symptoms of paraesthesiae in the thumb, index and middle fingers at night, relieved by moving the hands about or putting them above their head. This condition is relieved by decompression or, in mild cases, by the injection of steroids into the flexor retinaculum or splinting with the wrist in the neutral position.

ANTERIOR INTEROSSEUS NERVE

Involvement of this nerve produces a characteristic clinical picture with weakness or paralysis of pronator quadratus, flexor pollicis longus and flexor profundus of the index and, occasionally, the middle finger. There may be patchy sensory loss in the median distribution. Causes include compression from fractures of the forearm bones, direct violence, ganglia and involvement in viral neuritis – neuralgic amyotrophy.

TYPES OF LESIONS

There are three main types of nerve lesion, classified according to the amount of damage sustained: neurapraxia, axonotmesis and neurotmesis.

Neurapraxia

Neurapraxia is defined as loss of conduction in a nerve without degeneration. The signs of a neurapraxia are paralysis in muscles supplied by the nerve with minimal wasting, and electrical signs showing that there has been no denervation. It may often be possible to stimulate the nerve below the point of block and thus show that there has been no extensive damage to it. Stimulation above the block does not cause contraction of the muscles supplied by the nerve except in a few cases when a very high current might penetrate through the block. Common causes of neurapraxia are blows and pressure on the nerve, insufficient to cause damage to the nerve structures resulting in denervation.

Careful electrical investigations into cases of neurapraxia have revealed that a pure neurapraxia is very rare. Almost always there is some slight evidence of degeneration. This, however, is seldom sufficient to be obvious clinically when the block recovers, but it is of interest to know that injuries which cause a neurapraxia almost always produce some denervation, however slight.

Usually, one of the functions of the nerve is spared to some extent. Very often there is not as complete a sensory loss as would be expected in a complete lesion of the nerve, though motor paralysis is usually complete. Within the sensory modalities the proprioceptive fibres are most vulnerable. A neurapraxia usually recovers completely within 6 weeks after onset and often within 4 weeks. Patients have, however, been seen in whom a neurapraxia has persisted for up to 3 months. Careful electrical tests will relieve the patient's anxiety. Although electrical signs of denervation do not appear for 5–7 days after injury, the presence of nerve conduction with a comparable electrical threshold to the normal side at 5 days is highly suggestive of simple block to conduction without degeneration.

Axonotmesis

Axonotmesis is defined as injury to the nerve in which the axon is damaged to such an extent that wallerian degeneration occurs. The damage is not sufficient to affect the nerve sheath; the fact that the sheath is intact means that the nerve fibres can grow down their own tunnel. Suture is therefore not needed and recovery is usually almost perfect. Re-education is, theoretically, not required because the fibres make contact with the correct end-organs, but in our experience it is advisable for the best results. Surgical exploration may, of course, be necessary in axonotmesis if there is pressure by some agent such as callus or tumour, or if the nerve is under tension due, for example, to a neuroma.

Case 3.1 A farm worker caught his arm in moving machinery, sustaining fractures of both humeri and a posterior dislocation of the left shoulder. Four months later he was referred for intensive rehabilitation and an opinion on the site of complete median and ulnar nerve lesions in the left arm. The painful stiff shoulder responded dramatically to intra-articular steroid injection and intensive active exercises. The Tinel sign was positive for the median nerve 20 cm above the olecranon, being 16.5 cm below the tip of the shoulder and thus consistent with a regenerating lesion of the median nerve injured at the shoulder. A strong Tinel sign for the ulnar nerve was 12.5 cm distal to the medial epicondyle, while a weaker Tinel sign was present 19 cm proximal to this. It was felt that this indicated a regenerating lesion of the ulnar nerve sited at the level of the fracture. EMG studies showed highly polyphasic units in flexor digitorum profundus of the ring finger with latencies of 7.9 ms from elbow and 25.6 in axilla, giving a motor conduction velocity of 18 m/s in the regenerating segment. Similar findings were noted in flexor digitorum sublimis, thus confirming regenerating lesions. No surgery was therefore indicated and the patient returned to work with a lively splint and, being a sensible man, understood how to avoid trophic lesions in his anaesthetic hand.

On review, 4½ years later, the left upper limb was entirely normal. The grip on the left hand was the same as on the right, all the intrinsics worked independently grade 5 and sensation was nearly normal – localization being perfect; no hypersensitivity was experienced but he had slight difficulty in recognizing textures of thin paper and cardboard. Muscle bulk was only slightly less than on the unaffected side.

Neurotmesis

Neurotmesis is defined as an injury to a nerve involving both axis cylinder and sheath. Suture is essential to provide the growing axon with a tunnel, otherwise it will grow in a haphazard fashion and very few nerve fibres will achieve their destination. Re-education is vital, as only a small proportion of axons return to their original end-organs.

As discussed under neurapraxia, there may well be a condition in which part of the nerve is blocked and part is actually degenerated.

The classic signs of nerve degeneration, both clinical and electrical, are seen in both axonotmesis and neurotmesis; these are discussed in detail in Chapter 4.

The indications for surgical exploration in nerve injuries depend on whether the lesion is open or closed and on the type of injury that originally caused the nerve damage.

In complete lesions, exploration is indicated when there is an open wound, and in closed injuries if recovery is delayed longer than would be expected after waiting for the nerve to grow at a rate of 1 mm a day, or if there is obvious compression of the nerve by callus, tumour or aneurysm.

PATHOLOGY

After section of a nerve, certain changes take place in both muscle and nerve. The changes in nerves are known as wallerian degeneration. The nerve degenerates to the proximal node of Ranvier, the axis cylinder disintegrates and the debris is cleared away by macrophage activity. The empty tube is left, along which the large cells of Schwann proliferate. If the lesion is a neurotmesis, there is, of course, no tunnel present.

In the muscle some change in the arrangement of the fibres is seen by the end of the sixth week. Subsequently, there is progressive kinking of the fibres, the coarse striation becomes less obvious and finally they begin to disrupt after 3 years. By the end of the twelfth week, connective tissue elements increase and invade the terminal Schwann tubes. Gradually, the muscle is replaced by fibrous tissue. If reinnervation does not occur, the muscle becomes fibrotic after about 2 years.

The significance of these changes is that nerve suture must be carried out as early as possible in order that the best muscle function will result. As the muscle becomes fibrotic by 2 years after denervation, it is essential to perform nerve suture so that reinnervation occurs within this period. Good function cannot be expected in muscles a long distance from the site of lesion. For example, repair of the median nerve at its origin in the neck would be unlikely to give good function in the thenar muscles, as it would take longer than 2 years for the nerve to grow down to them; consequently, many surgeons carry out tendon transfer as an immediate procedure.

CLINICAL PICTURE

Certain changes common to all peripheral nerve injuries are seen; they can be divided into motor, sensory and sympathetic effects.

Motor

The obvious result of damage to the motor part of the peripheral nerve is motor paralysis. However, there are certain trick movements which may well confuse the examiner in his assessment of the extent of paralysis, and may also be confusing when assessing reinnervation. These trick movements do not seem to be well known and will therefore be discussed in detail under the appropriate headings.

Wasting is an inevitable accompaniment of axonotmesis or neurotmesis, but not of neurapraxia. It first becomes obvious in about 4–6 weeks after the lesion; 2 months after damage, wasting develops rapidly and becomes maximal about 3 months after injury. It is important to explain to the patient that the wasting will become more progressive, otherwise he may feel that the treatment he is receiving is doing him harm and he will naturally be worried to see a progressive loss of muscle bulk. The deep reflexes will, of course, be diminished and finally lost altogether with muscle paralysis. Tone is absent. Deformities will arise as a result of the muscle paralysis due to overaction of the antagonist muscle groups; these are described in detail later.

Sensation

In a complete lesion all modalities of sensation, except joint position sense, are lost. In many cases the nerves subserving joint sensation travel via the tendons and not through the large nerve trunks at the wrist. If there has been an isolated nerve lesion without tendon damage, position sense may be retained. It will usually be a coarse appreciation but it will be present. This may cause confusion and suggest a partial lesion, but only if the underlying anatomical facts are not realized. There will be the appropriate anaesthetic areas of skin. It is important to realize that sensory supply by no means always follows the description given in the textbooks.

Various common anomalies have been described in Chapter 1; the most common concerns the radial nerve which may well subserve no sensation at all. It is very rare in a patient with a radial nerve lesion to have any part of the skin completely anaesthetic.

Soon after injury the area of complete sensory loss contracts, due to the adjacent nerves taking over sensation in the periphery of the affected area. It is not to be taken to mean that there has been a partial nerve lesion only.

The skin becomes scaly, the nails brittle and curved, and the soft tissues become atrophic so that there may be as much as 0.6 cm loss in circumference of an affected finger.

Vasomotor disturbance

The changes in circulation are clearly divided into two phases. In the early stages after denervation the affected skin is warm – this appears to be due to paralysis of the vasoconstrictor nerves. Some 3 weeks later the skin becomes cold. Usually only the area of skin supplied by the affected sensory nerve becomes cold, but sometimes the whole hand is colder than the normal side. The temperature of the denervated skin depends very much on the climate – the colder the weather, the colder the denervated area. At this time, too, the skin takes on a characteristic reddish colour which becomes purple when cold. There is a clear-cut division between the affected and the normal skin.

Trophic lesions are most likely to occur in these early stages before the patient has learnt that he must be extremely careful with the anaesthetic skin; burns and blisters which may become infected are commonly caused by cigarettes and leaning with the hands behind the back on a radiator. It is very important to warn patients about the possible dangers of anaesthetic skin and they should always be encouraged to wear gloves whenever the weather becomes cold.

Later, the scaliness of the denervated skin disappears, the texture becomes smooth and shiny, and the skin creases, causing ridges to become much more obvious.

The vasomotor changes are not fully understood. Barnes (1954) suggested that the loss of the axon reflex may well be an important factor; this may be necessary to normal defence and nutrition of the skin.

It must not be forgotten that there are general effects of localized lesions of the hand. Later, the lack of use of the hand due to paralysis may produce stiffness in other joints of the limb.

The psychological effect of the paralysis must never be forgotten.

In peripheral nerve injuries, particularly severe ones involving the hand, it is more important than ever to explain to the patient exactly why he has the deformities, the paralysis and the loss of feeling, what is being done to help and what the ultimate result is expected to be. Such patients require continual encouragement throughout the long months of waiting for nerve regeneration.

DEFORMITIES IN SPECIFIC NERVE LESIONS

Median nerve lesions

Lesions of the median nerve, at whatever site, produce some deformity in the hand.

DEFORMITIES AT THE WRIST

The deformity of median nerve paralysis at the wrist is commonly known as the monkey hand, because of its flat appearance due to wasting of the thenar eminence and lack of opposition. The thumb is held beside the index finger because the internal

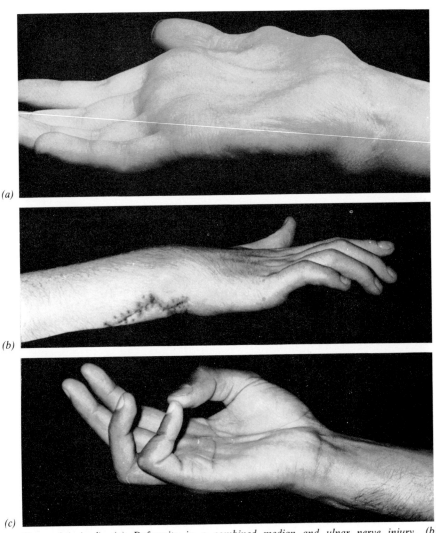

(a)

(b)

(c)

Figure 3.1 (a–d) (a) Deformity in a combined median and ulnar nerve injury. (b) Hyperextension deformity in ulnar palsy. (c) Attempted opposition—note inability to flex metacarpophalangeal joints with interphalangeal joints extended

rotator muscles of the thumb, the abductor brevis and opponens are paralysed and, therefore, their antagonist, the extensor pollicis longus, exerts an unopposed action in pulling the thumb round beside the index finger in extension. There is paralysis of the first and second lumbricals so there may be a hyperextension deformity at the metacarpophalangeal joints of the index and middle fingers, due to the overaction of the extensor digitorum (*Figure 3.1a*).

LESIONS AT THE ELBOW AND NECK

Lesions in the elbow or in the neck will result in motor paralysis of the flexors of the fingers and wrist and of the pronators, but not in any more marked deformity than is seen with lesions at the wrist joint. The only extra deformity seen with damage at the elbow is that there may be hyperextension of the wrist due to overaction of the wrist extensors unopposed by the paralysed wrist flexors.

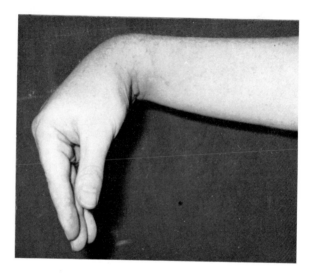

Figure 3.1 (cont.)   (d) Deformity in radial nerve palsy. Note extension of interphalangeal joint of thumb due to action of abductor and flexor pollicis brevis

FUNCTIONAL DISABILITY

Bowden and Napier (1961) described a number of objective tests for function for patients after peripheral nerve suture. These involve the ability to use precision grip when assessing weights and sizes of objects and the ability to carry out power grip, with varying sized cylinders and with various functional activities such as putting electric light bulbs in sockets. It cannot be overemphasized that the only way of assessing results of peripheral nerve suture is by the function to which the patient is able to put his hand.

Most patients with a median nerve lesion find difficulty in picking up both big and small objects, and are generally clumsy, finding that they cannot hold objects with confidence, nor can they tell what is in their hands unless they look. They cannot fasten buttons or shoelaces, or cut their finger nails or cut up meat. To hold a fork is difficult, as is shaving.

The main reason for their clumsiness is the loss of sensation. Some grip can be obtained by action of the flexor pollicis longus and adductor pollicis against the radial side of the index finger.

Interference with precision grip is a most serious disability in a median nerve lesion and power grip is affected also, due to loss of the stabilizing action of the thumb.

Ulnar nerve lesions

The classic deformity due to ulnar nerve paralysis is the 'claw hand'; this will occur whether the lesion is present at the wrist, the elbow or in the neck (*Figure 3.1b*). The metacarpophalangeal joints of the ring and little fingers are held in hyperextension (usually about 30 degrees). This is due to the overaction of the extensor digitorum communis and the extensor digiti minimi whose main action is at these joints, and the lack of the brake to hyperextension normally supplied by the lumbricals.

The interphalangeal joints of these two fingers are held in flexion (25 degrees at the proximal interphalangeal joint and 10–20 degrees at the terminal interphalangeal joint) due to the overaction of the flexors profundus and sublimis, which are unopposed by their paralysed antagonists, the interossei.

If the lesion is at the elbow, there will be paralysis of the flexor profundus to the ring and little fingers, and consequently there will be only a slight flexion deformity of the interphalangeal joints due to the sublimis action, there being none at the terminal interphalangeal joints. Paradoxically, a sign of satisfactory regeneration of an ulnar nerve lesion at the elbow, or in that region, is a gradual increasing deformity of flexion of the ring and little fingers, due to the recovery of the profundus muscle. The paralysis of flexor carpi ulnaris does not produce a deformity, although on attempted ulnar deviation the wrist will go into extension due to unopposed action of the extensor carpi ulnaris.

The claw hand in an ulnar nerve palsy mimics the position adopted by the 'refined' when drinking tea.

FUNCTIONAL DISABILITY

Most patients with an ulnar nerve lesion have a functional disability which prevents them from holding a knife properly: they usually hold it between the index and middle fingers.

Writing is difficult, due particularly to the loss of sensation in the little finger and hypothenar eminence with the hand on the paper. Pulling tight and tying shoe laces is awkward; there is difficulty in fastening buttons and cutting finger nails; shaving is also difficult.

Pinch grip is poor – attempts at which produce slight flexion only at the metacarpophalangeal joints of the fingers, 90 degrees' flexion at the proximal interphalangeal joints due to overaction of the flexor sublimis and hyperextension of the terminal interphalangeal joint. The thumb is usually flexed at the interphalangeal joint and hyperextended at the metacarpophalangeal joint.

Power grip is more affected than precision grip in ulnar nerve lesions. Three features responsible for the inefficiency of the grip are as pointed out by Bowden and

Napier (1961): inability to wrap the fingers fully round an object; failure of elevation of the hypothenar eminence; and ineffective clamping action of the thumb due to paralysis of adductor pollicis. Precision grip is affected to some extent, resulting from a lack of spread of the fingers due to interosseus paralysis.

A few patients, however, learn to carry out almost all activities, and some 10 per cent do not regard the lesion as any disability at all. We have had patients with complete ulnar lesions who have been able to play the saxophone or guitar, and fly fighter aircraft, and aircraft technicians who, with a lively splint, have been able to carry out the highly skilled work of servicing engines.

Patients with a median and ulnar nerve lesion combined, together with adherence of flexor tendons at the wrist, are seriously handicapped. They have crude grip, but are incapable of any fine co-ordinated hand activity.

Radial nerve lesions

The characteristic deformity in a radial nerve palsy is a wrist-drop. The wrist is held in some 45 degrees' palmar flexion due to the overaction of the wrist flexors unopposed by their antagonists – the paralysed wrist extensors. The thumb is held in palmar abduction and slight flexion, due to the unopposed action of the short flexor and short abductor, their antagonists – the long abductor and short and long extensors – being paralysed.

The metacarpophalangeal joints are held in about 30 degrees' flexion due to the unopposed action of the lumbricals, the extensor digitorum being paralysed. There is only slight flexion at the interphalangeal joints as the interossei extend these joints and are, of course, unaffected; the slight flexion is that due to the wrist and metacarpophalangeal joints taking up a position of flexion which automatically results in slight flexion at the proximal interphalangeal joints (*Figure 3.1b*).

Attempts at ulnar deviation result in increased flexion and deviation due to the overaction of the flexor carpi ulnaris unopposed by its paralysed antagonist – the extensor carpi ulnaris. Wasting of the extensor muscles of the forearm is obvious.

FUNCTIONAL DISABILITY

Patients with a radial nerve lesion cannot hold a knife or fork easily, nor cut their finger nails. They have difficult in fastening buttons and brushing their hair. Shaving and tying shoe laces are also difficult to manage. Generally they have a poor grip and cannot put objects like glasses or cups down flat on a table.

TRICK MOVEMENTS

When the prime movers are paralysed, other muscles may take over their function and produce so-called 'trick movements'.

It is important to know what trick movements should be present in nerve paralysis. Ignorance of them may lead to diagnosis of a partial lesion when, in fact, it is complete; knowledge of them allows the provision of lively splints so that they may be harnessed for function.

As a result of our experience in patients with nerve injuries, we recognize the following types of trick movements.

DIRECT SUBSTITUTION OF FAVOURABLY PLACED MUSCLES

Full abduction and elevation of the shoulder are possible, despite paralysis of deltoid, by using muscles which cross the shoulder joint – the long head of biceps and triceps, the pectoralis major and the spinati.

ACCESSORY INSERTION

The abductor pollicis brevis and the flexor pollicis brevis insert into the extensor expansion of the thumb. It is thus possible to extend the interphalangeal joint of the thumb when the radial or posterior interosseus nerves are paralysed. The abductor digiti minimi can be inserted into the volar aspect of the proximal phalanx and can thus flex the metacarpophalangeal joint.

TENDON ACTION

This is the shortening of a tendon when its antagonist, which is longer, contracts strongly and is seen in muscles which cross two joints. In paralysis of the long flexors of the fingers, extension of the wrist is associated with a tendon action of flexion of the interphalangeal joints as the flexors are shorter than the extensors. This is deceptive, for it can look very much as if the long flexors are contracting actively.

REBOUND

When the antagonist to a paralysed muscle contracts strongly and then relaxes quickly, it may seem as if there is active contraction in the paralysed muscle. Strong contraction of the extensor pollicis longus and sudden relaxation may look as if the long flexor is working. Similarly, in a lateral popliteal palsy, a strong contraction of the plantar flexors of the toes, followed by relaxation, may look as if the toe extensors are contracting.

ANOMALOUS NERVE SUPPLY

Anomalous nerve supply in the hand occurs in 20 per cent of all normal subjects (page 20).

GRAVITY

Wood-Jones, in his classic book, *The Principles of Anatomy as Seen in the Hand*, pointed out that muscles will always allow gravity to effect a movement if given the chance. When the triceps is paralysed and elbow extension is being tested, the patient will depress the shoulder so as to allow gravity to extend the elbow.

Trick movements in specific nerve injuries

RADIAL NERVE PALSIES

In radial nerve palsies the wrist extensors are paralysed, but after strong contraction of the wrist and finger flexors their relaxation can give the impression of an extensor action.

To be certain that there is no action in the wrist extensors, the patient's wrist should be supported in full dorsiflexion, and the tendons felt at the back of the wrist while the patient is asked to try to dorsiflex. In the absence of any action in the wrist extensors the wrist will be felt to flex instead of extend. In the early stages of recovery of the wrist extensors the patient will be unable to institute dorsiflexion of the wrist even when thus examined. If the patient is asked to grip an object, however, a flicker is often felt in the wrist extensors; this is because a muscle contraction is more easily detected in the early stages of recovery when it acts as a synergist rather than as a prime mover. Again, a sign of early recovery is apparent when the patient is asked to dorsiflex the wrist in the inner range; he no longer flexes first – that is, the lack of trick movement is an indication of recovery even though the prime-mover action may not be obvious. The extensors of the metacarpophalangeal joints are paralysed, but extension of the fingers is possible because this is performed by the interossei. If the patient is asked to extend the metacarpophalangeal joints, flexion will be seen at these joints, as the intrinsics contract in an effort to produce extension. When the metacarpophalangeal joints are supported in almost full extension and the patient is asked to extend the fingers, extension of the interphalangeal joints will be seen as the interossei contract but at the same time the metacarpophalangeal joints will flex, and it is this metacarpophalangeal flexion which is the key to the trick movement.

The earliest sign of recovery in the extensor digitorum is the lack of flexion at the metacarpophalangeal joints, rather than the obvious prime-mover action, on attempted extension.

Extension of the terminal joint of the thumb is possible in all patients with a radial nerve palsy because the short abductor always, and the short flexor sometimes, have an insertion into the extensor expansion. When the patient is asked to extend the interphalangeal joint of the thumb, the thumb goes immediately into palmar abduction, due to the short abductor action (*Figure 3.2*). To demonstrate that this is a trick action, the patient's thumb should be kept against the index finger and prevented from abducting. Extension of the interphalangeal joint will then be impossible without palmar abduction.

An early sign of reinnervation of the extensor pollicis longus is the lack of abduction when the patient attempts to extend the thumb, even though there may not be prime-mover action.

Extensor carpi radialis longus

This is the first extensor muscle to recover in a radial nerve palsy, so attempted dorsiflexion results in radial deviation because the extensor carpi ulnaris is still paralysed and cannot, therefore, exert its action to bring the wrist into neutral dorsiflexion. The early sign of recovery in extensor carpi ulnaris is therefore a lessening of radial deviation when the wrist is dorsiflexed.

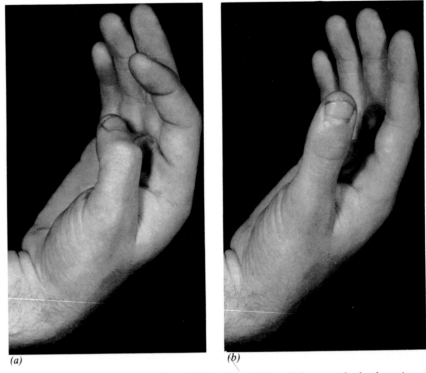

(a)   (b)

Figure 3.2   Extension of interphalangeal joint of thumb in radial nerve palsy by the action of the abductor pollicis brevis which can be seen contracting, bringing the thumb into palmar abduction. (a) Starting position. (b) Extension of interphalangeal joint of thumb — note palmar abduction

MEDIAN NERVE PARALYSIS

It was shown in Chapter 1 that opposition of the thumb to the fingers involves four separate movements – palmar abduction, flexion, rotation and adduction. In median nerve lesions at the wrist the palmar abduction is lost but radial abduction is present through the action of abductor pollicis longus and attempts at palmar abduction result only in radial abduction. Sometimes some fibres of abductor pollicis longus insert into abductor pollicis brevis, so some palmar abduction may be possible despite paralysis of abductor pollicis brevis. Flexion is present, of course, by the long flexor, but rotation is lost. Adduction is possible through the adductor (supplied by the ulnar nerve); consequently, when the patient is asked to oppose his thumb to the little finger, the thumb first goes into radial abduction but, as the long flexor brings the thumb across the palm, the thumb collapses into the palm through lack of palmar abduction. If the short flexor has no ulnar supply, then the interphalangeal joint of the thumb is flexed by the flexor pollicis longus in an attempt to carry the thumb across the palm; the adductor keeps the thumb well into the palm (*Figure 3.3*).

The basis of the lively splint in median nerve paralysis is to bring the thumb into palmar abduction and use the combined flexion and adduction action of flexor pollicis longus and adductor pollicis to simulate opposition.

The paralysis of the first two lumbricals means that when the patient attempts to bend the metacarpophalangeal joints, the interphalangeal joints are hyperflexed, thus attempting to use the long flexor action at the metacarpophalangeal joints. If the patient is asked to flex the metacarpophalangeal joints but keep the interphalangeal joints extended, he will be unable to do so for the lumbrical action of preventing hyperextension at the metacarpophalangeal joint is lost and a 'clawing' movement is produced. Nor will he be able to keep the interphalangeal joints extended and the metacarpophalangeal joints flexed at 90 degrees against any resistance, owing to interosseus paralysis.

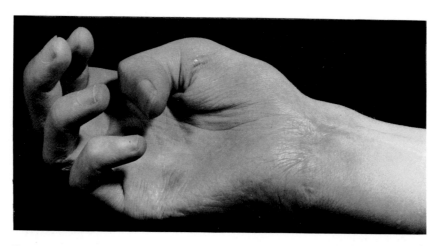

Figure 3.3   *Attempted opposition of the thumb to the little finger in a combined median and ulnar nerve palsy. Note the trick action of the flexor pollicis longus, lack of palmar abduction of the thumb and inability to elevate the fifth metacarpal*

The first sign of recovery in a median nerve lesion at the wrist is the ability of the patient to rotate the thumb. This should be tested in the inner range, supporting the thumb in palmar abduction and slight flexion.

Later, the patient will be able to hold the interphalangeal joints extended and the metacarpophalangeal joints flexed at 90 degrees against slight resistance without the metacarpophalangeal joints 'collapsing' into extension. This test is more sensitive than asking the patient to initiate this 'intrinsic' position, which requires much greater muscle strength, and therefore a more advanced degree of reinnervation.

ULNAR NERVE PARALYSIS

The paralysis of the interossei means that the interphalangeal joints cannot be extended unless the metacarpophalangeal joints are supported so that the long extensor can act on these joints. Without the metacarpophalangeal joints supported, it will be seen that the patient can extend the interphalangeal joints only by flexing the metacarpophalangeal joints as well. This is the principle of the lively splint which supports the metacarpophalangeal joints, thus allowing the long extensor to act on the interphalangeal joints.

The paralysis of the interossei also means that abduction of the fingers is seriously hampered. However, the long extensor can easily trick this action. This is particularly noticeable in the index and little fingers which each have an extensor of their own as well as a tendon from the extensor digitorum communis. Adduction can be tricked by relaxation of the extensors and by contraction of the long flexors.

When the patient tries to abduct the fingers in an ulnar nerve palsy, the long extensor tendons can be seen to stand out on the back of the hand, and the metacarpophalangeal joints go into extension (*Figure 3.4*). Similarly, in adduction, the metacarpophalangeal joints can be seen to go into slight flexion. To emphasize this trick movement the patient should place the hand palm down on the table and be asked to lift the middle finger off the table. This involves the long extensor tendon in maintaining the finger in the air against gravity, and it is now no longer free to act as an abductor. The patient is now asked to move the finger from side to side, when it

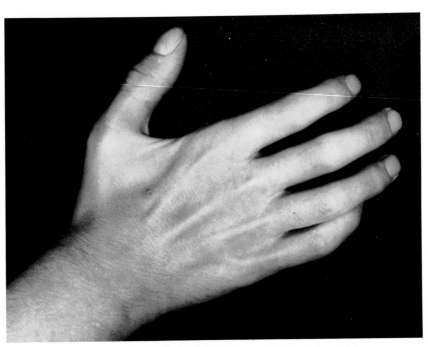

Figure 3.4   Trick abduction of the fingers in ulnar nerve palsy

will be found that it is impossible for him to do so. Instead, the whole palm and wrist joint are seen to move from side to side in a quite characteristic fashion (*Figure 3.5*). This sign is absolutely consistent and is to be seen in all cases of interosseus paralysis. The sign is positive for the ring finger as well. It is not advisable to use it for the index and little fingers as they have two extensors, and one can support the metacarpophalangeal joint in extension while the other produces some trick abduction.

The paralysis of the adductor means that true adduction of the thumb to the index finger is difficult. It is still possible, of course, to obtain a combination of relaxation of the abductors and, most important of all, gravity to bring the thumb down to the index finger. If, however, the patient is asked to bring the thumb to the index finger

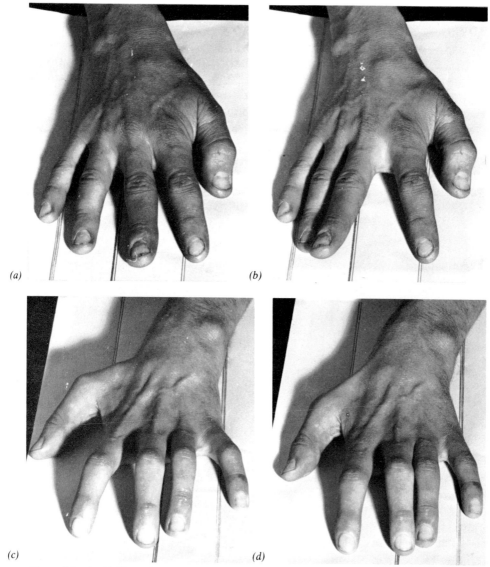

Figure 3.5 (a, b) Normal abduction of fingers. (a) Middle finger raised off the table. (b) Middle finger abducted to the ring finger — note that the wrist has not moved. (c, d) Trick movement in abduction of the fingers in ulnar paralysis — note the wasting in the interosseus spaces. (c) Middle finger raised off the table. (d) Patient attempting to abduct towards the ring finger — note the movement of the wrist that has occurred. Compare the relation of the ulnar border of the wrist to the double ruled lines on the paper in each case

with the radial border of the hand facing directly downwards, he cannot adduct the thumb against gravity without flexing the interphalangeal joint of the thumb. At the same time the long extensor can be seen to be contracting vigorously so that these two muscles are effective adductors. They are, however, unable to adduct the thumb against any degree of resistance. With the thumb fully adducted, the patient is asked to try to adduct against gravity and against the slight resistance of, say, a sheet of card;

immediately the interphalangeal joint of the thumb goes into acute flexion (Froment's sign) (*Figure 3.6*). In many patients this attempted adduction of the thumb with gravity resisting shows trick action of the long extensor as the interphalangeal joint is flexed. In a few patients the long extensor performs this trick action entirely and no flexion at the interphalangeal joint is seen at all. In these circumstances the metacarpophalangeal joint of the thumb goes into hyperextension and the characteristic sign of this trick movement is the pushing of the thenar eminence across the palm.

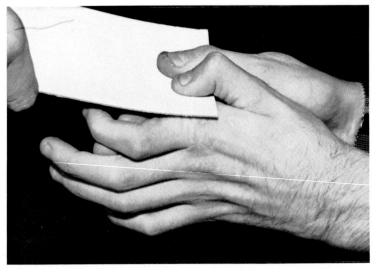

Figure 3.6   Trick adduction of the thumb in ulnar palsy. Note the action of the flexor and extensor pollicis longus

The paralysis of the third and fourth lumbricals means that when the patient attempts to flex the metacarpophalangeal joint he cannot do so without acute flexion of the interphalangeal joints. The paralysis of the hypothenar muscles results in a characteristic posture of the little finger in opposition of the thumb to that finger. Normally, when one opposes the thumb to the little finger, the fourth lumbrical supports the metacarpophalangeal joint in slight flexion and the proximal interphalangeal joint is usually extended by the interossei. In ulnar paralysis, attempts to oppose the little finger result in acute flexion at both interphalangeal joints (see *Figure 3.3*). The fifth metacarpal is depressed instead of being elevated.

In ulnar nerve paralysis the patient is unable to maintain a pinch with the thumb against the index finger and make a good 'O'. This is due to the paralysis of the adductor.

The early signs of recovery in the ulnar-supplied muscles are as follows. The first muscle to recover after a lesion at the wrist will be the abductor digiti minimi; contraction in this muscle is best looked for when the patient opposes the thumb to the little finger – a flicker is invariably seen in this circumstance before the prime-mover action is detected.

As recovery proceeds, in many patients the little finger becomes progressively abducted.

The first sign, clinically, of recovery in the interossei is the absence of the trick movement in abduction. When the patient raises the middle finger off the table and attempts to move it from side to side, there may not be actual movement of the finger, but the trick action of the lateral movement of the palm and wrist is not seen. This indicates that the interossei are beginning to work. If the interosseus spaces are carefully observed, a little flicker can be seen but the finger itself remains absolutely still. The only way to decide whether the interosseus is working or not is by asking the patient to move the finger when the palm is flat on the table and the finger raised off it by the long extensor. Any other method, including testing the ability to hold a piece of paper between the fingers, is not sufficiently reliable.

The clinical signs of recovery in the adductor of the thumb are very difficult to detect; therefore the earliest sign of recovery in this muscle is best seen by the absence of trick movement, so adduction without flexion of the interphalangeal joint or hyperextension of the metacarpophalangeal joint indicates that the adductor is working.

Recovery in the lumbricals is shown by the ability of the patient to flex the metacarpophalangeal joint with the interphalangeal joint extended, and as soon as these muscles begin to work the power of grip increases rapidly.

Treatment by lively splints

If the deformities are not prevented by splintage the muscles may be permanently stretched and function inefficiently after reinnervation. The need for corrective splintage in peripheral nerve injuries has been recognized for a long time, but only relatively recently has it been appreciated that a good splint should do more than merely prevent deformity, it should also encourage function.

Many of the splints in common use – for example, the 'knuckle-duster' splint for ulnar nerve palsy – only prevent the deformity, they are not designed to encourage movement and, indeed, they often deter it.

Many so-called trick movements are available in these nerve injuries, and if a splint is designed both to prevent deformity and to make use of these movements for function, the patient will make much more use of his hand. By this means movement patterns are not lost in the brain during the many months of paralysis, the circulation is kept at its best and, most important of all, the patient can often go back to work. The type of splint that performs both of these functions is known as a lively splint and should always be considered in patients with peripheral nerve injuries.

Each splint must be made specially for the individual patient, and the fitting must be reviewed at regular intervals. The splint must be altered or a new one made should increase in wasting make it too loose or recovery of bulk make it too tight.

It is essential that lively splints in nerve lesions be light, simple, cheap to make, easy to clean, durable, and made accurately to measure to ensure comfort. We have seen many patients who have come from different institutions with bulky splints which were only produced to please the doctors; many were covered in dust, indicating that they may have been left on top of a wardrobe. Patients will not wear a splint that is bulky, uncomfortable and rigid (*Figure 3.7*).

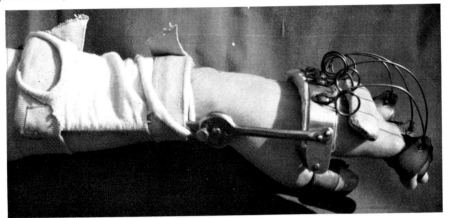

Figure 3.7   Bulky splint for radial nerve palsy, which patients find unpopular because of restricted movement

The test of the usefulness and good design of a splint is whether the patient wears it voluntarily. There is a tendency among some workers to invent a theoretically brilliant contrivance with all manner of springs to substitute for loss of function, but which becomes a lively splint in the most literal sense of the word. Often the patient becomes merely an appendage to his splint. They represent a triumph to the engineer, but a prison for the patient.

Our splints use piano wire (spring steel wire) which was the material originally used by Capener (1949) for finger splints. This material is easier to work, cheaper and more durable than rubber bands, and eliminates any need to make up metal hinges because the coils form their own hinges. These splints can be worn under a glove for they are much less bulky than previous models, are easier to put on and are much lighter in weight.

ASSESSMENT OF FUNCTION

Examination for muscle power

The study of muscle action in peripheral nerve injuries should always include the response to stimulation of the nerve trunks in order to demonstrate any anomalies of innervation. These are much more common in the hand than is generally realized and are dealt with fully in Chapter 1.

When recovery is well advanced, the assessment of muscle action is best done functionally rather than in an attempt to chart the muscle accurately on the Medical Research Council (MRC) scale.

It is very difficult to isolate some of the muscles in the hand. It is best, therefore, to assess the function of the hand in certain activities, such as opposition of the thumb, flexion of the fingers, various types of grip, and the ability to carry out crafts and workshop activities without using trick movements. To this end, careful supervision in the occupational therapy workshops is of great value.

Regular measurement of the grip, using a dynamometer, should be made and a quantitative estimate of the progress in various activities is most helpful to the examiner and encouraging to the patient, as, for example, the ability to play the piano for increasing periods, or to increase production in whatever crafts the patient is performing.

Assessment of sensation

TESTING

The response to cotton wool, von Frey hair, pin-prick and hot and cold are all used to assess the extent of sensory loss and test recovery.

As discussed in detail later ('Sensory re-education', page 115), testing for stereognosis is the only realistic way of assessing function. The abilities to identify objects and textures and to correctly localize touch are used when sensation returns to the distal phalanx.

Two points need special emphasis:

(1) In the early stages after nerve section, the area of sensory loss diminishes slightly as neighbouring nerves take over its function.
(2) The most reliable way of getting an accurate idea of the area of sensory loss is to ask the patient to map out the area with the index finger of the other hand.

Tinel's sign is the classic way of assessing the progressive regeneration of a peripheral nerve. The test has become rather denigrated in recent years, but in our experience, if it is performed carefully, in most cases it is reliable.

The tapping should start distally and work up proximally. Many people perform the test incorrectly by starting to tap over the suture line, rather than working *distally to proximally* from the periphery. This causes a sensory discharge which may have a long after-period and easily confuses the patient, leading to an incorrect level. The limb must be supported carefully so that the tapping does not jar and thus cause a false positive result, and both the proximal and distal sites where the response is obtained must be noted.

Henderson (1948) carried out the most extensive analysis of Tinel's sign yet reported. He pointed out that if the sign was strongly positive at the site of injury but persistently absent distally, there was no regeneration. If strongly positive at the level of injury, but weak distally, there was poor regeneration. The best evidence of recovery was when the sign was strongly positive at the site of injury but gradually diminished as the degree of response at the distal site increased. Our results bear out Henderson's findings completely. In a few cases it was found that the slightest tapping anywhere produced tingling and thus the sign was of no value, but in the great majority of patients it has been found that the Tinel sign is most reliable and well worth performing carefully.

The regular performance of sweat tests for assessing sympathetic recovery does not add any information to that obtained by the motor and sensory tests already described. Some workers like to use it in children, and though we have no experience of this, we feel that it would be a sound indication for its use. Recovery of sympathetic function is seen by the presence of sweating, and the patient notices that the hand does not respond so violently to changes in temperature. Several workers have shown that there is insufficient correlation of sensory and sudomotor reinnervation to make sweat tests worth while.

It is surprising how often patients predict recovery in both the motor and the sensory nerves by stating that they feel recovery is about to occur. Many patients have said that they feel as if a muscle was about to function even though there was no clinical sign, and almost invariably they were right.

SURGICAL TREATMENT

A complete lesion of a nerve (that is, neurotmesis) must be sutured. In general the common practice is to delay nerve suture for 3 weeks after injury unless the wound is clean, soft tissue damage is minimal and the best conditions for nerve suture are available.

Pulvertaft and Campbell Reid (1963) presented the case for secondary suture most cogently. They pointed out that damage to the nerve is almost always more severe than appears at first inspection, and intraneural fibrosis wider than expected. It is thus necessary to resect both nerve ends until unscarred nerve is reached. This is both unwise and unsatisfactory at primary operation, if there is any doubt as to the extent of damage, as the precise level of resection necessarily cannot be known. It is now clear that there is a place for primary suture – if the wound is clean, caused by a sharp direct cut, seen within 6 hours of injury and a highly skilled hand surgeon is available.

The conventional technique of repairing nerves is by epineural suture.

With the advent of the operating microscope there is a hope that better functional results can be obtained through the accurate apposition of the two nerve ends so that regrowing nerve ends can find their way to their correct destination. To this end, fascicular suture has been introduced whereby individual fasciculi are sutured or, if there has been loss of more than 2.5 cm of nerve, grafts are used. Millesi, Meissl and Berger (1972, 1976) favour grafting rather than epineural suture. They regard the most important factor influencing the results of nerve repair as tension at the suture line. The amount of connective tissue proliferation and the size of the gap between the stumps are directly related to the amount of tension, for degeneration of regenerating axons may occur as a result of shrinkage of scar tissue.

Millesi, Meissl and Berger also report that in 40 per cent of 38 median nerves treated by interfascicular nerve grafting, recovery to S3+ was achieved and S3 in 58 per cent. They compare these with 23 per cent S3–4 and 38 per cent S3 in the World War II series reported by Nichols and Seddon (1957). The actual function to which the patients put their hands was not recorded – the criterion being two-point discrimination. The war series comprised some high lesions and many had vascular damage as well, and the two series are not stricly comparable.

Owen (1976) has said, 'It is already evident to the informed enquirer that the results of meticulous microscopic funicular nerve repair in practised hands must show a vast improvement over our past methods'. Dickson and his coworkers (1977) state that 'The development of microsurgical techniques has led to a great improvement in the results of peripheral nerve surgery. Restoration of interfascicular continuity is now the treatment of choice.' This is not true, for no comparative study has been made of epineural suture and interfascicular grafting using functional testings as an assessment of the results, and all the recent work on which these large claims are based were carried out on animals. Cabaud and colleagues (1976), however, have reported a comparative study between epineural and fascicular grafting in the cat, measuring muscular efficiency, the maximum tension of the flexor carpi ulnaris, the weight of reinnervated muscle and axon counts proximal and distal to nerve repair, and showed no difference between the two groups.

Bratton, Hudson and Kline (1979) took 36 monkeys and repaired them in three different ways: interfascicular nerve graft, interfascicular nerve repair and epineural repairs. Histologically, neither the interfascicular suture lines nor the grafted segments showed distinct fascicular patterns, which they point out should be the theoretical advantage of an interfascicular repair. The nerves repaired by an epineural technique fared better. These results might have been related to the loss of regenerating axons to interfascicular tissue. By closing the epineurium, the internal environment was re-established and potentially regenerating axons were available for the distal stump.

Bratton, Hudson and Kline state 'that tension of any sort on a repair is an adverse factor, for regeneration was not supported by the quantitative electrophysiologic data or qualitative histologic studies in experiments on monkeys. Use of short interfascicular autogenous grafts offers no advantage in functional nerve regeneration when compared with end-to-end non-graft sutures done either by interfascicular or epineural techniques. Furthermore, data available to date also suggest that interfascicular or fascicle-to-fascicle repair offers no advantage over end-to-end epineural repair. None the less, it is equally clear that short interfascicular grafts, when properly prepared and placed, do work. Despite extrafascicular loss of axons at each suture interface and delay in reaching end-inputs because of graft transit time, sufficient numbers of axons reach the distal nerve to produce some degree of functional reinnervation. Thus, after using the classic methods for making up length such as mobilization, transposition, sacrifice of tethering branches, and some flexion of the extremity, the remainder of the interstump gap, provided it is short, can be spanned by interfascicular grafts with some hope for successful reinnervation.'

Sunderland (1979), in a masterly review of the various options open, suggests that each technique has its place, according to the circumstances.

As Sunderland (1944) has shown, there is branching and alteration of funicular pattern continuously down the nerve, and with a nerve graft it is impossible to obtain correct axonal alignment. No one can predict the funicular pattern distally if there has been loss of 2 cm or more of nerve.

Even with perfect alignment in which in experimental animals the suture was carried out *before* division of the nerve, 20 per cent of axons were lost (P.D. Wall, 1979, personal communication). It is therefore unreasonable to expect correct alignment when there has been any loss of nerve. It is likely that successful sutures provide the means for the maximum number of axons to gain the periphery. Resulting function depends greatly on the patient's motivation and response to an intensive rehabilitation programme.

Before surgery is undertaken, it is essential that the hand be in an ideal condition; there should be a full range of passive movements in all the joints, minimal or no tendon adherence, good skin condition and muscle power, and function as good as it is possible to obtain. It is wise to postpone surgery for a few weeks if these conditions are not present, so as to give intensive rehabilitation to obtain full range of movement, correction of any deformity and improve function as much as possible. Because the hand must be immobilized for a few weeks, any stiffness before operation will of necessity be aggravated, and full function may be difficult or even impossible to restore under such circumstances.

The management of peripheral nerve injuries can thus be divided into preoperative, the operation, postoperative treatment during the stage of paralysis and treatment during the recovery stage.

Treatment during paralysis

The principles of treatment during the stage of paralysis are: (1) to obtain and maintain full range of movement in all joints; (2) to maintain and improve the circulation; (3) to correct deformity; (4) to prevent deformity; (5) to encourage function; and (6) to increase power and function of unaffected muscles in the limb.

GENERAL PRINCIPLES OF PHYSIOTHERAPY

Patients who have had suture of the median or ulnar nerves will generally have a flexion deformity of the wrist when they commence active rehabilitation 3–4 weeks after suture. This is because the wrist must be flexed to allow approximation of the nerve ends. There will often be a tough scar and a variable amount of oedema on the dorsum of the hand which, if severe, may spread up the arm.

The following general principles apply to all nerve injuries, though the remarks concerning the scar will not, of course, apply to closed nerve injuries.

The doctor will already have explained to the patient the simple anatomy of the hand, its function, and the reasons for treatment in his particular case, and this will include a discussion on the rate of growth of a nerve, the importance of realizing that wasting will increase in the early stages, the expectation of recovery and the ultimate function expected. It is, however, a good plan for the physiotherapist to repeat the salient features of these explanations when she first sees the patient, and we encourage our patients to understand the functional anatomy of their hands; the patient thereby obtains a considerable insight and interest into his condition and is much more likely to be co-operative.

Immediately rehabilitation starts (usually 3–4 weeks after surgery), the hand and forearm are put in a warm (36.7°C, 98°F) saline bath, so that the patient can carry out active movements for 5–10 minutes. Wax baths are too hot for anaesthetic areas and we have abandoned their use; moreover the skin is left oily and rather smelly. They are, of course, contraindicated when open wounds are present. Special care must be taken with skin grafts and burns to avoid any excess temperature. Such skin is more easily damaged than normal skin and at a lower temperature. The patient must also be warned against the danger of repeated friction causing blisters. Light massage with hydrous ointment or oil is given to remove scaly skin. The nail and nail beds suffer from trophic changes and it is advisable for the therapist to cut the patient's nails.

As with all hand problems, the slightest sign of oedema must be treated with elevation in a sling by day and on a stand by night. If there is undue scarring due to adherence of tendons, massage should be given fairly gently at first to avoid blistering of newly growing tissue. Later, after 6–8 weeks, the tissues will stand deeper massage with lanolin. The skin is lifted up on either side of the scar and massage given deep to it. The patient should flex actively while the massage is given if flexion is limited, and extend during massage if extension is limited.

In the case of severe scarring and adherence, several sessions of intensive massage daily, followed by slow stretches and serial plasters, are indicated, as described in full on page 37. These should not begin until 8 weeks after suture.

Movements

As soon as possible, active unresisted movements should start to regain full range of the tendons that have been sutured or become adherent. The whole arm must be treated, as weakness of upper limb muscles and stiffness of the shoulder are not uncommon after hand injuries. Passive movements must be given to maintain range and increase movement, if limited due to immobilization. No stretch is allowed for 8 weeks after nerve suture. As each joint is moved passively, the proximal or distal joint is slackened by flexing it, and the hand and fingers are supported so that only one joint is passively moved. The interdigital webs of the fingers and thumb must be fully stretched and full opposition of thumb and little finger maintained, so as to preserve the palmar arch.

When there is adherence of the structures at the wrist, only flexion and deviation are given for the first 6 weeks after suture; gentle wrist extension can then be added. A resting plaster, worn between treatment sessions, is useful to maintain movement gained.

Deformity

The most common deformity in peripheral nerve lesions is adherence of the flexor tendons to the skin, to the scar or to each other. This leads to a flexion deformity of 90 degrees at the proximal interphalangeal joints due to shortening of the flexor sublimis. This is a severe disability and, unless corrected, will prevent full function of the hand. Moreover, the intrinsic muscles, when they recover, will be unable to extend the interphalangeal joints properly, because not only will they be weak anyway for some time after regeneration, but they will be unable to act functionally against the deforming action of the long flexors at the joints at which they work. The treatment of this condition is described fully in Chapter 2, pages 37 *et seq.*

Encouragement of function

During the stage of paralysis, the patient must be encouraged to maintain the strength of all the unaffected muscles, by general exercises, specific exercises and games of all kinds. Trick movements, or rather substitution movements, can be enlisted in the cause of encouraging maximum use and function by the application of lively splints. In an ulnar nerve lesion, for example, when wearing the lively ulnar splint described on page 193 the patient can use the long extensors throughout the finger, thus acting on the interphalangeal joints through the stabilization by the splint of the metacarpophalangeal joint. In addition, in a median nerve lesion, a lively median splint described on pages 196 and 198 will bring the thumb into palmar abduction and thus allow the long flexor to oppose the thumb and the index finger. The strength in the unaffected muscles is maintained by active resisted exercises, using adapted proprioceptive neuromuscular facilitation (PNF) techniques, and games, which must be closely supervised for the first 8 weeks after rehabilitation starts.

Electrical stimulation

It used to be the custom to give patients with paralysed muscles, electrical stimulation of the galvanic type twice daily, provided there was a reasonable chance of reinnervation before the onset of fibrosis.

This general use of electrotherapy has now been abandoned by us for two reasons. First, there is so much to do in severe peripheral nerve injuries that there is not really time to devote to electrical stimulation twice daily. This is particularly true where there are gross deformities to correct. Second, we were so impressed with the functional results in patients on full-time treatment who did not receive electrical stimulation that we have felt that, empirically at any rate, such treatment is not really necessary. No one has ever shown in a control series that electrical stimulation improves function in man, and in the majority of our cases not only was excellent function restored but muscle bulk was often little less than on the unaffected side.

In the early stages of reinnervation, however, electrical stimulation may be useful as a means of re-education if the patient cannot get the feel of the recovering muscle. One should then use a pulse duration which is comfortable for the patient and gives the best contraction. This may well be a long-duration current, even though the patient has shown voluntary movement. It is important not to assume that because the muscle is recovering, a faradic type of current (short-duration current) must be used when, in fact, a long-duration current, say 30 ms, may be more comfortable and more efficient.

RE-EDUCATION

There are two aspects of re-education in peripheral nerve injuries: re-education of motor function, and re-education of sensory function.

MOTOR FUNCTION

The muscles may be re-educated as prime movers, as synergists or in group movements. The conventional methods of re-education involve the techniques that are well known to physiotherapists of retraining the muscles as prime movers, and the more functional techniques of proprioceptive neuromuscular facilitation (PNF). The conventional techniques of re-education as prime movers and synergists will now be described for each peripheral nerve lesion in turn, and then the rationale and techniques of PNF will be discussed.

Median nerve lesions

In a high lesion of the median nerve there will be involvement of the wrist and finger flexors, which are re-educated with progressive exercises starting with assisted active exercises, progressing to PNF and finally with resistance; the re-education of these muscles is discussed in detail in Chapter 2.

THENAR MUSCLES

Abductor pollicis brevis
The patient holds the hand in the mid-prone position, with the ulnar border of the hand on the table, and attempts to hold the thumb in palmar abduction. As the muscle improves, resistance is given and the movement is executed through an increasing range.

The patient is asked to try to crease the thumb. At first the thumb is inclined towards the ground and is assisted by gravity. Later, it is held in a neutral position and then inclined against gravity and resistance so that the movement is being carried out in full supination. Perhaps the most important function of the short abductor is opposition of the thumb. The patient is encouraged to bring the thumb across the palm touching each finger in turn. He makes an 'O' against each finger in turn and the physiotherapist attempts to pull her fingers through.

Flexor pollicis brevis

The thumb is held in flexion at the metacarpophalangeal joint with the interphalangeal joint extended to prevent trick action of the long flexor. The flexion of the metacarpophalangeal joint of the thumb is trained, at first in the inner range with the thumb level with the ring finger, and moving to the little finger, and later, as recovery progresses, in an increasing range until it is carried from well outside the index finger to the little finger.

A pen is laid along the line of the short abductor and the patient attempts to roll the thumb over it.

OPPOSITION

Opposition is a combination of short flexor, short abductor and opponens action. Apart from the exercises already described for the short flexor and abductor, the following exercise for rotation of the metacarpal is used.

With the thumb lying in palmar abduction against the index finger the patient is encouraged to rotate the thumb, bringing it across the proximal phalanges so that the nail points vertically upwards.

The opponens is most active in holding the position of extension, whereas the short abductor is most active actually in opposition. The extensor of the thumb must be trained, as it is essential for the pinch grip in opposition. All forms of grip are also trained.

Radial nerve palsies

In the early stages of recovery synergic action is encouraged. The patient's hand is supported in the mid-prone position and he is asked to squeeze the physiotherapist's fingers. Muscles may be re-educated individually, as described below.

BRACHIORADIALIS

With the forearm in the mid-prone position, the patient is asked to lift his wrist off the table, when brachioradialis will contract synergically. The patient is then asked to flex the elbow, while the forearm is held in mid-position, in the outer range and without resistance. As recovery occurs, the range is increased and resistance added.

EXTENSOR CARPI RADIALIS LONGUS AND BREVIS

These muscles may be re-educated as prime movers, contracting with extensor carpi ulnaris to produce wrist extension, or with flexor carpi radialis to produce radial deviation. To extend the wrist, the patient supports his forearm in the mid-prone position, and with his wrist flexed he tries to move his hand back into extension. For radial deviation, with palm on the table, the patient is asked to move his hand in the radial direction. As these movements increase in strength, gravity is added as a resistance and the range increased. Springs are a useful form of resistance; the patient grasps a handle attached to the spring, twisting a broom handle between fingers and thumb, and all gripping movements work the wrist extensors synergically. Palmar abduction and adduction also produce a synergistic contraction of these muscles.

EXTENSOR CARPI ULNARIS

The muscle is trained as a prime mover in wrist extension as described for the extensor carpi radialis longus. It also contracts as a prime mover for ulnar deviation of the wrist when contracting with flexor carpi ulnaris. The patient is asked to move his hand from radial deviation towards ulnar deviation, and resistance and increasing range are added as soon as possible. The patient is asked to abduct the little finger against resistance, when the extensor carpi ulnaris will be felt to contract synergically.

EXTENSOR DIGITORUM COMMUNIS

With the forearm in mid-position and his fingers fully flexed, the patient is asked to extend the metacarpophalangeal joints, while maintaining the interphalangeal joints in flexion. When his power improves he attempts to perform this movement with the palm facing downwards. Next, the hand is supported so that the metacarpophalangeal joints are flexed and the interphalangeal joints are extended, and the patient is asked to extend his metacarpophalangeal joints so that his whole wrist and hand are in extension. Resistance is then gradually increased. The muscles may be re-educated synergically by asking the patient to abduct and adduct his fingers, as a group movement, with increasing resistance, and then each finger individually. The patient extends the metacarpophalangeal joint and then moves the finger from one side to the other.

As the actions of the intrinsic muscles of the hand are so closely linked with the action of the extensor digitorum, they become weakened, for their proper function depends on a stable extensor mechanism and therefore exercise should be given to the intrinsics in all cases of weakness of finger extensors. Yo-yo, jacks, dealing and shuffling cards, making card houses and cardboard boxes, and bouncing tennis balls are suitable for function of the extensors of the fingers. Playing the piano and other musical instruments, conjuring, miming and flicking beer mats are all excellent activities.

EXTENSOR POLLICIS LONGUS AND BREVIS

Synergically these muscles are best trained by asking the patient to make a 'O' with fingers and thumb, and to prevent the physiotherapist from pulling her finger through. Successively larger objects are then held between the fingers and the thumb. The prime-mover action is trained by supporting the hand, palm upwards, and the thumb flexed across the palm. The patient extends his thumb, first at the interphalangeal joint, then the metacarpophalangeal joint, and finally at the carpometacarpal joint, at first without and later with increasing resistance. Games previously described for the extensors of the fingers are also appropriate for the thumb, especially those involving precision movements.

ABDUCTOR POLLICIS LONGUS

The tendon can be felt to be contracting if the patient and physiotherapist grasp each other's hand, thumb to thumb. Increasing resistance may be given as recovery occurs.

In the normal hand, whenever extensor carpi radialis longus and extensor carpi ulnaris contract, the abductor pollicis longus automatically contracts synergically. It also works with the extensor pollicis longus; therefore all movements of thumb and wrist extension are appropriate.

For prime-mover action the patient is asked to take his thumb away from his index finger into the radially abducted position. Resistance is gradually added.

Ulnar nerve lesions

If the lesion is high, the flexor carpi ulnaris and flexor digitorum profundus to the ring and little fingers will be affected; consequently these muscles must be re-educated – the flexor carpi ulnaris in the same manner as the extensor carpi ulnaris only in flexion; the profundus as described in Chapter 2.

Hypothenar group

Opposition of the thumb to little finger involves synergic action of these muscles, so the patient is asked to grip a folded newspaper between thumb and little and ring fingers while the physiotherapist attempts to pull it away.

Each muscle is re-educated in its prime-mover action of flexion, abduction and opposition, starting in the outer range with no resistance and progressing to full range with resistance.

ADDUCTOR POLLICIS

The patient holds both hands together in the prayer position and a folded newspaper is placed between his thumbs and index fingers. He attempts to grip the paper with fingers and thumbs while the physiotherapist attempts to withdraw it. Later, progressively thinner objects are introduced until a card can be held. The patient should not be allowed to make use of the trick action of flexor pollicis longus and should keep his thumb straight.

From the abducted position the muscle will act as a prime mover to take the thumb up to the index finger, against gravity and with increasing resistance. The muscle will contract synergically with flexor pollicis longus, particularly in a strong pinch grip.

Interossei and lumbricals

ABDUCTION AND ADDUCTION OF METACARPOPHALANGEAL JOINTS

With the palm down, the patient lifts each finger in turn off the table and attempts to abduct and adduct. Increasing resistance is later given. In the early stages trick abduction and adduction, by the use of long extensors and long flexors, is encouraged as weak interossei will contract at the same time and gradually a normal movement will take over. The patient is asked to grip a towel or, later, a piece of paper between his fingers and prevent the physiotherapist from withdrawing it, and also to cross one finger over the other. Coins can be flicked over the fingers.

FLEXION OF METACARPOPHALANGEAL JOINTS AND EXTENSION OF INTERPHALANGEAL JOINTS

With the palm upward the patient is put into the position of metacarpophalangeal flexion and interphalangeal extension and asked to hold this. When there is no contraction in the intrinsics, the fingers collapse as the physiotherapist releases her hold. As recovery appears in these muscles, the patient can hold the position for a moment before the fingers collapse. This movement is repeated several times with the physiotherapist placing the fingers in the intrinsic plus position, and as the patient improves he will hold the position longer and will eventually be able to initiate the movement himself. With the palm down on the table, the patient is asked to pull the finger tips back towards the heel of the hand by flexing the metacarpophalangeal joints, and to maintain the interphalangeal joints in extension, gradually adding resistance.

All cupping movements, such as playing with balls, and fine movements as needed with pick-a-stick, picking up lead shot with forceps, playing shadow games and crumpling up several sheets of a newspaper one-handed, all provide strong work for these muscles.

Proprioceptive facilitation techniques

The rationale of these techniques is to make use of all physiological principles available to achieve muscle contraction more easily. The strength of contraction of a muscle depends on the number of motor units serving it that are stimulated. This in turn depends on the degree of excitation of the anterior horn cells supplying those muscles. In the early stages of recovery after nerve lesions, the threshold of those anterior horn cells will be very high and they are much more difficult to excite than normally. Successful exercise techniques therefore utilize the principles of trying to obtain maximum activity of the anterior horn cells by using measures to produce maximum excitation. It is a fundamental principle of behaviour of the central nervous system that maximum sensory input produces maximum motor output. Thus, if it is required to obtain maximum contraction in a muscle, maximum stimulation of the sensory afferents should be produced. This can be done by the following:

(1) Putting the muscle on a stretch, and thus stimulating the stretch reflex;
(2) Traction or compression to the joints which the muscle moves;
(3) Pressure on the skin over the muscles in the direction of movement and the maximal resistance which can be given to those muscles;
(4) The patient watching the movement, and the effect of the physiotherapist's voice.

Another means of obtaining increase in the sensory input is by the principle of irradiation. This involves stimulation of muscles whose cell columns in the spinal cord lie adjacent to those of the muscles to be exercised. Thus, for example, in wishing to obtain maximum contraction of the quadriceps muscle, the patient is asked to dorsiflex the ankle because the cell columns supplying the tibialis anterior lie adjacent to those of the quadriceps in the spinal cord. Another principle commonly used is that of successive induction. This means that when there has been maximum voluntary movement of an antagonist, the agonist is facilitated. Thus, if there is weakness of the flexors of the wrist, maximum activity is encouraged in the extensors of the wrist and then, without allowing relaxation, wrist flexion is encouraged.

Kabat (1961) was instrumental in pointing out that in normal function, muscles work in spiral and diagonal patterns. The functional movement of bringing the hand to the mouth from the position where the hand is at the side of the body demands a diagonal pattern of movement. Similarly, muscles tend to work in the upper and lower limbs in mass action patterns. For example, extension of the upper limb involves extension of wrist, fingers and thumb, extension of the elbow and extension of the shoulder. To obtain maximum activity in a weak triceps, for example, proprioceptive techniques employ mass extensor patterns; the patient is therefore asked to extend the fingers, wrist, thumb and shoulder. This will bring in the triceps more efficiently than the simple prime-mover action of extension of the elbow. Functional spiral and diagonal patterns have been worked out for all movements in the body and these techniques are being introduced more and more into routine physiotherapy. They are particularly valuable in the early stages of recovery in lower motor neuron lesions, such as the early stages of reinnervation after peripheral nerve suture.

GENERAL PRINCIPLES

The advantage of giving multiple joint movements, rather than one isolated to a joint, is that many more muscles are activated at the same time and, by using the stronger muscles in the same movement patterns, the action of the weaker muscles is reinforced. Maximal reinforcement is gained when the limb is first rotated and then moved in the diagonal plane. Maximal resistance is used to gain proprioceptive stimulation and the muscles are put on the stretch to increase sensory inflow. The resistance guides the patient in learning the diagonal patterns. Traction and approximation are used as joint stimuli; traction for flexion movements and, in painful joint conditions, compression during extension. The hands of the physiotherapist are placed on the surface in the direction of the movement and, when possible, over the muscle and tendons which are contracting, giving added sensory stimulation.

The patient is directed to follow the movement of his arm with his eyes, and his neck muscles are brought into the pattern. The commands to the patient are given precisely and firmly, so that maximal cortical stimulation is achieved, and the patient makes the maximum effort. It may seem obvious, but if a patient is asked to move in soft soothing tones he is unlikely to be galvanized into strong activity. All the techniques to be described can usefully be divided into relaxation and strengthening techniques, and frequently one will follow on the other.

STRENGTHENING TECHNIQUES

Repeated contractions, slow reversals and rhythmical stabilizations are used as strengthening techniques. Repeated contractions may be used isotonically or isometrically according to the patient's strength. When weak, the patient is asked to make the movement through a small range, and when he tires the physiotherapist gives an increasing resistance to produce stretch of the contracting muscles and he then continues the movement. This can be repeated several times. As he becomes stronger an isometric contraction is used. The patient moves through the range and is instructed to hold the position against resistance. The physiotherapist then builds up her resistance at the weakest pivot, eventually giving a stretch which stimulates the limb to move further through the range. This procedure should be repeated several times.

Slow reversals are based on Sherrington's law, which states that a muscle will contract more strongly if that contraction is immediately preceded by a contraction of the antagonist. The antagonists are made to contract through their full range; the therapist then changes her hands to the opposite surface and, without giving the patient the opportunity to relax, the movements of the agonist are carried out. Rhythmical stabilizations may be performed in any part of the range, and are therefore useful for increasing stability where it is most needed. The patient is asked to maintain a given position against increasing resistance, until the maximum build-up of power has been gained. Then, without allowing the patient to relax the muscles, resistance is transferred to the opposite group until a co-contraction is achieved. This is very hard work for the patient and should not be repeated too many times.

RELAXATION TECHNIQUES

These are used to increase range of movement, and are based on reciprocal innervation. They are known as slow reversal, hold, relax; contract, relax; and hold, relax. In the first technique the patient makes an isotonic, followed by an isometric, contraction of the muscle limiting the movement (antagonistic pattern), voluntarily relaxes for a few seconds and then is instructed to move isotonically through any increased range. The techniques may then be repeated. Maximal relaxation depends on maximal resistance to rotation of the antagonistic component of movement.

In the contract–relax technique the patient is taken passively to the point where no further range can be gained. He is then directed to contract into the antagonistic pattern, but rotation is the only movement allowed isotonically. Then when maximum relaxation has been gained, the limb is moved passively into the increased range. This is useful for very marked limitation of movement.

The hold–relax technique is similar to the previous one, except that the patient is directed to hold the position and not to contract to produce movement. The limb is then passively moved through any increase of range and the technique is particularly useful when pain accompanies muscle spasm.

All these techniques can be applied in supine and prone lying or other suitable positions, and can be used as unilateral, bilateral, symmetrical or asymmetrical movements. They can also be adapted for use with springs and with pulleys. They are no substitute for functional activities, but produce the best results when combined with all forms of active work.

PATTERNS FOR THE UPPER LIMB

These should be used in conjunction with neck patterns and scapular patterns. Limitation of movement, often accompanied by pain and weakness, is frequently found in the head, neck, scapular and shoulder movements of patients recovering from hand injuries. Recovery of the hand can be assured only if the other joints and muscles of the arm work as normally as possible; it is therefore essential to assess and treat these proximal components as early as possible. Teaching the desired movements on the good arm will gain the patient's co-operation and give him the idea of what is expected of his affected arm.

SPECIFIC HAND MOVEMENT PATTERNS

Flexion and adduction of the fingers is consistent with flexion of the wrist and adduction of the shoulder. Grip action of the hand can therefore be re-educated in either of the patterns involving these two movements. However, the shape of the metacarpal arch and its effect on the direction of flexion of the fingers should be considered for more specific re-education of flexor digitorum profundus and sublimis.

For the index and middle fingers, the flexion, adduction, external rotation pattern of the shoulder, incorporating supination and wrist flexion and radial deviation, should be used. For the ring and little fingers, extension, adduction and internal rotation of the shoulder is used, combined with wrist flexion, ulnar deviation and pronation. Precision grip, when the metacarpophalangeal joints of the index and middle fingers rotate and adduct to oppose the fingers to thumb, should be re-educated with opposition of the thumb, as described on pages 107–108.

Finger extension occurs consistently with wrist extension and abduction of the shoulder, so may be re-educated as a group in the patterns involving these movements. More specifically the index and middle fingers will extend and abduct maximally in the pattern of shoulder flexion, abduction and external rotation, combined with wrist extension and radial deviation and supination. The pattern for maximal extension of the ring and little fingers is extension, abduction and internal rotation of the shoulder with wrist extension and ulnar deviation and pronation.

THUMB MOVEMENTS

Flexion of the thumb across the palm is combined with shoulder flexion, adduction and external rotation patterns. Extension of the thumb is part of the pattern of flexion, abduction and external rotation of the shoulder.

Palmar abduction should be incorporated with the shoulder pattern of extension, abduction and internal rotation.

Opposition is combined with the pattern of shoulder extension, adduction and internal rotation. The thumb may be opposed towards the little finger, or towards the index and middle fingers if improvement in precision is required. Adduction of the thumb is part of the shoulder flexion and external rotation pattern, and radial abduction combines with shoulder extension and internal rotation.

Occupational therapy

In the early stages of peripheral nerve injuries some form of activity is required to encourage the patient to use his hand and in particular to start moving flexor tendons which have invariably been divided. Printing using a padded spongy handle shaped to the deformity is most useful. Type-setting with padded tweezers, guillotining with different shapes and size of handles, also covered in springy material, are repetitive and require a large number of movements in a relatively short time. Stool-seating, packing and mosaic work, rug hooking and knotting are all useful for nerve lesions and particularly for median nerve lesions.

In ulnar nerve lesions printing, which involves abduction and extension, basketry and rug making are used. For dexterity of intrinsic muscles, piano playing, typing or playing musical instruments are all valuable. In radial nerve lesions we use printing, brush making, rug making and stool seating.

In these early stages, lively splints are worn during treatment. In the later stages when power grip is required, all types of carpentry, using chisel, mallet, saw, plane, hammer and screwdriver, are most valuable and engage the patient's enthusiasm. All workshop activities – lathe work, wrought iron, soldering, radio assembly – are appropriate.

For children, useful pastimes are bead threading, using Plasticine, bouncing putty, clay modelling, brick building, finger painting, glove puppets, card building, and games such as halma, bagatelle, draughts and spillikins; later on Meccano, darts and carpentry may be indicated.

The games described in detail in Chapter 6 are all suitable once recovery has started – beat the clock, blow football, magnetic draughts, etc.

SENSORY RE-EDUCATION

While reasonable return of motor function is expected after nerve suture and much attention is paid to restoration of maximum power by splintage exercises and occupational therapy, less attention has been paid to restoration of sensory function. It is usually believed that only protective sensation can be expected after secondary suture of the median nerve in adults, stereognosis is poor or non-existent and two-point discrimination (2-PD) over 10 mm in the finger tips.

Onne in 1962 pointed out that, after median nerve suture in adults, the 2-PD is never less than 10 mm, often 30 mm or more, and in general is the same in millimetres as the age (in years) of the patient. Thus, a 25-year-old man might expect a 2-PD of 25 mm at his finger tips. As the normal 2-PD is 2 mm, this falls very far short of normal.

Two-point discrimination has been regarded as the touchstone of sensory assessment.

However, we have shown (Wynn Parry and Salter, 1976) that 2-PD does not correlate with sensory function. We have measured 2-PD in 40 patients after secondary median nerve suture and correlated this with sensory function as judged by the ability to recognize textures and objects by our standard assessments. In all cases, 2-PD, as Onne rightly stated, was well over 10 mm and yet function as judged by recognition and the patient's prowess in work and hobbies was excellent. *Tables 3.1* and *3.2* show some representative results.

We have been using formal sensory retraining procedures for 15 years (first reported in the second edition of this work) and been much impressed by how a few weeks of retraining can produce spectacular improvement in function. While workers

Table 3.1 Lack of correlation between sensory function and two-point discrimination in a patient 19 months after median and ulnar nerve suture at the wrist

Recognition times (in seconds) of objects

String	17	Small bottle	8	Match	7
Pencil	3	Nail brush	4	Shuttlecock	2

Two-point discrimination (in mm)

	Index	*Middle*	*Ring*	*Little*	*Thumb*
Proximal	9 (2)	10 (3)	9 (3)	10 (3)	9 (1)
Middle	10	8	11	11	–
Distal	8 (2)	9 (2)	15 (2)	13 (2)	12 (1)

(Figures in parentheses are 2-PD on equivalent site on normal hand)

Table 3.2 Lack of correlation between sensory function and two-point discrimination in a patient 22 months after suture of the median nerve at the wrist

Recognition times (in seconds) of objects

Bulldog clip	11	Nail brush	7	String	4
Can opener	8	Pencil	10	Screw-top	9
Matchbox	8	Shuttlecock	2		

Two-point discrimination (in mm)

	Index	*Middle*	*Thumb*
Proximal	16 (4)	6 (2)	11 (1)
Middle	12 (2)	12 (2)	–
Distal	15 (2)	11 (2)	10 (1)

(Figures in parentheses are 2-PD on equivalent site on normal hand)

continue to assess results by 2-PD and do not use realistic functional tests, we shall not be in a position truly to judge the efficacy of their various surgical techniques. The serious criticism of the use of 2-PD is that it is a static test. When one wishes to ascertain the nature of an object or texture without the use of one's eyes, one instinctively moves it between one's fingers and thumb, thus setting up spatial and temporal patterns of impulses which are the coding mechanisms for sensation. It is impossible to tell the nature of an object if it is placed on one's finger tip and allowed to rest there.

Two-point discrimination probably measures fibre density, and as such may be a valuable means of judging the number of fibres reinnervated – it is of great academic interest to know how many nerve fibres have crossed the suture line, but this is not an assessment of function. Confirmation of this view has been produced in the fascinating paper by Jabeley and colleagues (1976).

He and his workers took biopsies from the ulnar side of the index finger and the radial side of the little finger in 17 patients with nerve lesions, 24 months after suture. A battery of tests was used to assess function, including Moberg's (1958) pick-up test and object recognition. Independent examiners were asked to judge histologically if any nerve tissue was present at three levels – the deep reticular dermis, the superficial reticular dermis and the papillary dermis – and to report if many, an occasional or no Meissner's corpuscles had been reinnervated. There was no discernible correlation between the subjective appraisal and histological interpretation of the biopsies.

A 19-year-old college student, after median and ulnar nerve repair, could identify all of 15 objects; however, he had 2-PD of only 15 mm at the tip of the index and 20 mm at the tip of the middle finger, and at biopsy little nerve tissue was seen and only a few Meissner's corpuscles had been reinnervated.

In contrast, a 22-year-old domestic worker who had her median nerve sutured under the microscope with interfascicular suture could recognize only 6 of 15 objects, took 60 seconds in the pick-up test and did not use her hand at all because it felt as if it did not belong to her. At biopsy there was an abundance of visible nerve tissue and many Meissner's corpuscles had been reinnervated.

Thus it does not matter so much how many nerve fibres regenerate, but what one does with what recovers.

Jabeley *et al.* concluded that a number of factors are involved in the end-result other than axonal regeneration, including age, scarring, intelligence, motivation and rehabilitation.

Another prejudice against expecting good sensory function is the belief that misrouting of axons is inevitable and that, however careful the surgical technique, some motor fibres will innervate sensory receptors and *vice versa* or that sensory fibres destined for touch receptors will innervate temperature receptors or pain endings. Sensory function will thus be seriously impaired. Patients will not only mislocate stimuli to the wrong finger or part of the finger, but will also misread the modality of sensation. This, too, is founded on a misunderstanding of sensory physiology.

The classical concept of sensation assumes modality-specific receptors first put forward by von Frey, with the four modalities of cutaneous sensation – touch, heat, cold and pain. Each receptor had its own fibre tract to the cental nervous system (CNS) and relayed to the cortex in a specific manner, much as an electric cable with different coloured wires. We learned that pacinian corpuscles relayed pressure, Meissner's end-organs touch, Krause's end-bulbs heat and free endings respond to pain.

As Melzack and Wall first pointed out in 1962, this concept is wrong, and although evidence for its refutation has repeatedly been reported, the classic theory is still taught and is still in most of the textbooks. No one has ever found specific endings at spots in the skin where a response to temperature has been noted. The pinna of the ear, the cornea, lips and tongue respond to all modalities of sensation but only free endings are found there.

Mountcastle (1968) pointed out that it has been repeatedly confirmed that in spots of skin subjected to careful sensory testing and then marked and excised, histological study revealed no organized endings – only free nerve endings. He further pointed out that the perception of the size and shape of an object grasped in one's hand results from the combination of input from cutaneous mechanoreceptive afferents with that from position detectors in the finger joints.

Weddell (1961) stated that receptors cannot be considered unique entities and that they merge into one another at morphological level. Nor are they static; they are constantly being replaced and their precise morphology is determined by the stress patterns to which the hand is subjected. Immobilization of the hand results in retrogressive changes in the receptors.

Wyke (1979, personal communication) has shown that pacinian corpuscles disappear in a joint which is kept immobile; furthermore, they are not present in the soles of the feet in a newborn child, appearing only when the child starts to walk.

Thus the stimulus of normal use helps to differentiate new sensory receptors. Although it is known (Dellon, Curtis and Edgerton, 1974) that Meissner's corpuscles can be reinnervated 6–9 months after denervation in monkeys; all the evidence suggests that after 2–3 years the receptors disappear totally and growing nerve terminals must create the receptor system in the periphery. Brooks, from our hospital (personal communication), has seen protective sensation return in the hand 25 years after median nerve suture.

Receptors can be shown to respond to more than one type of stimulus. Large thermal stimuli initiate activity from several types of sensory elements which usually behave as mechanoreceptors (Andres and von During, 1973).

Iggo (1977) has stated that it is now clear that no cutaneous receptors have an absolute specificity. They have a high degree of selective sensitivity; that is, a low threshold to a particular form of stimulus (e.g. light touch or pressure) and a high threshold to other stimuli. Free nerve endings are organized into receptor fibre units with variable thresholds. Wall (1961) found these thresholds to vary from low to high in a continuous distribution with no sign of any subdivision. Moreover, Mountcastle (1968) has shown that the Meissner's corpuscles and Merkel's discs are linked to mechanoreceptive afferents and that they are likely to determine the dynamic response characteristics of those fibres, rather than their mode specificity. A given stimulus does not excite one and only one type of receptor. On the contrary, a stimulus from nature may excite several different kinds of receptor – and, conversely, each nerve fibre takes part in many different functions and a local stimulus falls at different positions in the overlapping receptive fields of a number of different fibres. The full range of qualitative sensitivities is represented in alpha delta, C and large diameter mechanoreceptive fibres – that is, there is multiplicity and redundancy in the nervous system.

It is not only the particular receptor which is stimulated that determines what is felt, but also the temporal and spatial patterns of activity in the various receptor types stimulated. Coding is dependent on the frequency of discharge along the nerve, the interval between pulses, the total duration of the discharge and the spacing of individual bursts. Variation in any or all of these will lead to quite different patterns on arrival at the spinal cord. Moreover, when one considers the firing of a group of fibres, further variables are given by the actual number of nerve fibres firing, the density of those fibres within the receptor field and the sequential activation (i.e. the pattern of rotation of fibres firing in that group).

Impulses can, of course, be inhibited or modified during transmission both pre- and postsynaptically.

'Specific modality and patterning theories are supplementary. The recognition of receptor specialisation for transduction of particular kinds and ranges of cutaneous stimulation does not preclude acceptance of the concept that information is coded in a pattern of impulses.' (Wall, 1961).

Moreover, there are no modality-specific cells in the dorsal horn. There is a different firing pattern in a single cell in the cord when activated by touch, temperature, skin damage or hair movement.

So it is seen that convergence and divergence, summation and pattern discrimination all go on in a dynamically changing CNS, itself subject to descending inhibition and disinhibition – a far cry from the simplistic theory of a specific receptor for a particular form of sensory experience.

This is of great significance for the management of patients with nerve lesions. The facts that the physiological basis of sensation is dynamic, that sensation depends on patterning, that receptors can vary according to the demands made on them all indicate that re-education is possible. This is the basis of our techniques – to try to teach the patient to learn a new code.

At 6–9 months after nerve suture, the patient will have protective sensation but poor, if any, stereognosis (*Table 3.3*). He is trying to feel with fewer fibres per unit area (i.e. his 2-PD is much greater than normal) and his conduction speeds are much lower – we know that conduction velocity never returns to normal. Thus the patterns, both temporal and spatial, will be distorted. The patient has to relearn sensation with slower conduction along fewer axons. The code in the CNS laid down in early life (or even possibly preprogrammed *in utero*) no longer resembles the information transmitted from the periphery.

Table 3.3 Time taken to give correct description of texture. (Median nerve lesion, April 1972; textures tested, May 1975; 2 out of 10 correct)

Object	Time (s)	Object	Time (s)
Carpet	No idea	Cotton wool	Sponge
Sandpaper	11	Plastic	No idea
Canvas	No idea	Rubber	5
Leather	No idea	Silk	Plastic
Sheepskin	Velvet	Wool	Foam

We know from the work of Paul, Goodman and Merzimch (1972) that, following nerve regeneration after traumatic lesions in the Macacus monkey, there is a marked disturbance of cortical representation of sensory nerve fibres in the hand. By stimulating the animal's paw and recording electrical activity in the contralateral parietal cortex, they were able to make a map of the cortical representation of peripheral sensory receptors. Following nerve division and primary suture they were able to show that when regeneration had occurred there was marked misrepresentation of the peripheral sensory field in the cortex. Sensory retraining must therefore involve reorganization of central connections.

By retraining, the patient can learn to lay down a new code centrally. This is the rationale underlying our techniques, and we have shown over many years that they do succeed in patients who are co-operative, well motivated and need their sensation for everyday activities. It is well known that children regain almost perfect sensation after nerve suture, and this must be due to their great capacity to reorganize their central connections.

Once the patient has appreciation of sensation in the fingers – usually 6–8 months after suture at the wrist – training starts with large blocks of wood of different shapes: square, rectangular, round and hexagonal. The patient is blindfolded and a selected block put into his hand. He is asked to describe its shape by feeling around it and to state if it is heavier or lighter than another block put into his other hand. If he fails to identify the shape or weight correctly the blindfold is removed and he repeats the manoeuvre relating what he feels to what he sees and comparing it with the normal hand.

The procedure continues with various different shaped blocks. Once this has been mastered, blocks are used with different textures on one surface (e.g. sandpaper or velvet). The patient is asked if all surfaces are the same and, if not, which texture is different from the wood.

Next he is asked to try to identify the nature of a number of textures – sheepskin, leather, silk, canvas, rubber, plastic, wool, cotton wool, carpet, sandpaper; finally, objects used in daily life are presented to him, still blindfold. Again if he fails to identify the texture or object, he opens his eyes and tries to relate what he felt to what he sees – large objects are used first and then, as progress is made, successively smaller objects.

Training sessions are made short so that patients do not become tired or frustrated. We found two or four 10-minute sessions a day to be of more value than one long session. Training is varied by using games; for example, objects are hidden in a bowl

Table 3.4 Average times taken by 50 normal subjects to recognize shaped blocks

Object	Test	Time taken (s)
(1) 170-g square wood block	To describe the shape and nature of object, its approximate weight and if all sides had the same texture	23
(2) 510-g oblong wood block, with one side covered with sandpaper	To describe the shape, and if it was heavier or lighter than object (1)	14
(3) 56-g rectangular block	To describe the shape, and if it was heavier or lighter than object (2)	4
(4) 282-g cylindrical wood block	To describe the shape, and if it was heavier or lighter than object (3)	9
(5) 113-g slim cylindrical block	To describe the shape and texture of the object	7
(6) 396-g octagonal cylinder, with one surface covered with lint	To describe the shape, the different texture of one side and the weight relative to object (5)	30

The aim and method of the test were explained carefully at the start and the subjects blindfolded. The blocks were presented in the same order for each subject, being placed in the hand and removed as soon as the answer was given.

Table 3.5 Average time taken at first and second attempts at recognition of materials by 20 male and 20 female normal blindfold subjects

Object	Male		Female	
	1st attempt (s)	2nd attempt (s)	1st attempt (s)	2nd attempt (s)
Velvet	6	5	3	4
Felt	2.5	3	4.5	3
Silk	2	4	4	4
Plastic	5	4	2	4
Hessian	5	4	4.5	3.5
Leather	3.5	2	3	3
Wool	4.5	5	3	5
Sandpaper	2	2	2	2
Cotton wool	3	1.5	4	2

Table 3.6   Time for recognition of objects in 40 normal blindfold subjects (no difference between males and females, or between dominant and non-dominant hands)

Object	Time (s)	Object	Time (s)
Cotton reel	2	Three-point plug	2
Spanner	2	Screw	2
Eraser	2.5	Safety pin	2
Rubber band	1	Cork	2
Matchstick	2	Key	2
Bulldog clip	2		

of sand and the patient is asked to retrieve a named object. Wooden shapes are fitted into a board and the time taken to complete the operation recorded. At a later stage wooden letters are given to the blindfold patient so that he can assemble words into a message.

Tables 3.4–3.6 show the times taken for recognition of the blocks, materials and objects in 40 normal subjects.

Localization

Incorrect localization is invariable when reinnervation occurs after nerve suture. However, it is almost always possible to retrain patients so that localization is near-perfect.

The patient is blindfolded and the therapist touches a number of places on the volar surface of the hand, avoiding several brushing movements over the area to prevent adaptation. After each contact the patient is asked to point with the index finger of his normal hand to where he felt the touch. If localization is incorrect, the patient is asked to look at the point where he was touched and to relate where he felt the touch to where the stimulus was actually applied, in order to retrain localization (*Figure 3.8*).

In order to test any change in sensory function as a result of training, assessments are made at various times after the initial examination – usually at 1 month, 3 months, on discharge from treatment and at follow-up (normally at 6 months and then yearly for 5 years). Three parameters are tested – time to recognize objects, time to recognize textures and time for correct localization. In order to avoid a training effect, different objects from those used in training are employed for the tests; it is not possible for all the textures to be different, but a number of new materials are introduced.

The patient is never told if his answers are correct, either at the time of testing or subsequently, in order to avoid a training effect. At each test, the number of objects or textures recognized and the time taken to achieve recognition are recorded. If the time exceeds 60 seconds, a failure is recorded.

Some objects are particularly difficult to recognize. Those most frequently identified wrongly at first testing are – in order of frequency – can opener, electric

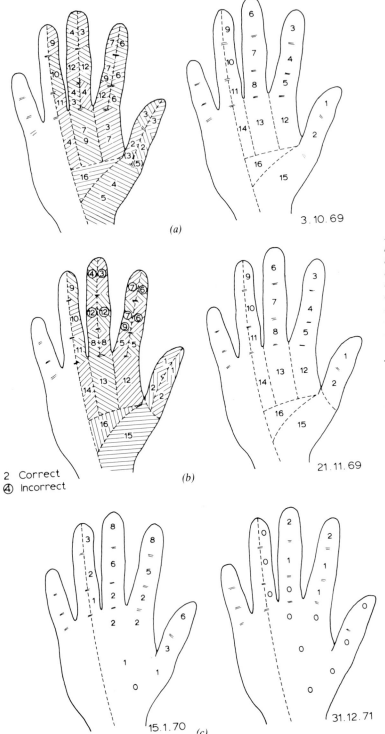

(a)

3.10.69

(b)

21.11.69

2 Correct
④ Incorrect

(c)

15.1.70

31.12.71

Figure 3.8 Training of localization. (a) The illustration on the right shows the regions of the hand supplied by the median nerve numbered for reference. On the left is the incorrect localization on starting training. For example, 3 on the thumb signifies that the patient, when touched on the thumb, felt the touch on the tip of the index. (b) Improvement after 7 weeks' training. (c) Localization now normal but slightly slower. Figures indicate time taken (in seconds) to answer correctly—on left, 14 weeks after starting training, and on right, normal values (0 = instantaneous)

plug, safety pin, purse, spanner, small bottle, screw, hook, nut and bolt. The objects most frequently identified correctly at first testing are – again in order of frequency – nail brush, bulldog clip, pencil, matchbox, Yale key, cotton reel, tennis ball, ballpoint pen, scissors, marble and string.

Textures most difficult to recognize at first testing are sheepskin, silk, plastic, wool and carpet. Those easiest to recognize are sandpaper, leather, cotton wool, canvas and rubber.

Figure 3.9 shows our techniques

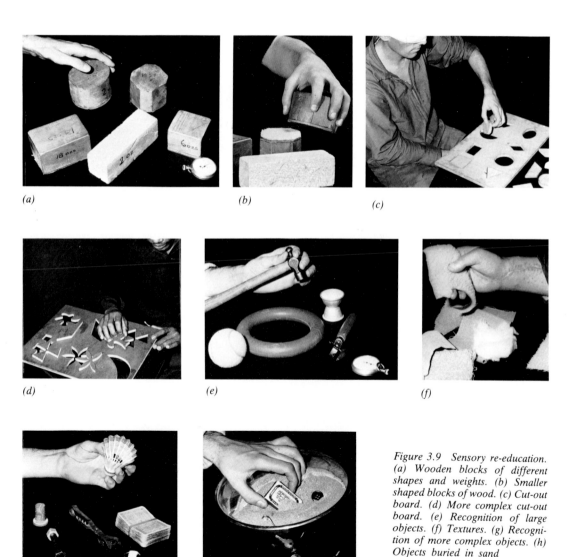

(a)

(b)

(c)

(d)

(e)

(f)

(g)

(h)

Figure 3.9 Sensory re-education. (a) Wooden blocks of different shapes and weights. (b) Smaller shaped blocks of wood. (c) Cut-out board. (d) More complex cut-out board. (e) Recognition of large objects. (f) Textures. (g) Recognition of more complex objects. (h) Objects buried in sand

Despite intensive training, most patients have difficulty in recognizing paperclips, playing cards, wool, canvas and plastic. *Tables 3.7–3.9* show examples of the results of sensory training, *Table 3.10* our composite results in 40 patients, and *Tables 3.11* and

Table 3.7   The results obtained by one of our earliest patients (1963), showing improvement in recognition time (in seconds) of (*1*) objects and (*2*) coins (now obsolete but of nostalgic interest). His median and ulnar nerves had been repaired at secondary suture 9 months previously

Object	1 Feb.	26 Mar.	20 May	26 June			
Elastoplast	35	15	10	7			
Light bulb	90	NR	35	20			
Overall button	10	20	6	3			
Paperclip	85	12	15	10			
Playing card	10	NR	7	3			
Thimble	28	10	8	5			
Yale key	20	12	3	3			
Coin	*30 Jan.*	*6 Feb.*	*21 Mar.*	*27 Apr.*	*20 May*	*28 May*	*26 June*
½d	30	8	8	6	7	7	5
1d	25	14	5	4	4	3	3
3d	8	18	20	3	3	5	3
6d	15	8	4	5	4	4	4
1s	10	6	5	10	3	3	3
2s	10	4	8	3	5	3	3
2s 6d	12	6	3	12	6	6	3

NR, not recognized

Table 3.8 Progress in recognition times (in seconds) of a patient after median nerve suture in September 1973

Object	13 May 74	18 Sep. 74	2 Oct. 74
Ballpoint pen	NR	8	3
Bulldog clip	13	9	3
Electric plug	NR	52	28
Handlebar grip	27	5	1
Nail brush	13	9	2
Safety pin	NR	30	8

NR, not recognized

Table 3.9 Results of sensory training, commenced July 1977, 3 years after secondary repair of median nerve

	July 1977	*September 1979*
Shapes	2/4 in 11 s	4/4 in 11 s
Coins	0/4	3/4 in 6 s
Textures	5/8 in 20 s	7/8 in 9 s
Large objects	2/6 in 15 s	7/7 in 9 s
Small objects	3/6 in 23 s	6/7 in 11 s

2-PD: 8 mm terminal interphalangeal index; elsewhere >10 mm

Table 3.10 Results of sensory training after median nerve division and suture in 40 adults

Average number of textures recognized:	before training	5/9 in 15 s
	after training	7/9 in 9 s
Average number of objects recognized:	before training	11/17 in 17 s
	after training	16/18 in 9 s

Localization almost perfect

2-PD: 10 mm or greater in all but 2 patients

3.12 details of some of those patients. *Table 3.13* indicates the value of these tests in other types of sensory loss than nerve disorder, and emphasizes their value in assessing the progression of disease. After an axonotmesis in which the nerve fibres grow down to their original receptors, sensory function is usually excellent and rarely needs training. *Table 3.14* gives the results in a patient after a brachial plexus lesion in continuity.

Dellon, Curtis and Edgerton (1974) have used sensory retraining with gratifying results. They noted that pin-prick is the first sensation to be felt, followed by the appreciation of the vibration of a 30 Hz tuning fork, then moving touch, then constant touch and finally the 256 Hz stimulus.

Before moving touch is appreciated at the distal phalanx, the therapist touches the skin with a blunt object at varying pressures and then moves it across the area being trained. Later, hexagonal nuts are given and the patient is asked to judge their relative size. For moving touch, four sides of a square nut or six sides of a hexagonal nut are used. They use 2-PD as a training procedure and report that 2-PD can improve considerably with training. It seems to us that, while their techniques of re-education vary from ours, we are both aiming at the same result: to help patients recognize objects and textures using the altered sensory profile resulting from slower nerve conduction and lower fibre density.

Table 3.11   Improvement in recognition times after training of patients following median nerve suture. Training commenced when the patient correctly identified the wooden shapes. Some patients (i.e. subjects 5, 10, 11, 12, 17, 19 and 22) had stopped training sessions some time before the second test

Subject	Before training		Time between	After training	
	No. of objects	Time taken (s)	tests (weeks)	No. of objects	Time taken (s)
1	4/10	20	16	9/12	11
2	23/33	18	8	30/33	6
3	8/11	30	3	11/12	9
4	8/21	21	7	12/16	9
5	22/28	13	24	22/24	5
6	10/14	18	5	12/12	9
7	13/26	12	5	17/25	8
8	15/23	9	8	23/23	2
9	2/10	7	8	19/22	8
10	13/19	11	20	12/14	5
11	4/8	42	28	13/14	11
12	12/37	36	20	39/40	7
13	14/19	16	3	15/15	11
14	20/41	15	5	20/20	12
15	9/20	11	3	18/19	9
16	2/10	43	4	7/8	23
17	7/9	11	16	9/9	11
18	8/16	10	6	14/18	13
19	17/20	13	28	11/15	11
20	10/14	5	16	12/14	11
21	12/15	9	5	8/9	3
22	12/13	10	16	14/16	6
23	3/12	36	4	12/13	9

Before training: 53 per cent of patients identified objects correctly in an average time of 18 s.
After training: 88 per cent of patients identified objects correctly in an average time of 9 s.
$P<0.001$

The problem of pain is discussed on pages 128–134, but it may be mentioned here that painful paraesthesiae can be a severe hindrance to sensory function. Transcutaneous electrical stimulation can often inhibit the abnormal discharges from the neuroma and allow sensory retraining which is otherwise impossible (*Table 3.15*).

PAIN

One of the most difficult problems in rehabilitation is pain. There are a number of conditions which give rise to such painful states that function is seriously impaired and the patient's life rendered a misery. One is speaking here not of pain after surgery – inevitable and temporary – nor after injury – which soon settles with appropriate definitive treatment – but of certain states of chronic pain which serve no useful purpose as warnings of damage nor of dangers of overuse.

The commonest disorders of chronic painful conditions of the upper limb are neuromata after peripheral nerve injuries, causalgia associated with partial nerve

Table 3.12 Progress in ability to recognize textures after training of patients following median nerve suture. Training commenced when the patient correctly identified the wooden shapes

Subject	Before training		After training	
	No. of objects	*Time taken (s)*	*No. of objects*	*Time taken (s)*
1	0/8	–	4/8	17
2	7/9	10	8/8	5
3	7/10	9	8/9	4
4	4/9	6	7/7	8
5	4/8	7	6/10	4
6	5/9	10	3/10	4
7	4/10	40	8/10	11
8	3/10	40	10/10	9
9	4/6	20	7/8	11
10	5/10	11	9/10	9
11	3/6	5	5/9	6
12	2/5	10	7/7	4
13	7/10	13	8/10	3
14	6/8	23	7/9	15

Before training: 53 per cent of patients identified objects correctly in an average time of 15 s.
After training: 74 per cent of patients identified objects correctly in an average time of 8 s.
$P<0.01$

Table 3.13 Severe deficit in sensory function (recognition of textures and objects) in a patient with cervical spondylosis, showing marked discrepancy between function and symptoms. Left hand, poor sensory function; right hand, symptom-free

Texture	Left Hand	Right hand
Cotton wool	12 s	5 s
Sandpaper	No idea	2 s
Rubber	No idea (metal)	No idea (metal)
Carpet	No idea (leather)	No idea (leather)
Wash leather	No (linen)	10 s
Canvas	No idea (hard)	No idea (hard)
Silk	10 s	No idea (fur)

Object	Left hand	Right hand
Cork	No idea (metal)	No idea (stamp)
Hook	No idea (small key)	12 s
Spanner	No idea (can opener)	15 s
Match	No idea (key)	No idea
Electric plug	No idea (padlock)	No idea (inkstand)
Rubber band	No idea (soft)	10 s
Cotton reel	No idea (metal)	No idea (rubber)
Key	No idea (metal)	No idea (metal)
Watch	No idea	No idea (metal and rubber)

Table 3.14   Sensory testing in a patient 9 months after complete right brachial plexus lesion in continuity

Object	Time (s)	Object	Time (s)	Object	Time (s)
Chalk	2	Egg cup	3	Nail brush	2
Ballpoint pen	2	Yale key	2	Playing card	5
Rubber band	1	Pencil	7	Tennis ball	1
Marble	3	Can opener	4	Eraser	6
Paperclip	13	Cotton reel	3	Nut and bolt	2
Button	7	Spanner	5	Matchbox	2
Safety pin	3	Purse	7	Electric plug	2

Table 3.15   Improvement in ability to recognize shapes and textures after primary repair of median and ulnar nerves (engineer, aged 50)

Date	Shapes	Textures	Coins	Small objects	Large objects
14 Sep. 1977	2/4	2/6	0/3	0/6	0/5
21 Aug. 1978	2/4	2/6	0/3	2/6	3/7
12 Sep. 1978, after TES	4/4	4/6	0/3	4/6	6/7

lesions, traumatic amputation stumps of the fingers, Sudeck's atrophy or reflex sympathetic dystrophy, phantom limb pain after amputation and the pain after avulsion of the brachial plexus.

Entrapment neuropathies can present with pain but are readily amenable to surgical release.

Neuromata

In most patients with nerve lesions, the nerve recovers at the rate of 1 mm per day. Protective sensation returns first, often associated with over-reaction to normal stimuli, such that warmth is felt as strong heat and cold as icy with a burning quality. Spontaneous hyperaesthesiae with a rather unpleasant feeling of pins and needles is felt for some weeks, gradually dying down to a background sensation to which the patient becomes accustomed. In due course, some degree of stereognosis may return.

In some patients, however, a painful neuroma may form at the site of injury despite meticulous surgery, causing severe burning and tingling sensations which stop the patient using that part of the hand. This is much commoner for the median nerve and thus the function of the hand is seriously affected. We have seen patients who have developed these symptoms after two or even three revisions of suture using grafts under microscopic control and yet the symptoms have recurred as fiercely as ever. In some cases there may not even be a palpable neuroma at the site of injury. It seems as if the recovering nerve is hypersensitive for reasons at present unclear and unpredictable. Dickhaus, Zimmerman and Zotterman (1976) have shown that after nerve crush the unmyelinated fibres regenerate most quickly; these are predominantly nociceptive, so there is a disproportion of nociceptive fibres. Similar symptoms are encountered after damage to the digital nerves and may recur despite resuture, crushing and burying the distal end of the nerve into soft tissue or bone. Sometimes transposition of the ulnar nerve at the elbow for ulnar neuritis is followed by persistence of painful tinglings shooting down the inner side of the forearm on even gentle use of the arm and even sometimes spontaneously. Most surgeons in this field are familiar with instances where they have carried out further exploration of the nerve, burying it deeper and freeing it from scar, and yet symptoms persist and even become worse with time.

Wall and Gutnik (1974) cut the sciatic nerve in rats and allowed the cut end to regenerate in a sealed tube. They showed that the terminal sprouts were spontaneously active, most prominent at 30 days after section. A tiny dose of noradrenaline administered to these sprouts produced a huge increase in activity. This may explain the success of sympathetic blocks in patients with painful peripheral nerve disorders. A high proportion of these sprouts were unmyelinated fibres that usually respond to damaging stimuli, and sympathetic fibres. This is a direct experimental analogy with the painful hyperaesthetic neuroma after nerve regeneration in man. Wall and Gutnik showed that proximal electrical stimulation of these fibres silenced the discharges, and this experiment led to their application of transcutaneous electrical stimulation to painful nerve lesions in man with such startling success.

Causalgia

The term 'causalgia' was originally used to describe the severe spontaneous burning pain following partial nerve lesions from bullet wounds but it is now widely used for any burning pain after partial nerve lesions, including neuromata and Sudeck's atrophy. The characteristic features in all cases of causalgia are:

(1) Severe, continuous, burning pain.
(2) Usually early onset after injury.
(3) Hyperpathia – the slightest stimulus or the lightest touch causes pain.
(4) Radiation of pain and hyperpathia outside the territory of the affected nerve.
(5) Exacerbated by emotional stimuli, noise, bright lights.
(6) Relief obtained by sympathetic block.

Weir Mitchell's classic description of one of his patients (reproduced by Melzack, 1977) deserves quotation.

'He keeps his hand wrapped in a rag wetted with cold water, and covered with oiled silk, and even tucks the rag carefully under the flexed finger tips. Moisture is more essential than cold. Friction outside of the clothes, at any point of the entire surface, 'shoots' into the hand, increasing the burning [pain]. . . Deep pressure on the muscles has a like effect, and he will allow no one to touch his skin, save with a wetted hand, and even then is careful to exact careful manipulation. He keeps a bottle of water about him and carries a sponge in the right hand. This hand he wets before he handles anything; used dry, it hurts the other limb. At one time, when the suffering was severe, he poured water into his boots, he says, to lessen the pain which dry touch of friction causes in the injured hand . . . He thus describes the pain at its height: "It is as if a rough bar of iron were thrust to and fro through the knuckles, a red-hot iron placed at the junction of the palm and [thumb], with a heavy weight on it, and the skin was being rasped off my finger ends".'

The debilitating effects of such prolonged pain have been described by Mitchell (reproduced by Melzack, 1977).

'Perhaps few persons who are not physicians can realise the influence which long-continued and unendurable pain may have upon both body and mind. The older books are full of cases in which, after lancet wounds, the most terrible pain and local spasms resulted. When these had lasted for days or weeks, the whole surface became hyperaesthetic, and the senses grew to be only avenues for fresh and increasing tortures, until every vibration, every change of light, and even . . . the effect to read brought on new agony. Under such torments the temper changes, the most amiable grow irritable, the soldier becomes a coward, and the strongest man is scarcely less nervous than the most hysterical girl.'

Melzack (1977) quotes the episode in World War II when the officer commanding a USAF hospital had to ask the director of a nearby air force flying base not to allow his aircraft to overfly the hospital because the noise and vibration caused such severe pain in his men with causalgia.

There must be some association with the sympathetic nervous system, for the limb is cold, sweating and discoloured and there is a dramatic response to sympathetic block. Indeed, Nathan (1972) has suggested that the true definition of causalgia is 'that pain relieved by sympathetic paralysis'.

It has been thought for some time that causalgia was due to an abnormality of the sympathetic nervous system; recently, however, Loh and Nathan (1978) have pointed out that it is unlikely that noradrenaline could change the characteristics of peripheral nerve endings or lower the threshold of non-myelinated nociceptors so that they could be excited by minimal mechanical stimuli. It is more likely that constant firing in the peripheral nerve produces changes in central activity, and this is how hyperpathia can spread and even involve the whole forequarter of the body.

Blocking the sympathetic fibres stops the emission of the sympathetic transmitter and this stops spontaneous firing of the peripheral nerve fibres; this in turn prevents abnormal function of the peripheral nervous system.

The abnormal state is maintained by large-diameter afferent fibres; it is a normal sympathetic system acting on these fibres which causes the input to the spinal cord with disinhibition and facilitation spreading from the original site of the input.

Wallin, Torebjork and Hallin (1976) have shown that transcutaneous electrical stimulation (TES) which relieves pain and hyperpathia has no effect on the sympathetic nerve discharge, showing that the sympathetic nervous system itself is normal.

Application of noradrenaline to an area previously painful before sympathectomy will produce recurrence of pain. Applying firm pressure over the nerve proximal to the site of damage – thus stimulating A fibres – stops the hyperpathia.

These authors also showed, using recording in the superficial radial nerve by microelectrodes, C fibre activity was unchanged as a result of the induction of hyperpathia by noradrenaline. These experiments show conclusively that it is the myelinated A fibres which are transmitting abnormal impulses. There thus appear to be a peripheral and a central component to this condition. Wall (1980, in preparation) points out that there are at least 12 effects of peripheral nerve section, many of which are central. These include changes in the central terminals of the axons damaged in the periphery, changes in the central terminals in intact neighbours of the peripheral damaged axons and changes in the reactions of spinal cord cells which have lost their normal receptor fields as a result of peripheral nerve lesions. This would explain the frequent finding that pain is felt over a much wider area than the autonomous territory of the affected nerve.

The tonic discharge of the sympathetic to viscera and blood vessels may summate with cutaneous input to produce pain. Cells in lamina V exhibit somatic and visceral convergence and are monosynaptically connected to visceral afferents. This is the basis of referred pain (cutaneous hypersensitivity over an inflamed appendix, for example) and would explain the summation of stimuli such that the slamming of a door can precipitate severe pain in the limb.

Loh and Nathan (1978) have shown that sympathetic blocking is much more likely to be effective if hyperpathia exists. It is true, however, that a number of patients with algodystrophy do not show obvious sympathetic over-activity yet sympathetic block can be effective and should therefore be considered in all cases.

In the early stages, pain predominates and this prevents the patient using the limb. We use sympathetic nerve block with guanethidine as a first choice; only if after three such injections this has proved unhelpful do we use stellate block (Hannington-Kiff, 1974).

Guanethidine acts by discharging noradrenaline from its storage sites. This immediately produces pain – but once all the noradrenaline has been discharged from its storage sites at the sympathetic nerve endings, a prolonged block is achieved. In practice, it is noticed that if the injection is given without an anaesthetic, the patient feels an immediate increase in pain but within 10 minutes, if the treatment is effective, the pain will be virtually abolished.

With a tourniquet applied proximally 20 mg guanethidine in 20 ml normal saline is injected slowly into a vein on the back of the hand. The cuff is left on for 20 minutes and then released. Half hourly blood pressure, pulse and respiration are recorded until the patient is completely recovered. No general anaesthesia is used as immediately after the patient's blood pressure is stable, intensive desensitisation with stroking the affected part and activities in physiotherapy and occupational therapy are begun.

If guanethidine is ineffective, stellate blocks are carried out at weekly intervals. If the effect is only temporary then sympathectomy may have to be performed. Some workers have found that the effect of sympathectomy is only transitory, lasting a mere few weeks due to the massive ability of the sympathetic nervous system to regenerate. They have therefore given up this operation, preferring to use repeated stellate blocks, with or without concomitant guanethidine injections as a reinforcer. Surprisingly, guanethidine can still be very effective after sympathectomy and is therefore well worth trying.

There is no doubt that some form of interference with sympathetic outflow can be dramatic in the relief of causalgia. Similarly, because all avenues of sensory input are capable of triggering nerve impulse patterns which produce pain, possible and known trigger points should be sought and treatment directed to them.

Hannington-Kiff (1979) has shown in 10 cases of causalgia that 80 per cent achieved relief if the treatment was given within 5 months, but only 50 per cent were helped if given at 15 months or later. Thus early treatment is imperative.

Because we know from Wall and Gutnik's work that spontaneous electrical discharges from a neuroma can be silenced by electrical stimulation, we also use the transcutaneous electrical stimulator in all cases for several hours a day (pages 139–142). Once pain relief is obtained, the patient is encouraged to use his arm as much as possible in the rehabilitation unit, both to restore function and to help replace abnormal central discharges with more normal neuronal patterns.

We have followed up 70 patients with painful peripheral nerve disorders in the upper limb, over a minimum period of 1 year – the majority for 3 years or longer. The patients comprised 20 with median nerve lesions at the wrist, 16 with digital nerve sections, 7 with lesions of the ulnar nerve at the wrist, 10 with ulnar nerve lesions at the elbow, 9 with amputations of digits, 3 with nerves involved in scar and 1 with crush injury.

The most effective treatment was TES, which afforded satisfactory relief in 38 (*Tables 3.16* and *3.17*). Nine were helped by guanethidine, 17 were unhelped by any

Table 3.16 Results in 18 cases of severe painful neuromata treated with transcutaneous electrical stimulation. Note that, despite very long-standing symptoms, relief was achieved remarkably quickly

Cause/Nerve	Duration of pain (years)	Surgery	Result	Time for relief (weeks)	Own stimulator
Bite/M	3	3 operations	Total	2	Yes
Cut/M	4	Graft	Total	1	Yes
Cut/UD	1	Resection	Total	1	Yes
Cut/M, U	2	Suture	Total	6	Yes
Cut/M	3	Suture	Total	2	Yes
Charcot elbow/M, U, R,	3	Nil	Total	6	Yes
Cut/M	1	Suture	Total	4 days	No need
Fracture of wrist/M	1	Arthrodesis	Total	1	No need
Cut/U	3	Graft	Total	1	No need
Neuroma in palm/M	2	Suture	Satis.	2	Yes
Ganglion/M	3	Excision	Total	5	No need
Cut/M	3	Suture	Total	9	No need
Cut/UD	1	Excision of neuroma	Total	2 days	No need
Traction plexus/M, U, R	2	Neurolysis	Satis.	2	No need
Ganglion/M	3	Nil	Total	2	No need
Osteoarthritis of elbow/U	3	Nil	Near total	3	No need
Ulnar neuritis	4	2 transpositions	Total	4	Yes
Ulnar neuritis	1	Transposition	Total	1	Yes

M. median;   U. ulnar;   R. radial;   UD. ulnar digital

Table 3.17 Pain relief obtained with TES following secondary suture of median nerve at the elbow 3 years previously (severe hyperaesthesia and hyperpathia in median zone)

Date (1978)	Intensity	Pulse width	Repetition rate	Time (hours)	Comment
5 May	3	8	6	1	Less pain in tips of fingers
15 May to 17 May	3	6	4	1½	Relief of pain in arm
19 May	3	5	5	1½	Feeling returning in fingers
22 May	3	6	5	2	Typing with little pain
27 June	4	1	5	2	Less hyperpathia; work in OT
3 July to 17 July	4	1	4	2	Steady progress
20 July	4	1	6	3	48 hours' total relief; discharged with own stimulator

Follow-up at 6 months: virtually no pain

form of treatment and 13 are left with severe intractable pain (7 of these last sustained wounds from glass). Our disappointing results are probably explained by the late state at which patients are seen, because we are a referral hospital and the majority of patients have been treated elsewhere for months or even years.

The single most unsuccessful treatment was further surgery. In 23 patients nerve grafts, transposition of nerve or nerve crush was carried out; 17 were made worse. It is always very difficult to decide whether further surgery should be attempted or should be abandoned on the grounds that further deafferentation will result, causing further central and peripheral changes – and more pain. The following case histories will illustrate this.

Case 3.2.   Mrs M cut her index finger, severing the digital nerves and flexor tendons. The nerve was repaired and a tendon graft effected. Pain persisted and, in July 1975, she had an amputation through the metacarpophalangeal joint. Causalgic pain persisted and a year later, because of severe hyperaesthesia and hyperpathia, she had an operation in which two neuromas were found in the scar and removed. The pain was worse after this procedure; stellate blocks, guanethidine, propranolol and TES were tried but none was of any value. She continues to have severe paraesthesiae and phantom pain.

Case 3.3.   Mrs B, aged 60, presented with a painful Heberden's node. An attempt at arthrodesis failed and left her with very severe pain in the finger and a full-blown Sudeck's atrophy. A repeated attempt at arthrodesis failed and amputation of the finger was carried out. She then developed severe phantom pain and severe causalgia in the normal middle finger. The standard treatments included stellate blocks, guanethidine, TES and drugs; none had any effect. The median nerve was crushed at the wrist in September 1976, and within 2 weeks the pain returned worse than ever. She was treated for depression. Repeated stellate blocks and, finally, a sympathectomy were carried out in November 1976 – with no effect. Repeated trial of TES worsened the pain. In 1978 a large neuroma was removed from the digital nerve and the stump was buried; she has had complete relief of pain ever since at 18 months' follow-up.

Case 3.4.   Mrs EK fell on a milk bottle in 1973 and cut her median nerve. Primary suture was carried out and she developed severe causalgia which persisted for 4 years. In 1977, scarring of the nerve was released and Silastic wrapped round the nerve. No relief of pain was achieved and the hand was useless. She responded dramatically to TES and was using her hand normally for some months. However, the pain recurred and she was treated with a radial digital graft to the median nerve. This produced some relief of pain, which was further reduced by TES and she has remained pain-free for 2 years. Following TES her sensory function improved dramatically and she was able to recognize all the standard shapes used in our sensory function tests in 7 seconds, 6 out of 8 textures in an average of 8 seconds, 4 out of 7 large objects in 17 seconds and 6 out of 7 objects in 12 seconds, and localization was perfect.

Case 3.5.   Mrs ES, aged 61, fell through a glass door and severed her median nerve, which was repaired as a primary procedure. She developed a large painful neuroma, severe causalgia and a useless hand. Three years later, sural grafts were carried out but pain returned after a further 3 years, with pain as bad as ever. She responded satisfactorily to TES 6 hours a day and regained full function of her hand. Two years later the pain returned at about 50 per cent of its previous intensity but responded dramatically to guanethidine injections and she has remained pain-free ever since.

These case histories underline the unpredictable nature of this condition but it seems clear that very careful assessment is required before repeated surgery is contemplated.

Over all, from a study of the literature, it seems that between one-third and one-quarter of patients are not helped by any form of treatment. There is no doubt that the sooner treatment is initiated, the better the results.

There may indeed be a good case for applying such treatments as TES and sympathetic blocks as a prophylactic procedure in any patient in whom it seems likely that causalgia will develop.

Phantom pain

Most patients who have suffered amputation of a digit or part or the whole of a limb will speak of a sensation that the limb is still present. Many of our upper limb amputees speak of the elbow being bent and the fingers flexed tightly into the palm; occasionally the position of the phantom alters in relation to emotional stress or a painful state elsewhere in the body. But a few patients suffer real, often agonizing, pain and the concept of how pain can arise in a structure no longer present has remained a mystery until recent neurophysiological research has enlightened us (see page 138).

Similarly, very severe pain can be felt in the paralysed arm – almost always the forearm and hand after avulsion lesions of the brachial plexus.

Avulsion of the roots of the brachial plexus

When there is an avulsion of the roots of the plexus from the cord, a very characteristic pain develops. The pain does not usually start until 3–4 weeks after injury, although it can be present within a few hours. The pain is described as burning, crushing, on fire, like the hand being compressed in a vice with, in addition, very strong electric shocks. Often the pain builds up to a crescendo over 10–15 minutes and the patient feels he is about to burst and thinks he can no longer bear it. Gradually it subsides to a background tingling or burning until the next crescendo occurs and there can be six or more of these attacks a day. During the acme of the pain, the patient will have to stop whatever he is doing and often seeks to be alone. Curiously the pain does not stop sleep. Usually these unfortunate patients have tried every form of analgesic available, but none has much effect. Occasionally codeine derivatives blunt the edge of the pain, but it is common to hear that nothing has any effect. A very few patients become addicted to 'hard' drugs and become pitiable wrecks, but it is inspiring to find that the overwhelming majority learn to live with the pain and get on with their daily life. In fact, distraction is about the only successful means of controlling the pain. When totally absorbed in work or hobbies they can put the pain at a distance and even forget it altogether for a few hours. Some grip their anaesthetic hand hard and move the paralysed limb about with their other hand and claim it gives some relief. Some learn that by sitting absolutely still and willing the pain away or relaxing into it, as it were, they can gain some relief.

The natural history of this pain is variable – mercifully the majority find that it gradually abates over a period of months, leaving behind a dull reminder of its once vicious nature. Some lose pain altogether, but most have a tingling sensation all the time, although this is quite bearable and has no effect on their life. Some 10–20 per cent, however, have their pain for life; it seems that the pain will be permanent if it is still severe 2 years after injury.

Table 3.18 shows the duration of pain in 98 patients with avulsion lesions of the brachial plexus. 'Severe' implies that the pain seriously affected their lives, and 'acceptable' that they had come to terms with it and it no longer worried them.

Table 3.18   Duration of pain in 98 patients with avulsion lesions of the brachial plexus

Duration (years)	Severe	Acceptable
1	14	15
2	5	12
3	5	4
4–10	7	7
11–15	4	5
16–20	6	5
20+	4	5

The mechanism of the pain is discussed on page 138. It seems as if the deafferentation releases spontaneous firing of cells in the dorsal horn. Experimentally such spontaneous firing can be recorded in the dorsal horn after section of nerve roots, reaching its peak at 30 days, and this relates well to the timing of the onset of pain in these patients.

We have recently completed a review of 108 patients who had evidence of avulsion of one or more roots. In 98 of these patients there was a significant degree of pain. There was a direct correlation between the number of nerve roots avulsed and the severity and duration of pain. Most severe pain lasting for the longest period was seen in patients with total avulsion of the whole plexus.

Unlike causalgia, there was no effect of external stimuli on the pain, so sudden banging of a door or noise had no effect. Most of them found that the pain was made worse by worry and emotional stress. In particular, these tended to increase the sudden severe paroxysms of pain. Almost all patients reported that when completely distracted with work or with an absorbing hobby they would be unaware of pain. Thus many patients feel that their pain is worse in the evening and at night when they have nothing to distract them. Very few patients were taking any form of analgesia although there were a few who took pentazocine (Fortral) regularly. Many patients found that alcohol gave them relief, but usually because it helped them to sleep rather than because of any direct effect on the pain; none of our patients could be described as a 'heavy drinker'.

Pain was very often increased by intercurrent illness, such as colds or 'flu, and this would characteristically make the paroxysms of pain very much worse. In about one-third of the patients the pain did not come on for some weeks after injury, and the longest intervening period was 8 weeks.

TES has been used in 37 patients. In 19 it was highly effective, in 6 of some help but in the remaining 12 of no help at all and in fact aggravated the pain for a few days in 3 patients. There was a clear correlation between the amount of remaining afferent input and the success of electrical stimulation; in those patients with total avulsion and no sensation over the C5 distribution, TES was ineffective.

The patients who are regularly using the stimulator find that it is most effective if used for several hours a day either at work or, if they do not suffer pain at work, in the evening when they are no longer distracted and the pain becomes obtrusive. As time goes on, they require the stimulator less and less, and many of them now use it for only an hour a day or perhaps 2 or 3 hours a week. There is no doubt in our minds that this treatment is well worth careful trial in all patients with avulsion lesions of brachial plexus.

Another approach has been that of Nashold, Urban and Zorub (1976), who coagulated the dorsal root entry zone in 4 patients with avulsion of the plexus, and achieved 50–80 per cent relief of pain at 1 year after surgery. This is theoretically reasonable because the operation is designed to destroy the spontaneously firing cells. However, a long-term follow-up is awaited, as procedures which destroy nerve tissue lead to further deafferentation and possibly more pain.

In severe intractable pain which is ruining the patient's life, the implant of a cerebral stimulator may be the only solution.

Case 3.6. This patient sustained avulsion of the C6, 7, 8 and T1 roots, but C5 was in continuity although severely damaged. *Table 3.19* shows the gratifying result obtained with TES in this case. Possibly the sparing of some fibres in the C5 root allowed a pathway for afferent modulation.

Table 3.19   Relief of pain with TES in a patient with avulsed plexus (burning pain in elbow–hand)

Date (1978)	Intensity	Pulse width	Repetition rate	Time (hours)	Comment
5 July	3	4	4	3	Relief in wrist and hand
7 July	4	4	4	2	Complete relief for 24 hours
2 Aug.	3	5	6	2	Total relief for 1 week
18 Sep.	3	4	6	2	Total relief by use three times a week

Case 3.7. This patient was involved in a car accident in May 1978, and presented with a complete paralysis of shoulder and elbow. Exploration by Mr G. Bonney revealed that C5 and C7 were avulsed, but C6 was in continuity; C8 and T1 were spared and there was normal function in the hand.

The patient developed the characteristic severe burning pain of the preganglionic lesion in the shoulder 28 days after the accident. A trial of TES was successful, reducing his pain to 50 per cent on the visual analogue scale and allowing him to return to his legal work. He used it for about 4 hours a day 8 months after the accident; at review in December 1979, he was using it once every 2 weeks for a few hours when the pain returned, but was virtually pain-free.

Pain mechanisms

Until recently, lack of knowledge and understanding about the mechanisms of pain production has tended to make patients with chronic pain the despair of the doctor, and all too often they have been dismissed as problems for the psychiatrist – 'The pain is in your mind' they are told. This is, of course, exactly true; but it is a real, not an imagined, phenomenon and these patients require all our concern, help and explanation.

Fortunately, the whole problem of pain is now taken seriously and is much better understood. The setting up of pain clinics and the collaboration of clinicians, physiologists and psychiatrists is a testimony to this. So important is this field of rehabilitation and so puzzling are some of the phenomena seen in the clinic, that we propose to review here the current concepts of pain and the mechanism of painful disorders in peripheral nerves.

It has clearly been pointed out by Melzack (1977) in his brilliant book, *The Puzzle of Pain*, that pain is not a modality of the same type as temperature, touch or pressure. Whether or not a stimulus is felt as painful depends on a variety of factors: cultural, ethnic, social, previous experience, the situation in which the potentially painful condition occurs, as well as the actual stimulus and the receptor system. The old concept of specific pain receptors with a private line through the spinothalamic tracts to the cortex is outdated.

Whilst there is undoubted specificity of peripheral receptors, there is much greater overlap than was once thought.

Peripheral receptors are divided into mechanoreceptors, thermoreceptors and nociceptors. Iggo (1977) has described the properties of nociceptors – by definition they response to potentially damaging stimuli, and have a high threshold and a small receptive field.

When the stimulus exceeds threshold, a persistent discharge is set up, providing continued information concerning the stimulus. Nociceptors are sensitized by prostaglandins, serotonins, histamine and noradrenaline. They relay to the cord via small-diameter afferents – the alpha delta and C fibres. Three-quarters of the small thinly myelinated alpha delta fibres respond to innocuous mechanical and thermal stimuli and one-quarter to strong damaging stimuli, so it is not true to state that these are 'pain' fibres.

Of unmyelinated C fibres in the dorsal roots, 50 per cent supply mechanoreceptors responding to innocuous stimuli, 20 per cent mechanical nociceptors, 30 per cent thermal nociceptors and some of each of these are polymodal. These polymodal receptors can go on firing for minutes after a single stimulus and their threshold is lowered for hours (Burgess and Perl, 1973). This is of great relevance for continuous pain states. It has been shown by Vallbo and Hagbarth (1968), using intraneural microelectrodes in man, that stimuli causing pain activate the C fibres, but these fibres also respond to other stimuli such as pressure and heat, though not to light touch.

At the same time, the damaging stimuli cause mechanoreceptors to discharge and so a complex pattern of impulses reaches the cord. It appears that there is no situation in which only nociceptive receptors are stimulated.

The total number of active fibres and their rate of firing may therefore be at least as important as the type of fibre stimulated.

Injury thus produces nerve impulses in small-diameter myelinated and unmyelinated afferents – these relay predominantly to laminas I and V in the dorsal horn. However, cells in lamina V also respond to low threshold afferents which, when stimulated, can inhibit the response of the alpha delta and C fibres (Cervero, Iggo and Ogawa, 1976).

Moreover, there is an incredible degree of modulation at all levels – excitation and inhibition from other afferents, both pre- and postsynaptically, and descending controls from higher centres. The transmission of information also depends on the state of activity in the dorsal horn at that time.

Melzack and Wall in 1965 introduced their gate theory of pain which, though criticized in detail and modified by its originators in the light of new findings, still helps to understand the mechanism of pain. They suggest that in the spinal cord, probably in the substantia gelatinosa, there is a form of gate which can close off transmission of nociceptive impulses centrally.

It was predicted by Wall and Melzack that, if the large-diameter afferents were stimulated by pressure, touch and vibration or electrical stimulation, it should be possible to prevent impulses travelling along the small-diameter fibres from being transmitted to the brain, and this indeed proved to be the case. We now know that stimulation techniques are sucessful in modifying or abolishing peripheral pain and are in routine use in pain clinics.

There is, however, firm evidence that many painful states are related to spontaneous central nervous activity. One can explain the pain of peripheral nerve disorders on the abnormal activity of sprouts and excess response to sympathetic discharge, but how can one explain phantom limb pain or brachial plexus pain when there is no afferent input at all?

The first clue to the explanation of this problem came in 1966 when Wall showed that if one cut one or more spinal roots in the cat, an abnormal rhythmic burst of firing occurred in the dorsal horn.

Loeser and Ward in 1967 cut the fifth (trigeminal) root of the cat and showed that there was a progressively increasing spontaneous discharge of cells in the cord. More recently, Loeser *et al.* (1968) recorded spontaneous discharges in the spinal cord of a patient with ankylosing spondylitis who, after an accident, suffered a paraplegia associated with severe painful flexor spasms. The spasms coincided with bursts of spontaneous firing in the cord. It thus seems that deafferentation of the cord releases cells from inhibition which then start to discharge spontaneously – a sort of sensory epilepsy. There is a further factor – denervation leads to sprouting of adjacent neurons and this may well lead to abnormal patterns of activity which are felt as pain.

Normally spinal cord cells have a resting discharge, but transmission of their messages is inhibited by afferent inputs along large-diameter fibres and descending inhibition. If these cells are released from such inhibition they start to discharge spontaneously.

Partial lesions are associated with partial deafferentation and this may explain the pain of neuromas and causalgia, for here two factors operate – the distal discharges of the regenerating sprouts and the lack of afferent input to the cord so there is spontaneous activity peripherally and centrally. Stimulation techniques thus act in two ways – suppressing the activity of fine sprouts and stimulating the large afferents to 'gate off' the small-diameter activity.

Foreman and colleagues (1976) showed, in monkeys, that activity in the cells of the spinothalamic tract was inhibited by volleys in the large afferent fibres of peripheral nerves or dorsal columns.

Why should some patients develop pain and others not? Some patients with avulsed plexuses do not suffer severe pain; others do for some weeks or months and then it abates – yet others have pain for life. Only a few patients (perhaps 5–10 per cent) develop painful phantoms after amputation. Sometimes it is possible to attribute this to the development of a lesion elsewhere whose painful impulses may trigger dormant spontaneous circuits to fire and reach consciousness.

Patients have described pain for the first time in their phantom limb – 25 years after the injury – following an episode of angina.

There is also a memory for pain. Nathan (1962) has described patients who, years after cordotomy when hypoalgesic areas were stimulated, relived pain of an incident such as a fracture sustained many years before. Melzack and Loeser in 1978 described five patients with paraplegia and severe pain in the trunk and legs in whom a whole section of the cord was removed – this made no difference whatsoever to their pain. Here the neuron pools were totally cut off from any peripheral input and were acting as pattern-generating mechanisms.

It has long been known that repeated blocks of painful peripheral nerves with local anaesthetic may relieve spontaneous pain. It is likely that when the limb is rendered painless it can then be used more normally. Normal patterns of activity can be established centrally and abolish the abnormal spontaneous firing. Certainly we have found it essential to encourage our patients to use the affected limb as much as possible when their pain is temporarily relieved by afferent modulation techniques.

Disappointing results of cordotomy are continually being reported. Section of the spinothalamic tracts relieves pain for a time, but almost invariably the pain returns – often more severe than before. It has been shown that nociceptive impulses can travel also up Lissauer's tract, by short links via non-myelinated and myelinated fibres in the substantia gelatinosa, via the posterior columns (division of these columns relieves the pain of distorted posture in amputees), by bilateral polysynaptic pathways and by short loops bypassing continuous columns of grey matter. There is a remarkable degree of redundancy in the central nervous system. Surgical ablation causes further deafferentation and thus sets the scene for the development of more spontaneous firing. Ablation of 'pain pathways' seems doomed to failure.

Afferent modulation

The principle of all these techniques is to stimulate selectively the large-diameter afferent fibres relaying touch, pressure and vibration in order to gate off the impulses travelling in the small fibres relaying nociceptive stimuli. When pain is relieved the patient must use the limb to restore normal patterns and suppress abnormal central discharges produced by partial deafferentation. A variety of techniques are used: vibration, acupuncture, electrical stimulation, even rubbing and massage. Probably the time-honoured way of rubbing a bruise is based on the effect of large-diameter fibre stimulation.

Which technique is tried first varies from one worker to another; all are agreed that one should try all – hoping to find the one modality which suits that particular patient. We have found in our practice that transcutaneous electrical stimulation (TES) is the most successful. This is possibly because we are dealing with painful peripheral nerve states which are very similar to the experimental models in which TES was effective.

It is known from Wall and Gutnik's work (1974) that electrical stimulation specifically damps down spontaneous firing of terminal sprouts.

There are a number of stimulators on the market, but all have much the same parameters. The pulse is a square wave of average duration 50–500 µs, the repetition rate can vary up to 60 pulses per second and the current is adjustable up to 60 mA. The correct electrode positions have to be found by trial and error. They must be proximal to the lesion – application over the painful area intensifies the pain – and it may take the therapist one or two sessions to discover the most effective siting. Generally speaking, application of one electrode just above the painful site is usually most effective with the other further proximal along the course of the affected nerve.

In amputation or in brachial plexus paralysis, they are placed across the neck as proximal as possible.

Despite careful follow-up of all our patients, perusal of the literature and discussion with colleagues working in this field, it is not possible to predict which patients will respond and which will not. Interesting, too, is the enormous variability of settings the patient chooses from one session to another.

Theoretically TES should work only if there is an afferent input to modulate, and it is certainly true that its greatest success is with neuromas, ulnar neuritis and partial nerve lesions. Yet we have had spectacular successes in patients with total amputation of the upper limb and even in patients with avulsed plexuses.

It is therefore always worth trying the stimulator – it is non-invasive, harmless and not unpleasant. We never raise our patients' hopes, but merely indicate that we are trying a technique which has been helpful in similar situations in the past.

Experience has taught us that originally we were using too short a treatment period; we now apply the stimulator for at least 2 hours at a time, two or even three times a day and often for period of 6–8 hours. The patient is given a stimulator to treat himself over the week-end. There is no doubt that there is a cumulative effect. Some patients find that 5 days' stimulation leads to complete relief for the sixth day and the pain only begins to return on the seventh day – as stimulation continues so the pain-free period increases. Patients are encouraged to use their hand in occupational therapy and workshops after the session when the pain is lessened and many can carry on their tasks in the home or even at work whilst actually wearing the device. They are encouraged to stroke the skin as the hyperpathia diminishes.

If there has been no significant diminution in pain by 2 weeks, there is no point in persisting with the treatment.

We prefer to admit our patients to the rehabilitation unit in order to integrate methods of pain relief into a comprehensive rehabilitation programme. Only thus can one determine the optimum parameters for stimulation, the time required and positioning of the electrodes. It is vital, in our view, that normal neuronal patterns are revived by use of the limb when pain is relieved.

In almost all cases we give our patients a stimulator to continue treatment at home after discharge because pain may recur if the treatment is stopped too soon. The length of time one needs to continue is a matter of trial and error. Usually it is weeks rather than days, and in severe cases it is advisable to continue use for months, gradually reducing the time of application.

The overall figures given by Long and Hagfors (1975) in their review of 3000 cases collected from the literature indicate that one-third of patients with chronic pain will respond to TES. Their cases included all causes of pain – chronic backache, trigeminal neuralgia and herpes as well as upper limb disorders. In our experience, 65 per cent of patients with peripheral nerve pain will obtain significant relief. Many will achieve this in a few sessions and the relief will be permanent; presumably normal central patterns have been restored. Others still have pain, but at an acceptable level, and may use the stimulator from time to time to damp it down. Occasionally a rash develops – a day or two's rest and liberal application of electrode jelly usually solves the problem. Others need it permanently and it will be interesting to see if a proportion of these eventually gain permanent relief. Many patients suffer severe paraesthesiae, burning and tingling as part of the recovery process in regenerating peripheral nerves. Treatment with TES can markedly reduce these symptoms and allow more normal sensory function.

We are currently investigating the effect of TES on sensory function as judged by object and texture recognition. So far the results are encouraging: in six patients marked improvement in sensory function followed relief of hyperaesthesia by TES. *Tables 3.20* and *3.21* show the results obtained in two such patients.

Table 3.20   The effect of transcutaneous electrical stimulation on the ability of a patient with hyperaesthesia following a median nerve lesion to recognize objects and textures and to localize a stimulus. The last entry shows a further improvement already effected by TES, by the patient's increased ability now to use his hand, having lost the hyperaesthesia. (Median nerve repair 4 December 1975; patient aged 12)

Date	Localization	Shapes (4)	Textures	Coins	Small objects	Large objects	2-PD
Re-education							
17 June 1977	18/35	14	6/8 in 18 s	3/3 in 11 s	1/6 in 22 s	3/6 in 16 s	>10 mm
23 July 1979	18/35	10	4/6 in 10 s	2/3 in 9 s	5/6 in 17 s	6/6 in 5 s	>10 mm
Hyperaesthesia: TES							
3 Sep. 1979	35/35	2	4/6 in 7 s	3/3 in 7 s	5/6 in 13 s	6/6 in 4 s	>10 mm
Use and TES							
8 Oct. 1979	35/35	3	4/6 in 6 s	3/3 in 8 s	5/6 in 5 s	6/6 in 4 s	>10 mm

Table 3.21   Effect of TES on the ability of a patient with hyperaesthesia following an ulnar nerve lesion to recognize objects and textures and to localize a stimulus. (Patient aged 61; ulnar neuritis for 3 years)

Date (1978)	Intensity	Pulse width	Repetition rate	Time (min)	Effect
24 May	5	7	4	30	Less pain on movement
25 May	4	8	4	60	No pain for 36 hours
2 June	4	6	1	60	Painless extension of elbow
12 June	4	10	5	60	Hyperpathia less
16 June	5	10	9	50	2½ days' relief
3 July	4	1	1	60	1 week's relief

There was a vogue for implanting cuff electrodes around the nerves by operation in chronic cases who needed permanent TES. These seem to have been abandoned as there were many complications, including infection and movement of the electrodes.

Similarly, dorsal column stimulation was very popular a few years ago for phantom limb pain and other intractable conditions, but on a recent review it was found that only 18 per cent had achieved excellent results and again there were many complications. This technique is very expensive and unpredictable, and most workers try to use only the transcutaneous stimulator.

Electrical stimulation

HISTORICAL BACKGROUND

Natural electricity was used in classical times and three electric fish are recorded: *Torpedo marmorata* (torpedo ray); *Malopterurus electricus* (Nile catfish); and *Symnotus electricus* (electric eel).

Nile catfish are seen in Egyptian tomb reliefs of BC 2750. The *Torpedo* (*torpere*, sluggish) was known to Aristotle.

Various parts of electric fish were long advocated as folk medicine to be taken orally. Scribonius Largus advocated piscine 'electrotherapy' specifically for the relief of pain.

'For any type of gout, a live black torpedo should, when pain begins, be placed under the feet. The patient must stand on a moist shore washed by the sea, and he should stay like this until his whole foot and leg, up to the knee, is numb. This takes away present pain and prevents pain from coming on if it has not already arisen. In this way Anteros, a freeman of Tiberius, was cured . . . Headache even if it is chronic and unbearable is taken away and remedied forever (*sic*) by a live black torpedo placed on the spot which is in pain, until the pain ceases. As soon as the numbness has been felt the remedy should be removed lest the ability to feel be taken from the part.'

It is interesting that characteristics of the stimuli from electric fish are similar to those produced artificially for electrical analgesia. In the USA, Francis, in 1858, used an electroanaesthetic apparatus which anaesthetized the pulp for tooth extraction. Robinovich in 1910 (reported in Gwathney, 1914) carried out amputations of legs at the St Francis Hospital, Hartford, USA, with electricity – optimal levels being 40 V using a 10 ms pulse width with a frequency of 100 impulses per second.

So it is curious that the value of electrical stimulation for pain relief has been dormant for almost 100 years.

ACUPUNCTURE

Acupuncture is held in high regard by many authorities and there seems no doubt that it should be part of the armamentarium of any pain relief service. It probably acts both peripherally and centrally, and it certainly does work in some cases. It has been our experience that patients with nerve pain such as we see in our service have often already tried acupuncture without success and many respond subsequently to TES.

We have been disappointed by the use of vibration, but some patients will respond and, if so, this is satisfactory for it is cheap and easy to use.

CENTRAL MECHANISM

We have spoken about central inhibiting pathways, and it is well recognized that people can suffer wounds which one would expect to cause pain yet, in the heat of battle, they can be totally unaware of their pain – if indeed they can be said to have pain if they do not feel it. Patients with severe pain from avulsion of the plexus can, by sitting quietly and concentrating, will away their pain for a time. Distraction and will power must therefore bring into play some inhibitory tracts that prevent impulses from reaching consciousness. The nature and behaviour of these central pathways have become much clearer in recent years.

In 1954, Olds and Milner were stimulating the reticular formation in rats. By chance they had their electrodes in the wrong place and noted that stimulation caused the animal obvious pleasure.

Heath, in 1963, stimulated the septal region electrically in patients with severe pain which completely abolished it. Then Reynolds in 1969 showed that electrical stimulation of the central grey matter or the adjacent central tegmental tract elicited profound analgesia in rats, so much so that he was able to carry out laparotomy on them without an anaesthetic.

The pathway is from the periaqueductal grey matter round the third ventricle in the mid-brain and passes via the raphe nucleus in the medulla direct to cells in lamina I and V which, as we have seen, is where the small-diameter fibres relay from the periphery that respond to noxious stimuli. Interestingly, stimulation of this tract, while abolishing pain in the particular area to which it refers, has no effect on other sensations nor does it affect the threshold for noxious stimuli.

Morphine acts at the same sites as those at which stimulation-produced analgesia (SPA) is effective and SPA is reversed by naloxone – a morphine antagonist. Hughes (1975) found a peptide in the brain that acts at morphine-binding sites and is antagonized by morphine antagonists.

It is possible that SPA acts by releasing endogenous opioid peptides which then become bound at the receptor sites. The search is now being intensified for these peptides – or enkephalins – in the hope that some day a naturally occurring chemical pain antagonist can be produced for human pain without the side-effects and addictive properties of morphine.

The discovery of these central mechanisms led to the trial of cerebral stimulation in patients with intractable pain. At first it was tried in terminal cancer patients who had failed to respond to any drugs and, often, ablative surgery.

Stimulation of the periaqueductal grey matter for a few minutes gave hours of total relief from pain.

Adams (1976) reported the case of a 54-year-old man with severe pain due to diabetic neuropathy. He implanted an electrode 3 mm lateral to the lateral wall of the third ventricle, and stimulation resulted in complete relief of his severe burning pain. One of the fascinating aspects of this report was that the effect of SPA was abolished by injections of the morphine antagonist, naloxone.

Mazars in 1976 reported on 17 patients in whom cerebral stimulators were implanted. He used a pulse of 2 ms duration, with a frequency of 10 Hz and an amplitude of 1 V. He obtained pain relief in patients with phantom limb pain, pain from complete plexus avulsion, X-ray fibrosis of the plexus and paraplegia.

These are exciting results and it may be that cerebral stimulation holds the answer to those patients with intractable pain unaffected by any other method. It is, of course, one matter to use this technique in someone with a limited life span and quite another to put an implant in a young person with 50 years of pain ahead of him. Selection of the patient will be all important. Only psychologically robust patients should be offered such a solution. There is always the dread thought that pain may be relieved for a time but then recur, and the last state of that man might be worse than the first.

Measurement and recording of pain

There is only one way to judge the effectiveness of any technique aimed at relieving pain and that is by seeking the patient's comments. He alone knows whether he is having pain and what it is like.

It is now accepted that the use of a visual analogue scale is a valid and reproducible means of assessing pain (Scott and Huskisson, 1976). In this, the patient indicates on a scale how bad is his pain. The scale can be numbered from 0 (no pain) to 10 (unbearable), and the patient marks the place along the scale that he feels is fairly represented by his pain. Alternatively, one can put descriptive words along the scale; for example, ranging from 'Severe' through 'Moderate' to 'Mild'.

Another method is to invite the patient to indicate which words in a pain rating scale describe his pain. These words all have a score and the total score is a good reflection of his pain and, most importantly, a change in the value will indicate alteration of his pain.

Melzack (1977) has validated these scores by showing that there was close agreement, in a group of doctors, nurses and patients, as to the extent to which these words represent intensity of pain.

A comprehensive pain profile will include an account of the patient's pain given verbatim, its effect on his life, work, hobbies, and social and domestic activies. Also noted are the length it lasts, any variation in intensity and effects of outside agents, anything he can do to modulate it (e.g. self-manipulation), any long-term effect on his health and the number of analgesics taken. Then an analogue scale and a pain rating scale are completed.

Thus comparison can be made before and after treatment and statistically significant results obtained. Psychological testing may be useful in certain situations, but a well motivated young person in active work and social life with phantom limb pain or a painful neuroma after median nerve suture will not need a professional psychological assessment – he has pain and wants to get rid of it. It is a different matter if some long-term implant surgery is contemplated where its effects may be unpredictable.

Case 3.8. This patient developed Charcot ankles 35 years ago. Both were arthrodesed – the right successfully, but the left became infected and the leg had to be amputated. Five years ago she fell and sustained a fracture of the elbow; as a result of this and the strain put on the joint by using a stick, the joint developed an extraordinary appearance with abnormally increased range of movement – a Charcot elbow in fact. She then developed entrapment neuropathies of all three nerves at the elbow.

Surgery was ruled out, but a polyethylene foam (Plastazote) gutter splint attached to a crutch allowed her to walk; however, because she suffered severe continuous pain in the distribution of all three nerves with characteristic skin changes she was unable to do so. Within 3 weeks of TES 4 hours a day, her pain had abated to less than 50 per cent and she was able to walk again. She uses her stimulator daily and 1 year later it is still effective.

Case 3.9.   This patient was run over by a car when she was 12 years old and sustained a traumatic amputation of the right upper limb. Ten years later, due to unequal growth, the amputation was revised. She had no pain at all in her phantom limb, until 51 years later she suddenly developed excruciating pain in the phantom limb. She could feel her fingers tightly clenched around the shilling she was carrying when she was run over by the car. This pain had been continuous and almost unbearable for the 6 months preceding her attendance at our pain service. After 2 weeks' TES over the shoulder for 2 hours three times a day, she completely lost her pain. The fingers are gradually uncurling and she has promised to send me the shilling if it drops out of her grasp!

It is likely that the sudden onset of pain was connected with severe cervical spondylosis stirred up by a fall.

ASSESSMENT OF RESULTS OF TREATMENT

Return of function after neurapraxia is perfect and in axonotmesis should be excellent (*Figure 3.10*). In this section, therefore, the results of neurotmesis only are discussed. In general, our experience has been the same as that of Seddon and Brooks (1954),

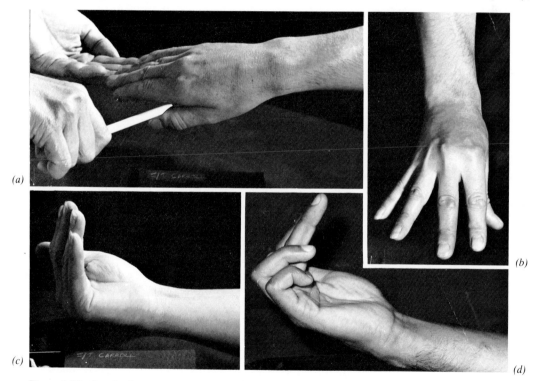

Figure 3.10   Result after axonotmesis of ulnar nerve. (a) Lack of Froment's sign when abducting thumb against gravity and resistance. (b) Abduction of the fingers. (c) Flexion of metacarpophalangeal joints with interphalangeal joints extended. (d) Same movement in a patient with complete ulnar palsy to contrast

that the rate of growth of the nerve is between 1 and 2 mm a day. It has been said that full recovery of independent action of the interossei is rarely seen. However, where full-time treatment throughout the recovery stage could be given, a small proportion of patients did recover independent intrinsic action.

Clarkson and Pelly (1962) stated that in only 54 per cent of nerve sutures is there return of independent intrinsic action. In 45 per cent of low median sutures there is useful motor return, and in 5 per cent useful sensory return with protective sensation. In only 10 per cent is there return to two-point discrimination and then only to 8 mm.

Highet (1954) described an assessment of motor and sensory recovery which is widely used.

MOTOR RECOVERY

(1) No contraction in any of the muscles supplied by the affected nerve.
(2) Perceptible contraction in the proximal muscles.
(3) Perceptible contraction in proximal and distal muscles.
(4) All muscles act against resistance.
(5) All synergic and isolated movements are possible.
(6) Complete recovery.

SENSORY RECOVERY

(1) No sensation.
(2) Deep cutaneous pain in the autonomic zone.
(3) Superficial pain and tactile sense in the autonomic zone.
(4) As for (3), with the disappearance of over-response.
(5) There is also recovery of two-point discrimination within the autonomic zone.

COURSE AND RESULTS IN NERVE LESIONS

Ulnar nerve lesions

The first sign of recovery of an ulnar nerve lesion at the wrist is a flicker in the abductor digiti minimi, and this is best seen in synergic action when the thumb is opposed to the little finger. When the lesion was at the wrist, the average time between nerve suture and the appearance of a flicker was 81 days in our series (extremes: 73–93 days).

When the suture was performed 2.5 cm above the wrist the average time was 111 days (extremes: 100–120 days). A number of sutures were performed at 3.8 cm above the wrist. The average time before a flicker was seen was 144 days, but there was a small group in whom the average time was 170 days. It will be seen from these figures that the rate of regeneration is roughly 2.5 cm a month as generally accepted. Taken in conjunction with the electrical signs, the combination is reliable enough to suggest that if there is no sign of recovery 2 months after it should be expected, something serious is preventing progress.

The average time between the appearance of a flicker in the muscle when acting as a synergist and a flicker when acting as prime mover was 3 weeks; 40 days later the muscle achieved a grading of 2 on the MRC scale, and by 60 days after the first appearance of a flicker a grading of 3.

The average time before obvious appearance of metacarpophalangeal flexion with interphalangeal extension was 140 days, and for abduction and adduction of the fingers between 150 and 200 days. These times are at least twice as long in our experience as for axonotmesis.

The average time for full function from damage to the nerve at the wrist causing an axonotmesis was 7 months. In the case of neurotmesis at 2-year follow-up 80 per cent achieved grade 4 but only a few regained independent interosseous action. Some patients achieve remarkably quick recovery – favourable factors being youth and previous high degree of skill. Our best result was a 30-year-old technician who had complete normal motor and sensory function 9 months after primary suture of the ulnar nerve at the wrist.

SENSATION

Using Tinel's sign as an index of speed of regeneration of sensory nerve fibres, it was found that the average rate of regeneration was 6 cm a month (extremes, 3–8 cm). After median nerve suture at the wrist, protective sensation was felt at the finger tips at 6 months.

Median nerve lesions

MOTOR RECOVERY

It is very difficult to judge the presence or absence of a contraction in the flexor pollicis brevis and the opponens unless the short flexor has a complete median supply, but this is unusual. Consequently, the only indication before a flicker appears in the short abductor is a general sign that the patient's function with his thumb has improved. If, however, complete relaxation of the thumb can be obtained, the medial aspect of the thumb can be seen, with progressive recovery, to lie along the index finger and an increasing distance from it, thus showing recovery of function in the short abductor. When the thumb is supported in palmar abduction, opponens can be felt rotating the thumb if put in its inner range. The average time between nerve suture at the wrist and response in the short flexor in those cases where one can be sure of this sign is between 70 and 90 days. For the short abductor the times are 72–140 days with an average of 91 days. One-half the cases achieve M4 at 2-year follow-up; one-quarter M3; and a few M1 and M0.

Most patients regain good function of the thumb, though only a small proportion regain completely full rotation. Abductor pollicis brevis often does not recover but only a small proportion of these require an opponens transfer because of good ulnar function. If sensation is poor, tendon transfers are pointless because patients do not use the hand if feeling is absent. Some patients find that they like to wear lively splints at work many months after recovery has started.

SENSORY RECOVERY

Sensory recovery as judged by stereognosis is, in our experience, usually poor unless special techniques of re-education are used – when excellent results can be obtained (page 119–126). The real test is whether they use that hand in daily activities. On the

Highet (1954) scale (which is not truly a functional test), one-half of our series achieved S5 and one-third S4. With training, 70 per cent of our patients really used that hand in daily life for most normal activities.

A few regained good sensation but no motor power. In such conditions there is no question of further surgery to the nerve. The patients therefore returned to work with the lively splint or had reconstructive surgery.

Some spectacular advances have been made in the surgical restoration of sensation in median and ulnar nerve lesions. Tubiana and Duparc (1960) pointed out that the most important situations in the hand where sensation is vital are the palmar aspect of the thumb and the lateral parts of the fingers opposing the thumb, and the medial aspects of the little finger. All these are the sites where restoration of sensibility is most important. Littler (1959) was the first to use a heterodigital cutaneous transplant with its neurovascular pedicle. This neurovascular skin island transfer corresponds to the terminal zone of distribution of the palmar collateral neurovascular pedicle.

Tubiana (1969) pointed out that two conditions must be observed in the choice of the donor finger. The flap must have perfect innervation and vascularization, and removal of the island must give rise to minimal disturbance. The donor sites that are used most are the medial aspect of the middle and ring fingers, where loss of sensation matters least.

In 10 cases reported by Tubiana (1969), the transplant conserved its viability and sensation, and the sensation was comparable in quality to the normal fingers. After a while the 2-PD becomes normal. Shortly after the operation the patient feels sensation as if it were coming entirely from the donor finger. After a few weeks, however, the sensibility of the grafted finger is added to the sensibility of the donor finger. This double sensitivity is gradually modified, and the patient becomes more and more aware of the grafted finger.

In permanent paralysis of the median nerve, the island is taken from the radial side of the ring finger and transferred either to the index finger or the thumb. In permanent paralysis of the ulnar nerve the transplant is taken from the medial side of the middle finger and transferred to the medial side of the little finger. There seems no doubt that this technique is of value in the restoration of sensation in patients with permanent loss of sensation after peripheral nerve injuries in the hand, although disappointing results are now being reported, some patients preferring their old anaesthetic thumb to the abnormal sensation in both donor and recipient areas. Sensory transfer should not be carried out until mobility has been restored by tendon transfers. The indications for this operation are a young, active, intelligent, mentally stable patient with a median nerve lesion, good ulnar sensation and a useful pain-free hand, and whose occupation demands sensation in the median zone.

There are certain situations, however, where not even such brilliant and complicated surgery can help. This situation arises when there is permanent anaesthesia of the whole hand as is found in leprosy. This is a very severe problem, particularly because the average person suffering from total anaesthesia of the hand due to leprosy lacks intelligence, and is therefore very prone to develop trophic lesions. The problem here is one of rehabilitating a patient with total sensory loss, and the principles are quite different from those involved in the re-education of a patient with altered sensation. The great dangers of a totally anaesthetic hand in leprosy to the worker are the cuts at work, damage to the hand in machinery, and to the housewife burning the hand when manipulating cooking implements and household activities such as ironing. Here the problem must be solved by careful education and demonstration of how to avoid situations which might lead to trophic lesions. This means teaching the housewife how to manipulate the hot utensils with tongs and to take care never to handle hot plates or dishes except with oven cloths or thick gloves. Similarly, a leper who is being taught to drive must be shown that it is not necessary to grip the steering wheel hard, a natural inclination owing to complete lack of proprioception, otherwise severe trophic ulceration will develop at the palmar aspect of the metacarpophalangeal joints and may ultimately lead to complete loss of the fingers. He must be taught to learn by experience the minimum pressure required to have confident handling of the steering wheel. Similarly, at work he must be taught all the dangers of machinery, proper use of guards and care in the treatment of superficial cuts and abrasions so that they do not become infected.

That normal function is possible, despite total anaesthesia of the hand, will be familiar to those who have had charge of patients with complete median and ulnar nerve lesions in the first few months after suture and before any form of sensation returns. If the patient is properly instructed and supervised, no trophic lesions will ever occur and the texture and colour of the skin should be normal. Similarly, with the correct education, publicity and propaganda, patients with leprosy can be taught to avoid trophic lesions and to carry out skilled function with totally anaesthetic hands.

Paul Brand has been a pioneer in the development of rehabilitation services for leprosy and the reader is directed to his chapter in Cochrane and Davey (1964).

Radial nerve lesions

The average time between nerve suture and the first response cannot be given as in the case of median or ulnar nerves because the conditions and levels of injury are so variable from one patient to another, but generally the rates were those expected assuming the rate of regeneration to be 1 mm a day.

In the stage of complete paralysis the grip is reduced to 25 per cent of that of the normal hand. When the extensor carpi radialis longus and brevis are working with power 3 (MRC scale) the grip is about 50 per cent that of normal. When the extensor carpi ulnaris and the extensor digitorum communis are recovering, the grip is between 60 and 70 per cent that of normal.

Normal grip as measured by the dynamometer does not return for many months after a good recovery is seen (grade 4 motor recovery).

SENSATION

The amount of sensory loss in radial nerve palsies varied greatly. In some there was loss over the radial part of the dorsum of the hand. In others there was sensory loss over the lower third of the forearm and fingers. There was slight diminution to pin-prick over the first dorsal interosseus space in some cases, while in others the loss was only over the medial side of the dorsal surface of the limb; in some there was no loss at all. In only one patient in this series was there complete sensory loss in the whole area supplied by the radial nerve and thus the sensory loss is not of importance in radial palsies, and careful testing is seldom necessary.

Case histories in nerve lesions

Case 3.10. Radial.   As the result of a motorcycle accident, this patient sustained a comminuted fracture of the left humerus at the junction of the middle and lower thirds, and developed a radial palsy at the same time. He was admitted to the rehabilitation centre 2 months after injury. Radiographs at this stage showed considerable callus

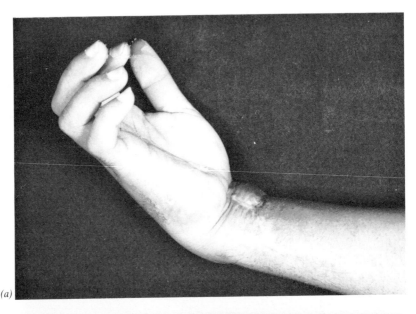

(a)

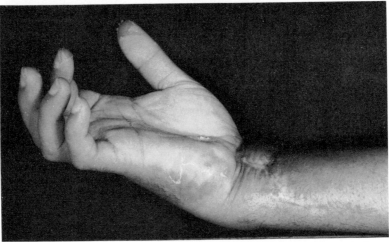

(b)

Figure 3.11   Lesion of the median and ulnar nerves and all tendons in the right wrist. Gross adherence of tendons 4 weeks after secondary suture of all structures, and at commencement of rehabilitation. (a) Maximum flexion, and (b) maximum extension possible at the wrist and fingers. (Case 3.11)

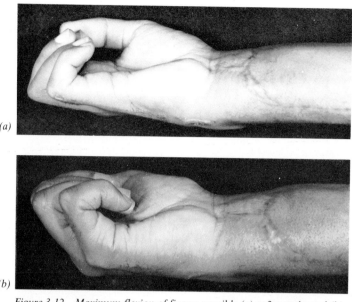

Figure 3.12 Maximum flexion of fingers possible (a) at 2 months and (b) at 4 months after commencement of rehabilitation. (Case 3.11)

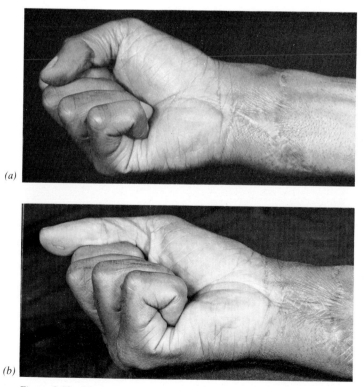

Figure 3.13 Maximum flexion of fingers possible (a) 14 weeks after that shown in Figure 3.12 and (b) 1 year after suture. (Case 3.11)

formation which it seemed might well be interfering with the nerve. Four months after the accident the nerve was explored and found to be fairly adherent to callus over a length of about 2.5 cm. It was freed and found to be thickened.

A flicker was observed in the extensor carpi radialis longus 166 days after the original injury, followed 21 days later by a flicker in the extensor digitorum communis. One month later the patient stated that he was sure the arm was increasing in bulk and that the muscles felt as if they were working properly. After a further 4 months there was full power in all the muscles except the extensor pollicis longus, which was still rather weak.

Case 3.11. Median and ulnar.   Severance of all the structures in front of the wrist joint was the result of this patient's putting his hand through a glass window pane when sleep-walking. Eight days after injury all the structures were sutured (all the flexor tendons of the wrist and fingers and both nerves).

He was admitted to the rehabilitation centre 1 month after operation, when it was found that all the tendons were just working. There was an open wound across the wrist 3.8 cm in length and the wrist joint was held at 30 degrees' flexion, there being no movement in it. The hand was very oedematous, so much so that the patient was instructed to wear a sling when not having treatment.

Two months after suture, stretch splinting was started to overcome both the gross scarring and contracture at the wrist joint and the severe degree of flexor tendon adherence at the wrist, which was now becoming obvious. Even 3

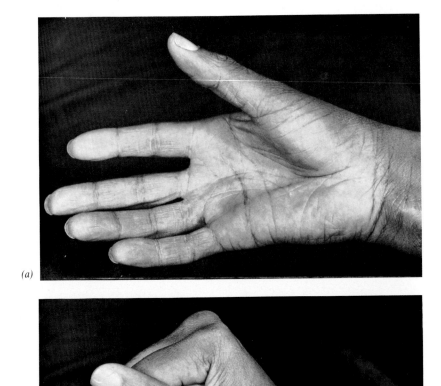

(a)

(b)

Figure 3.14   (a) Maximum extension and (b) full fist, 1 year after suture. (Case 3.11)

months after suture there was a 70 degree flexion deformity at the interphalangeal joints with the metacarpophalangeal joints extended, but with the metacarpophalangeal joints flexed, the interphalangeal joints could be fully straightened. New stretch splints were made twice a day in the first month, daily in the second month, and later twice a week. The splints were worn at all times when not having treatment, including at night. Stretch splinting continued for 6 months in all.

A flicker was seen in the abductor pollicis brevis 151 days after suture and in the abductor digiti minimi 100 days after suture.

When discharged 10 months after suture, examination showed a grip of 4.8 kg as compared with 5.9 kg on the normal side. All the thenar muscles were working well. The thumb could be opposed to within 5 cm of the tip of the little finger. All the lumbricals were working, power 3+. Independent action of the interossei had not been recovered. Touch sensation had returned throughout the hand except for the tips of the ring and little fingers. Pin-prick was felt normally throughout the hand; there was no overaction, and general function was extremely good.

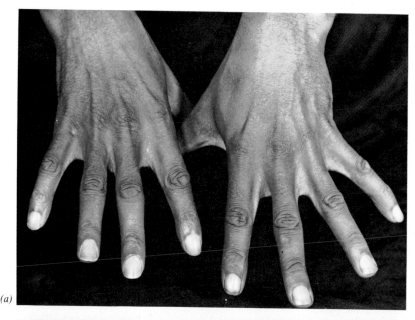

(a)

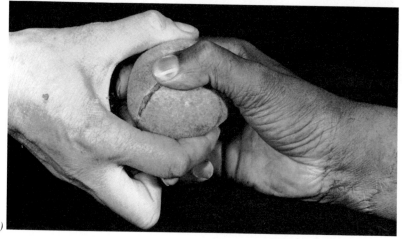

(b)

Figure 3.15   (a) Abduction of fingers and (b) thenar muscle function, 1 year after suture. (Case 3.11)

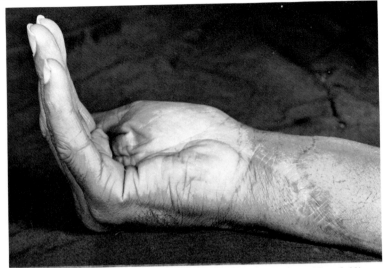

Figure 3.16 MP flexion and IP extension 1 year after suture. (Case 3.11)

At follow-up as an outpatient 24 months after suture, there was no hyperaesthesia, and 2-PD was the same as in the normal hand. The grip was only 0.5 kg less than normal, all the muscles worked well. The general function was assessed as grade 5 sensory and grade 5 motor; the interossei worked well. He was carrying out duties as a motor fitter with no difficulty, and had just passed with top marks at a fitters' course when last seen. He managed all heavy work and most fine work, such as handling split pins and screws, and did not need to use his sight to carry out fine work.

This case illustrates that, despite a very severe injury with the complications of gross flexion contracture due to tendon adherence at the wrist, an excellent result can be obtained. Full-time intensive treatment is essential in a case of this sort.

Being employed as a motor fitter, this patient required really good function of the hands; careful re-education was therefore essential. Furthermore, the gross tendon adherence cannot be overcome without daily stretch splints, as described in Chapter 2. Unless this is overcome, motor return will, of course, be hampered seriously by the deformity. Such a result can be expected only if the problem is accepted as being one that demands expert care, full-time if necessary, over a period of many months. Apart from stretch splinting, oil massage to reduce the scarring on the wrist is required several times a day, and re-education of function when the muscles begin to recover. All this takes time and cannot be done satisfactorily unless the patient is prepared to attend for treatment for the full day.

Figures 3.11 to *3.16* illustrate the progress of this patient from the early stages to the final recovery.

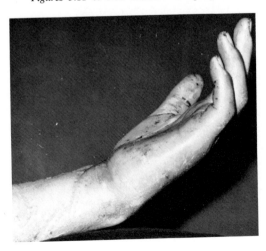

Figure 3.17 Appearance of hand 5 weeks after suture of median and ulnar nerves at the wrist. (Case 3.13)

Case 3.12. Ulnar. This patient cut his right hand when he fell on some glass and sustained a complete lesion of the ulnar nerve on 15 September 1960. The ends were approximated at primary operation but not sutured. An infected ulcerated wound developed which was treated preoperatively with ultraviolet light. On 9 January 1961 secondary ulnar nerve suture was carried out and the patient was admitted to the rehabilitation unit on 1 February 1961. At this stage a typical ulnar nerve deformity was present, grip was 3.6 kg on the affected side compared with 5.4 kg on the normal side. There was a certain amount of tendon adherence as a result of the infected wound before operation, which speedily stretched out with oil massage and plaster stretches. By 20 March 1961, 72 days after suture, the abductor digiti minimi was contracting and the lumbricals showed a flicker. Touch was felt 2 cm distal to the wrist. Grip was 5.9 kg on the left, 5.7 kg on the right.

The patient was assessed in his trade as air wireless fitter and found to be fully capable of doing all aspects of his job. He was therefore returned to duty 4 months after secondary nerve suture. He was reviewed again 2 years later, when there was no wasting and all the muscles supplied by the ulnar nerve, including interossei, were working normally. Grip was now 0.9 kg better on the affected side than on the original normal side. Localization to touch was normal throughout. Two-point discrimination was about 50 per cent of normal.

Electromyography showed on the third dorsal interosseus that almost complete recovery had occurred. His hand was in every way fit for his job and he regarded himself once again as completely normal.

Case 3.13. Median and ulnar. This patient sustained division of the median and ulnar nerves. Tendon adherence at the wrist required intensive physiotherapy (*Figure 3.17*). Primary tendon and secondary nerve suture was carried out, together with routine motor and sensory rehabilitation. The sensory charts (*Table 3.22*) show function 3 and 4 months after suture and 2 years after injury.

Table 3.22 Progressive recovery of sensation in Case 3.13

Object	Time (s)		
	27 Feb. 68	*25 Mar. 68*	*13 Nov. 69*
Sandpaper	4	3	2
Wool	20	NR	3
Canvas	NR	NR	10
Carpet	10	4	NR
Leather	NR	3	NR
Sheepskin	20	4	5
Cotton wool	3	2	2
Plastic	4	8	5
Rubber	NR	3	NR
Silk	30	5	10
Wood board	4 min 15 s	3 min 30 s	3 min 30 s
Soap	4	3	3
Chalk	5	NR	2
Ballpoint pen	10	5	2
Rubber band	10	3	2
String	7	4	2
Screw hook	11	NR	2
Paperclip	6	NR	2
Button (overall)	16	3	2
Safety pin (large)	18	3	2
Egg cup	15	2	2
Spanner	2	3	3
Bandage	5	3	2
Eraser	7	NR	2
Nut and bolt	10	5	2
Handlebar grip	15	2	2
Screw top	9	3	2

NR: not recognized

Case 3.14. Median.　This patient severed the right median nerve and flexor digitorum profundus to all fingers, flexor carpi radialis and pollicis longus. Secondary suture was carried out 3 weeks later. The opponens was supplied by the ulnar nerve and, by its use, opposition was possible (*Figure 3.18*). His motor function was normal; he only required a few weeks' after-care to restore full tendon function and he was able to return to duty as a steward, taking the usual precautions to prevent sensory trophic disturbances in the anaesthetic area of the hand involving thumb, index, middle and half the ring fingers. He was readmitted 5 months later, when sensation had returned to the finger tips, for sensory re-education. On discharge after 3 weeks' intensive training his charts showed reasonable function (*Table 3.23*). He was taught the techniques for continued sensory training as his unit. On review 4 months later, 1 year after suture, he had made further progress and sensation was now practically normal (*Table 3.23*).

Table 3.23　Progressive recovery of sensation in Case 3.14

Object/Texture	*Time (s)*	
	6 July 71	*17 Jan. 72*
Blocks Small Wood Circular	5	3
Wood Hexagon	45	10
Wood circular smooth	10	8
Light wood rectangle	25	20
Textures Sandpaper	9	4
Wool	3	2
Canvas	NR	NR
Carpet	4	3
Leather	6	6
Sheepskin	20	NR
Cotton wool	3	2
Plastic	5	6
Rubber	6	3
Silk	4	3
Soap	NR	8
Tape measure	4	2
Chalk	15	10
Ballpoint pen	NR	6
Rubber band	5	2
String	3	1
Screw hook	6	12
Marble	10	6
Yale key	11	9
Pencil	14	4
Screw top	15	4
Spanner	11	6
Tin box	7	3

NR. not recognized

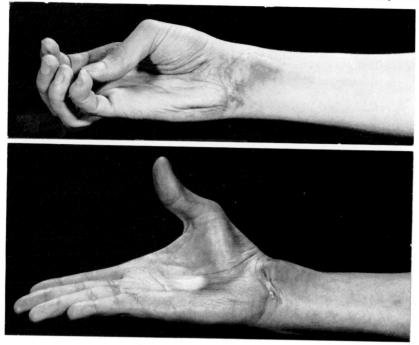

Figure 3.18   Activity of thenar muscles 4 months after repair of median nerve lesion by primary suture. (Case 3.14)

Case 3.15. High lesion of all three nerves.   This patient was on patrol in Aden in 1967 when a sniper shot him in the left axilla, severing all three cords and the axillary artery. As the patient was seen within a few hours of injury, primary suture was undertaken by an experienced surgeon. He was transferred to the MRU and received a year's intensive rehabilitation with passive movements to the paralysed joints, lively splintage to the hand and, as reinnervation proceeded, intensive physiotherapy, occupational therapy and games. He regained excellent function for, on discharge, there was power triceps 2, extensor digitorum communis 3+, extensor carpi radialis longus 5, extensor carpi radialis brevis 4+, extensor carpi ulnaris 3+, abductor pollicis longus/extensor pollicis longus 3+, wrist and finger flexors 4+. No return as yet in interossei, but sensation had returned to mid-palm.

On review 18 months after injury, pronation and supination had power 5, extensor digitorum communis 4, extensor carpi radialis longus 5, abductor pollicis longus/extensor pollicis longus 3+, abductor digiti minimi 2, medial lumbricals 2, abductor pollicis brevis 3−, opponens 3−. Opposition to ring finger was strong. Sensation was now present although altered to finger tips. He was able to pick up small objects and could drive a manually geared car.

BRACHIAL PLEXUS LESIONS

Traumatic lesions of the brachial plexus are unfortunately becoming more frequent. As the price of petrol rises, so more young men are taking to the motor cycle and it is accidents on these potentially lethal machines that make up by far the commonest cause, with car accidents a close second. These lesions almost invariably involve traction to the plexus. The common story is for the cyclist to hit an oncoming car or stationary object such as a lamp post or tree – his head and neck are stretched as the body moves on with the momentum developed and the hand retains its grip on the handlebars for a fraction longer. The mechanisms of the injuries are discussed in detail in a later section.

Not all lesions of the plexus are associated with traction and not all traction lesions are inevitably permanent.

Pressure lesions do occur – *Table 3.24* lists a number of causes of plexus lesions in which the pressure over a prolonged period of time caused damage to the nerves. In most cases, the pressure causes segmental demyelination; when the compressing force

Table 3.24   Pressure lesions of the brachial plexus (10 cases)

Cause and site	Recovery
Pack or rucksack (16–21 kg):	Full, within 8 weeks
1: C5	
1: C5, 6	
2: C5, 6, 7	
2: C5–T1	
Pallbearer's palsy, C5, 6, 7	Full, in 8 weeks
Compression, C5, 6	Full, in 9 weeks
Pernod palsy (complete)	Full, in 18 months
Whisky palsy (complete)	Full, in 15 months

is removed, however, the myelin re-forms and complete recovery occurs in weeks or a few months. Sometimes these lesions are associated with an underlying anomaly such as a cervical band or rib and the patient is then well advised to avoid the situation which gave rise to the palsy.

Two of our patients drank a whole bottle of Pernod and Scotch whisky respectively and succumbed to their soporific qualities. Eighteen hours later when they awoke they had complete paralysis of the whole arm – the lesion must have been totally degenerative for recovery took over a year, but was complete. (This small series suggests – *Table 3.24* – that British alcoholic beverages are less damaging than French!)

The paralysis associated with dislocation of the shoulder always recovers virtually completely – the lesion is infraclavicular and in continuity.

It is the traction injuries associated with high speed road traffic accidents which result in such devastating paralyses.

If the injury is not too violent, the nerves are stretched sufficiently to cause axonotmesis and a totally degenerative lesion, but the sheath is in continuity. If the injury is more violent, the nerve roots actually rupture between their emergence from the intervertebral foramen and the clavicle. This lesion has only been recognized in recent years. With greater violence, the plexus is avulsed from the cord. We thus think of three grades of injury: traction in continuity, rupture or avulsion. These can coexist – a common pattern being rupture of C5, 6 roots and avulsion of C7, 8, T1. Unfortunately, the situation is even more complicated, for there may be lesions at two or even three levels. It is not unknown for the roots to be avulsed from the cord, ruptured in the neck and the nerves torn distally.

This is doubtless because there are often two, three or even four injuries: one when the cyclist makes impact with the oncoming vehicle, a second when he hits the roof or bonnet and a third when he is thrown onto the road, or a passing vehicle may then hit him as he lies in the road.

Clearly the more information one can glean from witnesses and the patient himself, the better able one is to reconstruct the sequence of events, but this is rare – patients are almost always rendered unconscious and have no recollection of the accident nor are the witnesses able to help as these accidents occur with such suddenness.

Anatomical factors

There are some mechanisms that protect the plexus from being damaged in the normal activities of daily life which may put stress on the plexus.

The fifth, sixth and, to a lesser extent, the seventh cervical roots are held at the transverse processes in gutters of bone by invaginations of the prevertebral fascia, and these roots are linked together by bridges of fibrous tissue.

Below the clavicle, the cords of the plexus are firmly bound together and to surrounding structures, including the clavicle and coracoid, by layers of the clavipectoral fascia.

The integrated neurovascular cord is snubbed again by these fascial investments between the clavicle, the coracoid and the first rib; that is, in the apex of the axilla (Stevens, 1934).

The plexus gets stretched between its two firm points of attachment – the transverse processes and the clavipectoral fascia.

The roots do not always break; indeed they are the last to give. The forces of tension are disseminated via the blood vessels – which may break – and the fascia and the perifascicular connective tissue which is much more plentiful in the roots than in the nerves. The plexiform nature of the plexus, arranged as it is in a parallelogram, itself helps to disseminate forces of traction. It is much less vulnerable than if it consisted of five single nerve trunks.

The strong downward inclination of C5 compared with the almost straight direction taken by the first thoracic root makes it much less vulnerable – the fifth cervical root is almost twice as long as the eighth cervical root, and again makes for more protection against stress.

The posterior roots have a thick ligament attaching them to the cord, while the anterior rootlets are small and less well protected – this explains why one can suffer total motor paralysis with sparing of sensation. There are thus many built-in factors that protect the plexus from stretching. Otherwise, mothers would frequently give their children traction lesions of the plexus when pulling them away from enticing shop windows.

In the 1940s and early 1950s it was common for surgeons to explore lesions of the plexus in the hope of repairing the nerves. However, there was a unanimity about the futility of such procedures.

Stevens reported that at operation, 'The plexus seemed a mass of scar tissue – the cords were welded together in an inflammable mass – on account of the scar tissue nothing could be made out as to the exact location of the injury. Yet many such cases have recovered in whole or in part.'

Brooks (1949) rarely found a rupture of a root and in only 1 of 10 cases explored by Barnes (1954) was there a rupture. Despite the mass of scar tissue and depressing look of the plexus, a high proportion of such patients recovered. Drake (1964) pointed out that the fibrous encasement of plexus elements does not interfere with reinnervation; rather it is the intraneural disruption and fibrosis that prevent regrowth.

We reported (Wynn Parry, 1974) on 130 cases of traction lesions of the plexus treated conservatively, and the results are given in *Table 3.25*. Examination of the

Table 3.25   Results in lesions of the brachial plexus

Number	Site	Abd.	Ext. rot.	Elbow		Wrist		Finger		Average time to return to work (months)
				F	E	F	E	F	E	
Complete										
2	C5	2	1	1	–	–	–	–	–	4
22	C5,6	16	13	19	–	–	–	–	–	8
22	C5,6,7	8	6	14	5	–	4	–	–	8
31	C5–T1	0	0	5	0	0	0	3	–	11
4	C7–T1	–	–	2	2	2	3	2	–	11
Partial										
18	C5,6	16	16	16	–	–	–	–	–	–
4	C5,6,7	3	3	4	4	–	4	–	3	–
2	C7	–	–	–	2	–	2	–	2	4
2	C7–T1	–	–	–	2	2	2	2	2	–

Abd, abduction;   Ext. rot., external rotation;   E, extension;   F, flexion;   –, not affected

results in the upper root lesions shows that about two-thirds regain significant function. We might regard this as the natural history of lesions of the upper trunks. Narakas (1977) has reopened the whole question of surgery to the plexus and in 107 operations found that one-third showed actual ruptures of the roots.

It may well be that the reason why one-third of our series did not recover is that they had unrecognized ruptures.

Why are ruptures now so much more common than 30 years ago? One likely explanation is that the compulsory wearing of crash helmets has enabled the survival of more accident victims who have sustained violent injuries. Before, they would not have survived.

The outstanding problem is correctly to diagnose the nature of the lesion, for, if it is in continuity, there is a good chance of spontaneous recovery and surgery is not indicated. If there is a rupture, repair with nerve grafts may be indicated; if roots are avulsed they are irrecoverable and a definitive plan for reconstructive surgery or neurotization can be made. There are a number of clues from the history and clinical examination and some diagnostic investigations which can help in distinguishing these three types of lesions.

History

Knowledge of the speed of impact will give a clue as to the violence of injury. High speed accidents are clearly more likely to be associated with rupture or avulsion. An eye witness account of the sequence of events will indicate if there are likely to be multiple lesions at different levels. Associated injuries such as damage to blood vessels or fractures of the long bones or ribs suggest considerable violence.

Clinical picture

Table 3.26 shows the pattern of involvement of the roots in order of frequency in our experience. Paralysis of serratus anterior and rhomboids indicates a very high lesion, as the nerves to these muscles are the first to come off the plexus.

Table 3.26   Common patterns of traction lesions of the brachial plexus

Complete C5, 6 in continuity
Complete C5, 6, 7 in continuity
C5, 6 ruptured C7, 8, T1 in continuity
C5, 6 ruptured C7, 8, T1 avulsed
Avulsion of all roots

Partial lesions (i.e. complete lesion of C5, 6 but no involvement of C7, 8 or T1) are usually a sign of damage distal to the posterior root ganglion; this is not always so, however – workers with long experience of such patients have seen some in whom there has been avulsion of C5, 6 with complete sparing of C7, 8 and T1.

A total paralysis of the whole arm is a bad sign and usually, but not always, indicates avulsion. We have seen a few patients in which the C5–8 lesion has been postganglionic and only T1 preganglionic.

Scattered sparing of muscles supplied by different roots indicates a lesion in continuity. Extraordinary patterns do, however, occur. We have seen two patients with total avulsion of four roots and sparing of flexor sublimis to two fingers. So while general rules can be laid down that usually indicate the correct nature of the lesion, surprises do occur and it is wise to deploy the full panoply of investigations in all cases where the diagnosis is not obvious.

Long tract signs indicate cord damage and a bad prognosis.

The main distinction to be made is between pre- and postganglionic lesions. If the lesion is proximal to the posterior root ganglion, then the nerve is avulsed from the cord and no recovery can take place – no one has yet succeeded in implanting rootlets into the cord. If the lesion is postganglionic, then it will be either a rupture or a lesion in continuity, with the prospect of recovery either with surgery or spontaneously.

If the lesion is proximal to the posterior root ganglia (preganglionic), the following symptoms and signs will be present.

HORNER'S SYNDROME

The cervical sympathetic nerve travels along the T1 root in its preganglionic course and will be damaged, leading to constriction of the pupil, drooping of the eyelid (ptosis) and, occasionally, lack of sweating on that side of the face. The signs must persist for some weeks, for there can be a transient Horner's syndrome due to irritation by blood which does not indicate preganglionic damage.

PAIN

The characteristic pain after avulsion of roots of the plexus from the spinal cord is fully described in the section on pain (pages 134–136). The severe continuous burning pain with strong tingling sensations and periodic paroxysms of acute pain is virtually diagnostic of a preganglionic lesion and is never seen in postganglionic lesions. A careful history of the pain is therefore of great value.

CONDUCTION STUDIES

If the lesion is proximal to the posterior root ganglion, the axon is intact and living, and will therefore conduct an electric current normally. The demonstration of normal sensory conduction in the presence of total anaesthesia is thus a bad sign.

Conversely, absence of sensory conduction may indicate a postganglionic lesion, but it is possible to have a mixed lesion – pre- and postganglionic – when the electrical signs will be those of the postganglionic element because the nerve has degenerated.

MYELOGRAPHY

When the roots are avulsed from the cord, they pull some of the dura with them. If an opaque dye is injected into the cerebrospinal fluid they will show up as pouches on the X-ray (*Figure 3.19*). The myelogram is not infallible and tends to underestimate the severity of the lesion.

HISTAMINE RESPONSE

Introduced by Bonney (1954), this is based on the same principle as sensory conduction. If the axon is intact, a flare develops in response to pricking histamine into the skin. Thus, a flare reaction indicates a preganglionic lesion. It is still useful, though results can be equivocal and sensory conduction has tended to replace this test. If electromyography apparatus is unavailable, the histamine response will, of course, be most valuable but it suffers from the same drawbacks as sensory conduction if it is a two-level lesion.

ELECTROMYOGRAPHY (EMG)

The detection of fibrillation potentials in the posterior spinal muscles indicates a lesion proximal to the ganglion because the nerve supply to these muscles takes origin proximal to it; owing to the considerable overlap in nerve supply, however, it is not possible to assign an accurate level to the lesion, and fibrillation may not be detectable despite a lesion being present.

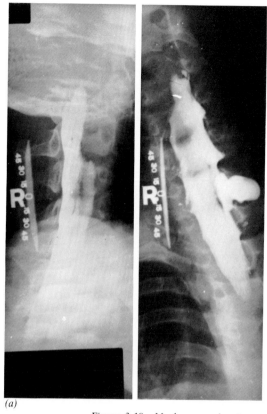
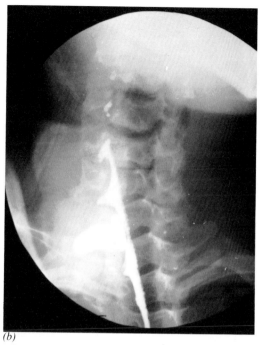

(a)   (b)

Figure 3.19 Myelogram, showing traumatic meningoceles at C7, 8 and T1

Two muscles supplied by each route are routinely sampled to detect any surviving units, which will indicate some fibres in continuity and a good prognosis.

We sample the infraspinatus and deltoid for C5, both heads of pectoralis major, sternal C8, T1, clavicular C5, 6, biceps and brachioradialis C6, triceps and extensor carpi radialis longus C7, flexors of the fingers and wrist C8, abductor pollicis brevis C8 or T1, and interossei T1.

Rhomboids and serratus are sampled if not clinically working, to confirm a high lesion.

Sensory conduction studies are carried out for each root.

C5 Stimulate lateral cutaneous nerve of the forearm just lateral to biceps tendon and record over axilla (Trojaborg, 1976).
C6 Stimulate in mid-forearm over radius and record over first dorsal interosseus space.
   Stimulate median nerve at wrist and record with ring electrodes around thumb (antidromic) or conventional orthodromic thumb to wrist.
C7 As for C6, using index and middle fingers.
C8 As for C6, using little finger.
T1 Stimulate ulnar nerve at wrist and record over ulnar nerve above elbow.
   Stimulate ulnar nerve at elbow and record over ulnar nerve in axilla.

SPINOGRAM

Jones (1979) has studied the sensory action potential evoked by stimulating the median and ulnar nerves at the wrist and recording over the supraclavicular region, over the neck at C3 and over the contralateral cortex.

The detection of a response over the plexus in the presence of anaesthesia in the stimulated part indicates a lesion proximal to the ganglion. If the N9 response (*Figure 3.20*) is present but attenuated compared with the normal side, this indicates a mixed pre- and postganglionic lesion.

TINEL SIGN

If the patient is seen some months after injury, it may be possible to elicit a Tinel sign in the neck at the site of injury and a distal Tinel sign consistent with regeneration at the appropriate distance distally for a recovery rate of 1 mm a day.

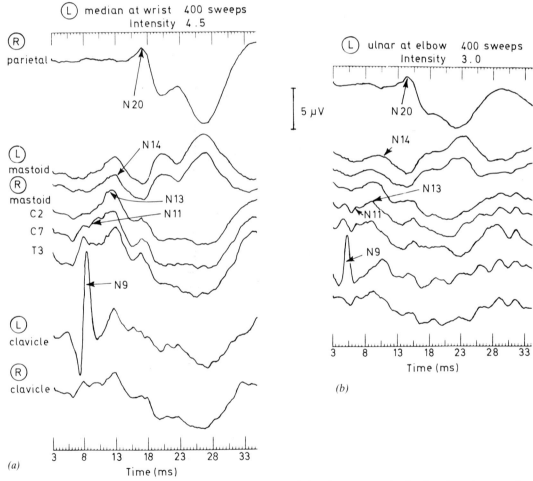

Figure 3.20 Spinogram. (a, b) Normal subject: (a) median and (b) ulnar nerves stimulated at the wrist; recording electrodes over the brachial plexus record a response at 9 ms (N9) over the cervical spine (N11), mastoid (N14) and contralateral parietal cortex (N20). (Continued opposite)

Copeland and Landi (1979) have shown that a strong painful Tinel sign, which they call a neuroma sign, is usually associated with a rupture of the root distal to the intervertebral foramen. The neck is tapped, and if the patient winces and complains of pain at that site and also referred to the root distribution, a rupture is likely.

X-RAY

The diaphragm is screened to determine whether or not the phrenic nerve (C3, 4, 5) is involved, and X-rays of the cervical spine are taken to exclude fractures or a slip forwards of a cervical vertebra.

SUMMARY OF BAD PROGNOSTIC SIGNS

Paralysis of serratus and rhomboids
Complete lesion of all roots
Horner's syndrome
Severe burning pain

Multiple injuries – vascular and bony
Retention of sensory conduction in anaesthetic areas
Positive myelogram
Positive spinogram

SUMMARY OF GOOD PROGNOSTIC SIGNS

Mild violence
No associated injuries
No pain
No Horner's syndrome

Sparing of serratus and rhomboids
Progressive Tinel's sign
Sparing of some muscles
Absent sensory conduction
Negative spinogram

A positive neuroma sign suggests a rupture.

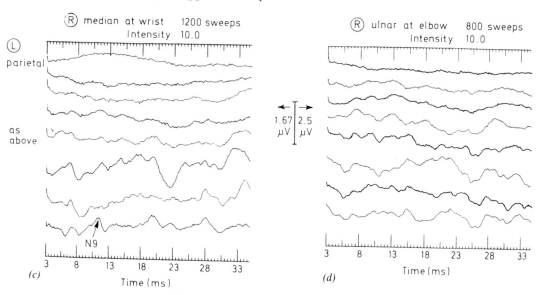

Figure 3.20 (cont.) *(c, d) Patient with avulsion of lower roots of the plexus and total anaesthesia of the arm. There is a response (N9) over the plexus although it is attenuated, due to postganglionic involvement also — no response is seen over the spinal cord or cortex. Thus the spinogram indicates damage both proximal and distal to the posterior root ganglion.*

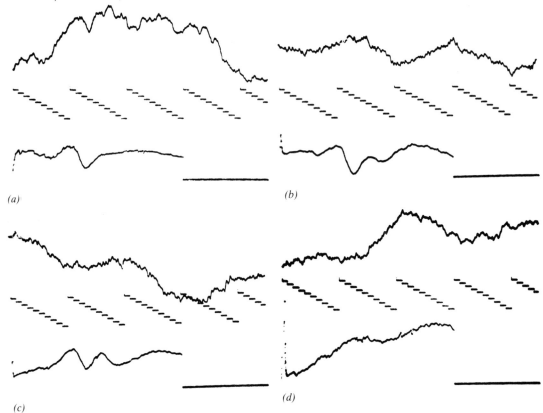

(a)

(b)

(c)

(d)

Figure 3.21   Peroperative recordings in a patient with a traction lesion of the brachial plexus. Clinically there was complete C5, 6 paralysis. At operation, the plexus was in continuity and recordings were made over the contralateral parietal cortex. (a) C8, (b) C7 and (c) lateral cord all show clear response, indicating that there is continuity with the spinal cord. The suprascapular nerve was caught in scar tissue and hooked back on itself. After release it was stimulated and a tiny response could be seen (d). It was therefore decided not to resect and graft this nerve. The next day a contraction was seen in the spinati. The peroperative electrical studies proved invaluable.

Decision as to surgery

The decision whether or not to explore the plexus in the expectation of finding a rupture is a difficult one. When all the investigations suggest that a complete lesion of C5, 6 or 7 is postganglionic and there is a strong neuroma sign, our surgical team will explore the plexus if there is a good prospect of obtaining reasonable function following grafting. Thus, there should be no gross stiffness of joints, nor such a degree of damage to the upper arm or forearm through vascular or bony damage as to make any return of muscle activity following grafting functionally useless.

If there has been rupture to a major vessel and multiple fractures to the bones of the forearm, fractures into the elbow joint, marked deformity or serious trophic lesions, surgery is not worth while. If the patient is not seen until 1 year after injury, it is doubtful whether surgery should be contemplated. It will be at least 18 months before recovery can be expected in the proximal muscles and by 2½ years after injury the muscles will be atrophic.

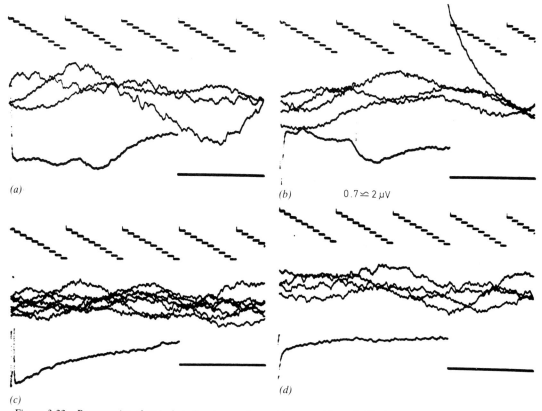

(a)   *(b)* $0.7 \cong 2 \, \mu V$

(c)   *(d)*

Figure 3.22   Peroperative electrical studies in a patient with an avulsion of C5, 6. The roots were stimulated and recordings made over the contralateral parietal cortex. (a) C8; (b) T1. Clear responses are seen, indicating that there is continuity with the spinal cord. (c) C6; (d) C5. No response — the roots are avulsed from the cord

The most one can hope for after surgical repair is elbow flexion, finger and wrist flexion, sometimes elbow extension and some protective sensation in the hand. Very rarely does abduction or external rotation return. It is never worth attempting repair of C8 or T1 because, long before reinnervation can occur, the muscles will have atrophied.

The indications for exploration can be summarized as follows: postganglionic lesions with a suspected rupture of C5, 6, 7, within 6 months (at most, 1 year) of injury, with satisfactory circulation, good passive range of movement and in a patient who needs and will use elbow flexion in his work or hobbies. It is very helpful if, as introduced by Landi and colleagues (1980), the proximal stump is stimulated at operation and recordings are made over the contralateral parietal cortex to ensure its viability (*Figures 3.21* and *3.22*). In three patients there was apparent continuity at operation, but the sensory-evoked potential (SEP) was absent, indicating an avulsion. In five patients there were normal SEPs, indicating that the stumps were in continuity; grafting was therefore carried out, with excellent results in four.

A careful preoperative assessment by physiotherapist and occupational therapist is vital to ensure that the patient needs the function the surgeon hopes to provide and that he is motivated to use it when it does return. We admit our patients to the rehabilitation unit for a careful assessment. If there is significant restriction of passive joint range, intensive physiotherapy is instituted – hydrotherapy and passive movements several times daily. Not only will this be needed if muscle function is to recover, but the surgical approach to the plexus demands at least 30 degrees' abduction and external rotation. The occupational therapist together with the rehabilitation officer will study the locomotor demands of the patient's job and hobbies in a realistic setting and, if necessary, visit his place of work.

Postoperatively, the arm is rested for 6 weeks, with no neck or arm movements being allowed in order to protect the grafts. Thereafter, gentle passive movements are started which the patient can continue at home with the help of a relative or friend. Whether recovery is expected spontaneously or after surgery, the patient is reviewed every 3 months; when the first sign of muscle activity appears, a short spell of intensive rehabilitation is given. We like to admit our patients for 5–10 days of intensive rehabilitation every 6 months or so to capitalize on reinnervation. It is all too easy for the patient to neglect to exercise his recovering arm, having been one-handed for so long.

All our patients are given a trial of functional splinting.

Functional splinting

Whatever the decision about surgery, it will be 12–18 months before recovery starts in the proximal muscles and much longer in the forearm muscles. During this time we offer – indeed urge – the patient to try a splint, for two reasons: first to offer him some function in that limb and, second, to maintain the arm as part of his body image in the nervous system.

We have seen many patients not treated with splints who have recovered function after 2 years, but never use their arm so completely one-armed have they become.

Most patients are virtually one-armed within 6 weeks and, remarkably enough, most have learnt to write with their non-dominant hand. If they are not encouraged to use their paralysed arm in some form, they will never become two-armed again and many jobs and hobbies may be closed to them. The decision as to whether or not a patient will be fitted with a splint will depend on his reaction when shown its capabilities and on the use to which he will put it. This trial period is also most valuable on deciding if a patient is likely to be a good candidate for surgery. If he rejects a splint designed to offer him function, he is liable not to use his arm after surgery.

TYPES OF SPLINT

In C5, 6 lesions, the patient cannot bend his elbow or abduct his arm. However, his hand is normal though he cannot put it in a functional position. The splint we use has an upper arm and forearm piece linked by an elbow ratchet lock (*Figure 3.23*). The patient can put the elbow in five or six different positions of flexion (in practice, only four positions are used in most cases), thus making his hand much more useful.

The lock can be automatic, so that he has only to extend it actively to unlock it, or it can be hand operated.

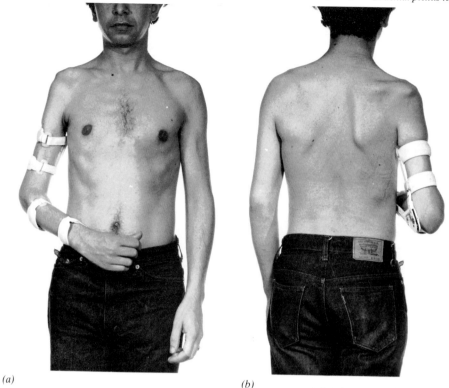

(a)   (b)

Figure 3.23   Elbow lock splint for C5, 6 palsy, to allow positioning of the elbow in one of four positions and thus facilitate hand function

In C5, 6, 7 lesions, a cock-up splint is added to support the wrist in extension with a spring at the wrist to allow active wrist movements. Sometimes a spider splint is incorporated to keep the fingers in extension, but this is not always accepted.

TOTAL PARALYSIS

In complete paralysis a flail arm splint is provided which is virtually an artifical arm over the paralysed arm. There is the same elbow ratchet, but the forearm piece is a gutter that extends beyond the wrist so as to stabilize it in the neutral position. A platform is provided at the distal end into which can be screwed any of the standard terminal devices for an artificial arm operated by a cable from the opposite shoulder. Support is provided either by a pelvic band and rod with shoulder cap posteriorly or by a shoulder piece which we are now favouring because the pelvic band can be cumbersome and uncomfortable. The patient thus locks the elbow and, by using the appliances appropriate to his work or hobbies, uses the flail arm as a prop or support (*Figures 3.24* and *3.25*).

If he has active adduction (i.e. the pectorals have been spared or have recovered), he can bring the splint across the body and the spring load at the shoulder will return it to the resting position. If he has recovered elbow flexion or the lesion was C7, 8, T1

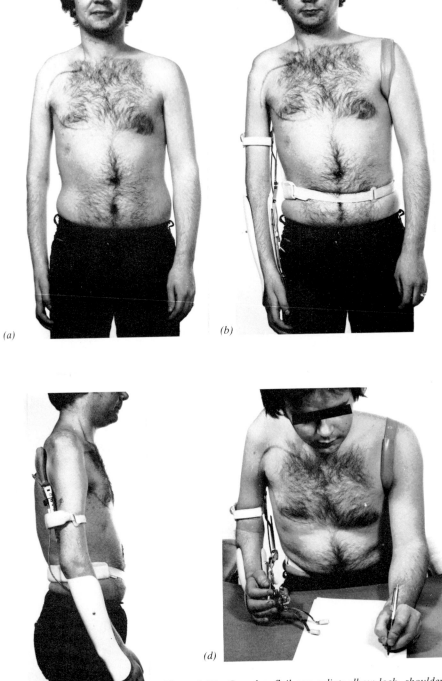

(a)

(b)

(c)

(d)

Figure 3.24   Complete flail arm splint: elbow lock, shoulder support, forearm platform for terminal appliances powered by cable from the opposite shoulder. The shoulder cap is not used, owing to scarring over the shoulder following grafting of the plexus

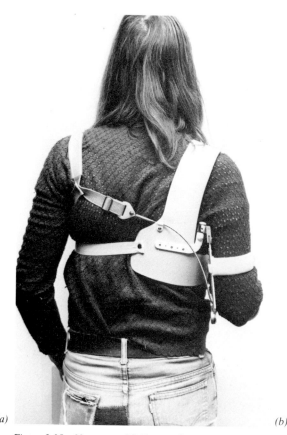

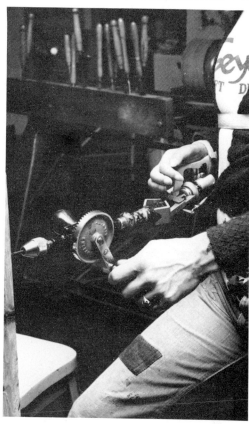

(a)   (b)

Figure 3.25   New type of flail arm splint with shoulder cap (designed by Mr J. Heritage). This is more comfortable and is well tolerated but cannot be used if there is any scarring over the shoulder. (Continued overleaf)

from the onset, then only the forearm piece with platform is needed and the patient powers it with his own flexion (*Figure 3.26*).

    The point to be emphasized is that these splints are ready-made, not custom-made. Our fitter attends the weekly clinic, selects one of the three standard sizes and makes any minor adjustments or alterations to give a good fit. The patient then learns to use the splint in the occupational therapy department and workshop for the next 3–4 days, and if any problems have arisen he attends the following week for further adjustments. The majority of patients are back at work using their splint within 7 days. We have fitted over 100 patients with these splints and at 6-month follow-up 70 per cent were using them either full-time or most of the time at work or play. Almost all prefer to wear the splint instead of having the arm hanging loosely from the shoulder, as it gives them more support. The splints are worn until such time as sufficient recovery has occurred to make them unnecessary. In some patients recovery may not take place and reconstructive surgery is impossible. It is then well worth while making a custom-built permanent splint such as that shown in *Figure 3.27*.

    This patient had a preganglionic C5, 6, 7 lesion. There was no question of providing a muscle transfer like a Steindler or a pectoralis transfer and so a permanent splint

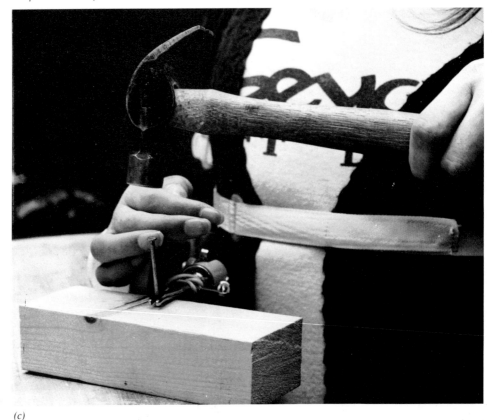

(c)

Figure 3.25 (cont.)

with ratchet elbow lock, rotation element for the upper arm and cock-up for the wrist was custom-made. The patient has been able to continue in his trade as engine fitter in the RAF for, with the splint, his function is as good as his able-bodied colleagues.

Reconstructive surgery

When it is clear that there will be no recovery, there are a number of reconstructive procedures available; in general, however, these are not undertaken until at least 18 months have elapsed.

SHOULDER

Arthrodesis of the shoulder joint can be useful in the flail arm if there is scapular control. It allows the patient to hold things between his arm and trunk and is cosmetically better. It is fused in the 'hand in pocket' position – 45 degrees' internal rotation, no flexion and only 30 degrees of scapulohumeral abduction.

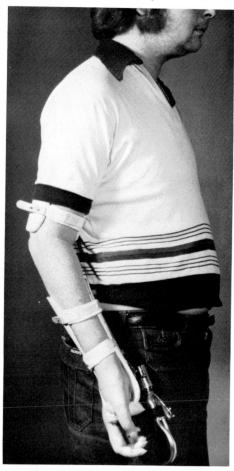

Figure 3.26   Forearm splint with split hook for total below-elbow paralysis (C7, 8, T1 palsy); the C5, 6 muscles were spared.

To restore elbow flexion in a permanent C5, 6 palsy either the Steindler or the Clark–Brooks transfer is available. In either case, if shoulder control is absent, an arthrodesis must be performed. The principle of the Steindler is well seen by studying the instinctive attempts of such patients to flex their elbow. They make a fist, extend the wrist and pronate the forearm, sliding the arm up across the chest.

Reinsertion of the origins of the common flexors and extensors higher up the arm into the intermuscular septa provides excellent flexion (*Figure 3.28*). For a Steindler to be successful, the patient must be able to hold the elbow at 90 degrees with the fingers clenched. If this is impossible (i.e. if the flexors or extensors are too weak), then the Clark–Brooks transfer is used, the pectoralis major being inserted into the biceps or the coracoid.

If flexion of the elbow is accompanied by too much adduction, an external rotation osteotomy of the humerus is performed and the elbow is then clear of the trunk in flexion. Very recently, the operation for transferring the latissimus dorsi – a whole muscle transfer – has shown excellent results. As in all muscle and tendon transfers, the power must be over grade 4 on the MRC scale because one grade is lost in the transfer.

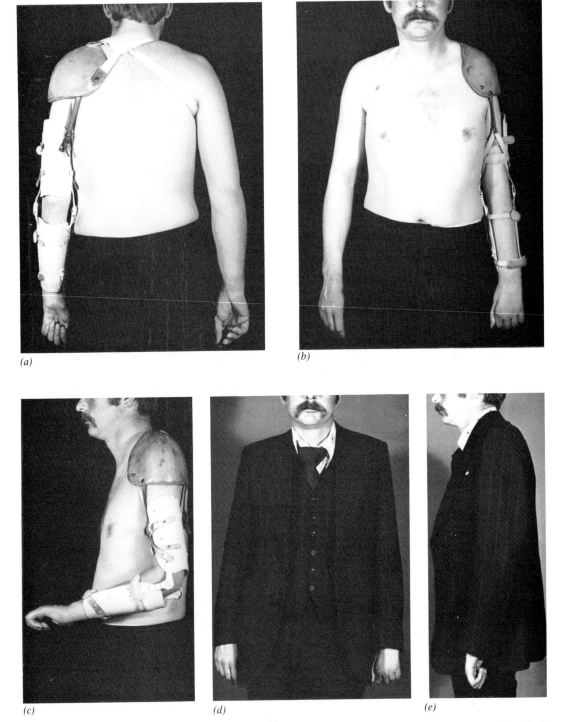

(a) *(b)* *(c)* *(d)* *(e)*

Figure 3.27   Permanent custom-made splint for a patient who had complete C5, 6, 7 paralysis. Note the elbow lock, rotation of the upper arm, the dropped wrist support and inconspicuousness of the splint under clothing. (Case 3.16)

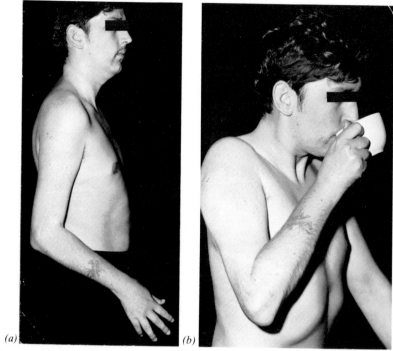

(a) (b)

Figure 3.28 Patient with complete C5, 6 palsy, after Steindler's flexoroplasty. (a) Extension. (b) Flexion. (Courtesy of Mr Donal Brooks)

Operations to provide elbow flexion can be done relatively early in order to provide function, though functional splinting has reduced the indications for such early surgery. If and when the biceps does recover, the situation has not been compromised.

Another alternative is transfer of triceps to biceps. This is indicated when both muscles have recovered, but cross-innervation has made co-contraction seriously interfere with function.

Very occasionally, it is possible to restore active abduction, for which external rotation is essential and which rarely recovers in plexus lesions. The latissimus dorsi and teres major are inserted into the infraspinatus – this is the Zachary transfer, but it needs a determined patient who will work really hard at his rehabilitation.

Many patients find the flail wrist a nuisance and are improved by arthrodesis; a trial period in a plaster or splint will help the patient and doctor to decide if this is worth while.

In permanent C7 paralysis, wrist and finger extension can be provided by the standard tendon transfers as for radial nerve palsy, provided, of course, that the C8 muscles are spared.

Amputation

At one time it was the custom in a patient with a flail arm to offer amputation above the elbow, arthrodesis of the shoulder and fitting of a prosthesis. There is no doubt that some patients are pleased with the results of this reconstructive surgery and find their limb very useful at work. However, the enthusiasm for this approach has waned – Randsford and Hughes (1977) found that only 2 of 16 patients actually used their limb, and in a recent follow-up we found that 18 of 24 patients fitted with a prosthesis never used it.

Most of our patients are opposed to the idea of amputation. This is for a variety of reasons – aesthetic dislike of a stump (on the beach, in the swimming pool), desire to keep the arm because it is part of them, feeling that recovery might occur and they might regret losing it, dislike of the prosthesis for being cumbersome and ugly, feeling that they would be unlikely to use it because they have learned to cope with one arm.

We believe that the flail arm splint offers a satisfactory compromise – an artificial arm yet allowing them to keep their own arm.

Some of the patients we have seen were told by their surgeons that they would lose their pain after an amputation. This is, of course, absolutely wrong and one can imagine the despair of a young man who has lost his arm, but still has the pain.

There are, however, circumstances when it is right to amputate – if trophic lesions are frequent, if there has been gross damage to the limb by multiple fractures and destruction of blood vessels and if it is clear that the patient would certainly be functionally better off in his job. Randsford and Hughes (1977) found that athletic men with a non-dominant injury and patients with involvement of the dominant limb who had difficulty in converting to non-dominant were the most likely to use a prosthesis. The wise approach of Ian Fletcher is described in Chapter 7.

What we do insist on is that the attitude of 20 years ago – that amputation is the routine treatment of the flail arm – is wrong. Quite apart from the reasons already given, we have seen recovery occur in proximal muscles 2 or 3 years after injury, which has been functionally useful and despite the gloomy prognostication of the various tests.

Amputation can be done at any time. There is no hurry, for function can be provided by splinting and the patient returned to work quickly.

In cases of avulsion of the upper roots, it is possible to offer some function by neurotization. The upper five or six intercostal nerves are mobilized from their ribs and put into the distal stump of the lateral cord or medial and musculocutaneous nerves. The accessory nerve has been used with or without a free graft, but with disappointing results. The aim is to provide elbow flexion, possibly finger flexion and some protective sensation in the median distribution.

It is necessary to check the viability of the intercostal nerves by conduction studies with EMG in the theatre in case they were damaged in the original injury.

Of 7 patients in whom Millesi (personal communication) carried out this procedure, 4 regained elbow flexion, wrist and finger movement and activity in pectoralis major.

The overall results in the series of Narakas (1977) who has unrivalled experience in this field, was that grafting or neurotization gave 7 good, 25 fair and 26 poor results. Cross-innervation is often a problem and needs intensive re-education.

Resettlement

We reviewed 130 patients in the armed services in 1974 with brachial plexus lesions, of whom 38 were invalided out at 2-year follow-up, but all were at work. Of 78 patients

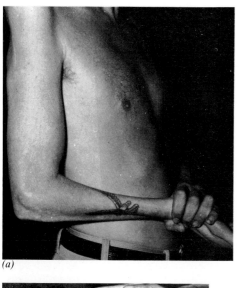

(a)

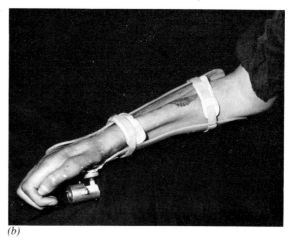

(b)

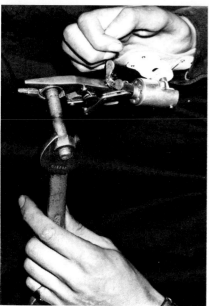

(c)

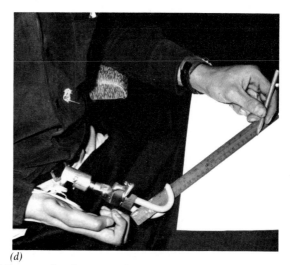

(d)

Figure 3.29   Complete postganglionic plexus lesion. (a) Four months after injury. (b) When elbow flexion recovered a flail arm below-elbow splint was provided to allow function, with various attachments. (c) Pliers. (d) Hook. (Case 3.18)

from the Royal National Orthopaedic Hospital followed up all but 1 were at work (the exception had retired).

The following were the most frequent occupations taken up by those with a total flail arm – clerical, welding, engineering, spray painting, draughtsman, storekeeper, messenger. The most frequent occupations taken up by those who had amputations of the flail arm were engineering, spray painting, welding, managerial, clerical, gardening, car park attendant and painter-decorator.

Case 3.16. This patient was involved in a motor cycle accident in March 1972. Initially, there was complete paralysis of the left arm. He also sustained crush fractures of the metacarpals and developed ischaemic contractures requiring Littler's release at a later stage. He was left with permanent complete paralysis of C5, 6 muscles. He had excellent finger flexion and extension, but no intrinsic function and very weak wrist flexion. Arthrodesis of the shoulder was performed in June 1974 so that he now has a good 30 degrees' abduction and forward flexion.

There could be no reconstructive surgery to restore active elbow flexion because pectorals and latissimus dorsi were paralysed and the wrist flexors were too weak for a Steindler procedure.

Figure 3.27 illustrates the permanent custom-made splint which gave him excellent function; he has remained in the RAF as a highly skilled aircraft engineer. (Surgery by Mr Donal Brooks.)

Case 3.17. This patient was thrown off his motor cycle onto the bonnet of a car in May 1977, sustaining a complete left plexus lesion. At operation, C5 was found ruptured and the rest of the plexus was avulsed. Mr G. Bonney grafted his C5 root to the musculocutaneous nerve. While awaiting recovery of elbow flexion, a flail arm splint was supplied which he was able to use in his job as a gardener.

In fact, he devised a number of ingenious attachments for the splint to enable him to dig, hoe and wheel a barrow.

Case 3.18. This technician was involved in a motor cycle accident in which he sustained a complete traction lesion of the right brachial plexus. Three months later investigations showed absent sensory potentials for median and ulnar nerves but the presence of a Horner's syndrome and T1 meningoceles on the myelogram suggested that there was a preganglionic element. However, no meningoceles were seen for C5 to C8, and the histamine test was negative for C6, 7 and 8, so it was decided to treat conservatively.

Five months after injury a 'Roehampton splint' was provided and in view of the patient's enormous enthusiasm for the RAF he was sent back to modified duty. The end-result was that the deltoid remained paralysed, but spinati recovered to 2, biceps to 4, triceps to 3, finger and wrist flexors to 3, and protective sensation in the whole of the palmar surface of the hand returned. During the 3 years after injury, he had reconstructive surgery as follows: Zachary transfer to improve control of the shoulder, external rotation osteotomy to prevent excessive adduction in elbow flexion, and arthrodesis of the wrist. He now no longer needs the splint, but it had allowed him to return to work at an early stage. During the recovery phase he came top of a highly demanding armament fitter's course (*Figure 3.29*). (Surgery by Mr Donal Brooks.)

Case 3.19. This patient sustained a C5, 6 lesion from a road traffic accident. During the stage whilst awaiting any recovery a lively splint was provided which allowed him active elbow flexion and he returned to work as a cook within 4 months of injury. Recovery did not occur and so a Steindler's operation was performed (*Figure 3.30*).

Case 3.20. This patient showed no recovery at all 18 months after a C5, 6, 7 lesion. Arthrodesis of the shoulder, pectoralis transfer using extensor carpi radialis longus to extend the tendon for elbow flexion and transfers to give active wrist extension provided sufficient function for him to be retained in the RAF as a general mechanic.

Case 3.21. This 65-year-old clerical worker sustained a direct violence injury to the left brachial plexus involving C5, 6 when a car ran into his car. The condition was complicated by severe cervical spondylosis at this level with much pain and stiffness of the neck. When first seen 1 month after the accident, there was complete clinical paralysis and electrical evidence of complete denervation in the deltoid, supraspinatus and infraspinatus and elbow flexors, and a stiff shoulder but no sensory loss. Intensive rehabilitation mobilized the shoulder using active assisted exercises, proprioceptive neuromuscular facilitation techniques, occupational therapy and graded games. As he lives locally he attended once or twice a week for a year. On review 4½ years later, he had recovered completely normal function – deltoid, spinati, elbow flexors were all 5. The only abnormality was a limitation of full elevation of the shoulder of 10 degrees, although the neck remained stiff.

Case 3.22. This patient sustained a complete C5, 6 paralysis in May 1974. He returned to work with an elbow lock splint. Eighteen months later there had been no recovery and a Steindler flexorplasty was performed. This worked well, but he had the characteristic excess adduction, making it difficult to bring his hand to his mouth or to clear his chest when flexing his elbow. An external rotation osteotomy performed 7 months later gave him excellent function and greatly improved the efficiency of his elbow flexion.

Muscle charting 2 years after injury was biceps 1, deltoid 4, spinati 0 and pectoralis major 4.

Case 3.23. In March 1976 this 20-year-old was involved in a motor cycle accident in which he sustained a compound fracture of the right humerus, avulsion of C8 and of T1 roots as shown on myelography and destruction of the radial nerve. The fifth and sixth cervical roots were intact. No recovery occurred below the elbow, as was to be expected. The patient was unwilling to have an amputation and prosthesis, so a flail arm splint was provided over his forearm with a platform for the insertion of terminal appliances worked by a harness from the opposite shoulder (see *Figure 3.26*). He was off work for 1 year.

The occupational therapy report after he had been wearing the splint for work and hobbies was as follows.

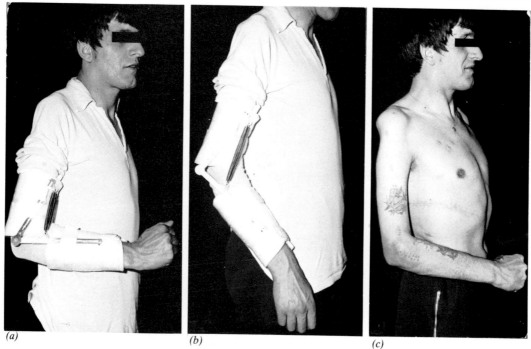

Figure 3.30 Lively splint for a patient with C5, 6 palsy. (a) Flexion. (b) Extension. (c) Recovery did not occur and a Steindler's operation was performed (Mr Donal Brooks). (Case 3.19)

FUNCTIONAL ASSESSMENT WITH RIGHT FLAIL ARM SPLINT AND ATTACHMENTS

Occupation: wood machinist

Diagnosis: (R) brachial plexus lesions

The patient is left-handed from birth. Has had splint about 3 months and has been back at work about 2 months. Has good muscle control at shoulder and elbow.

Work: involves sorting out wood in the wood store most of the time. He is unable to use splint attachment for this, as span width of hook is too narrow and he cannot get a good grip. Uses (L) hand only for this.

Cross-cut power saw: stabilizes wood with (L) hand and pulls saw across with splint hook. Unable to push this back so has rigged an elastic band device to return it to position.

For smoothing model aircraft pieces on a two-handed gig, he is able to steady the wood block at (R) side with splint.

Has some difficulty with (R) handed machines but can manage.

Unable to use power rip-saw as he cannot get a good grip with the hook – it is too round and not long enough to clear his fingers of the machine. He is going to draw up a diagram of the attachment he requires (roughly 25 cm long and T shaped) for the appliance officer at Stanmore.

Machinery vibrations tend to loosen attachment locking nut so he has to tighten and untighten this with pliers. Can a key/spanner be made to fit into a nut with socket for this purpose? At present the nut is getting very worn.

Driving: has knob attachment to steering wheel of father's car and socket attachment to splint. Manages well and is hoping to get a 'trike' [three-wheeled car] of his own soon.

Rides a push-bike to and from work, holding (R) handlebar with hook at horizontal angle.

Fishing: is now able to tie knots with hook attachment and goes fishing on his own.

Personal care: uses (L) hand mainly. Splint tends to make arm ache after a day's work and he removes it at home.

Eating: uses a Nelson knife.

Washing: takes shower.

SUMMARY

Splint is proving invaluable for work, hobbies and transport.
Further adaptations requested:

(1) T-shaped attachment for use with rip-saw (patient will specify).
(2) Key/spanner for locking nut.
(3) Hook with wider span (width of 15 cm?).

[These were provided and further review showed that the splint was now even more useful.]

Case 3.24. This patient sustained multiple fractures and a complete right-sided brachial plexus paralysis in May 1971. When first seen in January 1976, muscle charting showed pectorals 4, triceps 3, biceps 2+, finger flexors 3 and no action in the hand muscles. He could therefore just not bend his elbow against gravity owing to the greater strength of the triceps. In March 1976, triceps was transferred to biceps. In August, an external rotation osteotomy of the humerus gave him much more efficient elbow flexion, and an arthrodesis of the wrist in November increased the efficiency of his finger flexion.

Case 3.25. The strange clinical pictures that can occur are exemplified by this patient who sustained a severe plexus lesion when climbing. He had complete paralysis of all muscles except the flexor sublimis (3+) and abductor pollicis brevis (2). Myelograms showed meningoceles for C5, 6, 7 and T1. He has had intractable crushing pain in the hand and is currently being considered for a cerebral implant.

SHOULDER WEAKNESS

Apart from lesions of the brachial plexus, other conditions which can cause weakness of the shoulders are circumflex nerve lesions following dislocations or fractures of the shoulder joint, neuralgic amyotrophy (shoulder girdle neuritis), myopathies, motor neuron disease and poliomyelitis. Neuralgic amyotrophy is not uncommon but not widely enough known. Classically the illness begins with the sudden onset of intense burning pain in the root of the neck and over the shoulder joint, with fever and malaise. The pain is so severe that morphine derivatives may be required for the first 48 hours. Usually the pain subsides within 3 days or at the most a week. Some 10 days after the onset, weakness or paralysis of muscles is noticed. The most common muscle to be involved is the serratus anterior or deltoid, less commonly the spinati and deltoid, biceps and, rarely, the anterior interosseus nerve or radial nerve. The condition is believed to be due to a virus affecting the nerve roots or peripheral nerves. The C5 root has the largest diameter in relation to its bony canal, thus explaining why the C5-supplied muscles are the most commonly affected. In the armed services there was a minor epidemic some 22 years ago following TAB injections, suggesting an autoimmune component. We have had three cases in which close relatives or colleagues at work were similarly affected, giving added support to the infective hypothesis.

Prognosis for eventual recovery is good but may take up to 18 months, as reinnervation has to proceed from the root. We have a personal series of 130 cases – 85 per cent of whom made virtually full recoveries.

Circumflex nerve lesions are common and the deltoid does not often recover, but functionally this may well be unimportant as other muscles can take over its function.

There is a widespread belief that paralysis of the deltoid means loss of abduction of the arm. In 145 consecutive patients seen with paralysis of the deltoid alone, or a combination of teres minor and deltoid paralysis in a circumflex nerve lesion, every patient has regained full function, including full abduction and elevation against strong resistance without any recovery being seen in deltoid. In every case the finding of clinical paralysis was confirmed by electromyography. The key muscles that must be present before this compensatory movement can be obtained are the external rotators of the humerus. In the absence of the deltoid, abduction is initiated by the supraspinatus, if present, and carried to about 70 degrees by the long heads of the biceps and triceps. At the beginning of abduction, the humerus is externally rotated by the infraspinatus. At about 70 degrees the clavicular fibres of the pectoralis major act as powerful abductors because the axis of the shoulder joint has now rotated externally. Thereafter, the serratus anterior elevates the arm through forward and upward pull on the scapula.

It is our practice to teach patients this compensatory movement from the earliest stages after paralysis. First, it is essential to restore passive movements to the shoulder joint if these are absent. The re-education is carried out with the patient lying on his back and the arm supported in a sling with overhead suspension. Before any attempt is made to initiate abduction, the patient externally rotates the humerus. He is then asked to try to abduct the arm, and in so doing he will inevitably hitch up the shoulder by trapezius action. The physiotherapist directs the patient's attention to this bad habit and encourages him to obtain the movement entirely at the shoulder. A certain degree of swing is allowed at this stage to give the patient the idea of movement. When the first few degrees are obtained the patient is encouraged to think about each group of muscles, first the biceps and triceps, then the pectoralis major, and finally the serratus, throughout the various stages of movement. All the time he must keep the humerus in full external rotation if possible. As soon as the patient loses the hitch it will be found that the range increases rapidly.

In a small number of patients difficulty may be experienced in learning this trick. In these cases it is helpful to give specific resistance exercises to the long heads of biceps and triceps, and to break down the movements into isolated ones for each muscle involved. This is particularly helpful when there is associated weakness of the other muscles, such as the biceps and pectoralis major.

As the patient improves, the treatment couch is gradually inclined at an increasing angle so that gravity resists the movements more and more. A light weight of about 0.5 kg helps the patient to initiate and hold the movement.

The patient should watch his movements in a mirror in order to get the normal scapulohumeral rhythm restored at an early stage. In difficult cases, and particularly where there is much joint stiffness, re-education in a warm pool is most helpful.

The length of time required to learn these compensatory movements is approximately 4–6 weeks. In a few patients, however, this may be very much shorter, and the quickest success we have ever had was in a patient who sustained complete paralysis after shoulder dislocation. Re-education started 4 weeks after injury and he had regained full movement in all ranges at the end of a half-hour session in the physiotherapy department. It must be stressed that these movements providing full abduction and elevation are not trick actions in the sense usually associated with this word; all the muscles involved normally help to abduct the shoulder. The scapulohumeral rhythm is quite normal, and in the later stages of re-education the patient does not even need to rotate the humerus externally to initiate the movement. Furthermore, the power of abduction becomes by the end of treatment quite as strong as the normal side, and many of our patients have returned to full duty and have been enabled to manage the most arduous of tasks, including top class horse riding and parachute jumping. *Figure 3.31* shows the movements in a patient with a paralysed deltoid.

It has been found that about 20 per cent of these patients at follow-up had eventual recovery in the deltoid, but it was not possible to distinguish by power and by general function those who had from those who had not.

If the deltoid begins to recover during re-education, paradoxically the rate of progress in learning these movements slows down. It seems as if the body cannot cope with the two slightly different movement patterns at the same time.

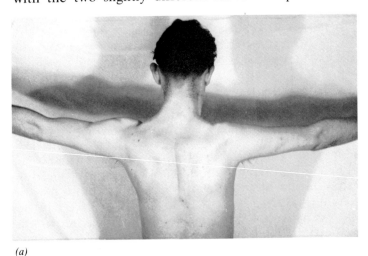

(a)

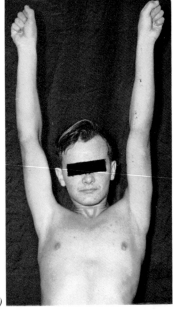

(b)

Figure 3.31 Paralysis of right deltoid. (a) Abduction to 90 degrees. (b) Full elevation

It is our firm opinion that no purpose is served by not teaching patients to learn these movements as early as possible, irrespective of whether they are likely to get recovery in the deltoid or not. Recovery of maximum function as soon as possible is the aim of rehablitation, and experience has shown that no possible harm is done in teaching these movements to patients who ultimately recover full deltoid action. We have yet to see a patient with deltoid paralysis, with or without teres minor paralysis, who has not been able to regain full function by learning these movements.

Deltoid paralysis and involvement of other shoulder muscles

When other muscles in the shoulder are affected, re-education is much more difficult. In the presence of complete paralysis of the infraspinatus, it is not possible to teach this action. If the paralysis remains permanent it is worth while considering reconstructive surgery, such as the Zachary transfer. The principle of surgery here is to enable the compensatory movements described above to be used by transferring the internal rotators to the back of the humerus so that they act as external rotators.

Provided the patient has the long head of biceps and pectoralis major, he will be able to abduct the arm. It is obviously an operation that is only done on rare occasions, but if the patient is prepared to work really hard, the results are well worth while.

It is not uncommon for patients to be seen with paralysis of the infraspinatus. A surprisingly small amount of muscle in the infraspinatus needs to be working for the patient to be able to abduct the shoulder. A number of patients have been seen who, at the commencement of treatment, were unable to abduct their shoulder at all, and who had paralysis of the infraspinatus, as well as the deltoid, due to traction lesions of the brachial plexus. Electrical investigations showed that there was definite activity in the infraspinatus, and accordingly re-education was started.

In a matter of 4–6 weeks good abduction resulted. Training starts with the patient lying on his back with the arm supported in a sling in suspension. Gentle rotary movements of the whole arm are encouraged first. Next the arm is bent to a right angle and held by the physiotherapist with the elbow right into the side and the forearm supinated. The patient is then encouraged to rotate the humerus externally, the physiotherapist giving very slight resistance at the lateral aspect of the mid-forearm and supporting the scapula posteriorly, feeling for the muscle contraction at the same time. By this means the physiotherapist can tell if the patient is tricking the movement or if he is genuinely using his infraspinatus. Sessions of six to eight attempts are interspersed with the same action on the normal side so that the patient then feels the correct movement.

Pattern re-education of all arm movements is carried out at each treatment session. This includes forward flexion with the elbow flexed and extended, and swinging movements with the patient standing and the trunk flexed.

The use of proprioceptive facilitation techniques are valuable in the re-education of shoulder function.

The principle of this technique is to bring into action muscle groups whose motor nerve cells adjoin those of the weak muscles in the spinal cord and, by irradiation, coax them into action. The following manoeuvres are carried our.

(1) Patient lying in prone position. The patient pulls the shoulder and arm posteriorly and inwards, drawing the scapulae together. Resistance is given to the whole arm by the physiotherapist. If the patient is too weak to produce significant movement (for example, as in a brachial plexus palsy), resistance is given to the neck, and the patient is asked to extend the neck as he tries to pull back the shoulder and arm.
(2) Patient lying in prone position. The patient rotates the arm inwards, at the same time pulling the arm back and the scapulae inwards as before.
(3) Patient lying on his back. The elbow is held firmly into the side at 90 degrees. The patient then tries to rotate the humerus externally, feeling for the infraspinatus contraction himself. The physiotherapist gives resistance, stabilizing the shoulders by pressing down on them on the plinth. The patient next crosses his arm over his body, the wrist and fingers being fully flexed. The patient then brings the arm across in an arc away from the body in an extensor thrust, the fingers, wrist, elbow and shoulder all being extended maximally against the physiotherapist's resistance throughout, a final hard resistance being given as the movement is completed.

(4) When the elbow flexors and pectorals are weak, the reverse manoeuvre is used. The arm is held extended fully at all joints, wrist, fingers, elbow and shoulder, and in external rotation. The patient pulls the arm across the body against resistance in a flexor thrust, aiming for the forehead.

(5) In addition to the special techniques outlined above, the general principle holds that any muscle which crosses a joint can be made to move that joint whether that is its prime function or not. Hence, muscles crossing affected joints are re-educated as synergists, with and without resistance, until eventually they can be urged to act a prime movers.

Case 3.26. This patient was involved in a road accident 14 September 1956. He sustained a traction lesion of the right C5 root, resulting in paralysis of the supraspinatus, the infraspinatus and the deltoid, and sensory loss over the lateral aspect of the lower part of the upper arm. In addition, the right scaphoid was fractured. Rehabilitation commenced 1 week after injury. Passive movements to the shoulder and general arm exercises were given. Electromyography (13 October 1956) showed complete paralysis of the deltoid, but a partial lesion only of the infraspinatus – many discrete normal motor unit potentials being seen against a background of fibrillation.

Re-education was started in earnest in the hope that enough of the infraspinatus was working to enable compensatory movements to be successfully taught. Treatment was complicated by the fact that the patient had the weight of the scaphoid plaster to work against on the affected side.

Within 2 days the patient could raise the arm above the head when lying down; 29 days after injury he could abduct to 40 degrees in a standing position.

Two months after injury (14 November 1956) he was able to abduct and elevate the arm with ease, despite the complete paralysis of the deltoid. The scaphoid plaster was removed 11 weeks after injury.

The patient was discharged to storeman's duties 6 February 1957, nearly 5 months after injury, with very strong power in the right shoulder, but the deltoid remained paralysed. The only detectable weakness was lack of full power in extension and forward flexion.

It is worth encouraging all patients with severe shoulder weakness or paralysis to learn the arm fling; this manoeuvre consists of the arm being swung briskly across the front of the body and relaxed very quickly, so that the momentum and the extra pull provided by the pectoralis major brings the arm above the head. The fling is useful both for lifting light objects from the shoulder above the head and as good pattern re-education for the early stage of recovery.

Serratus anterior weakness

Paralysis of the serratus anterior occurs after trauma, particularly traction injuries to the upper limb, and the long nerve of Bell is vulnerable to serum neuritis. It can, of course, be involved with the other muscles in traction lesions of the plexus, poliomyelitis and myopathies.

When the muscle is completely paralysed, disability is severe because the scapula cannot be rotated and, therefore, abduction is difficult over 90 degrees; provided there is some serratus action, however, good function in the shoulder is possible.

One of our pilots with such a lesion was able to fly a Hunter aircraft with no trouble. In myopathies the shoulder girdle muscles are weak and the patient cannot raise his arm more than a few degrees from the side. Although the hand is normal, function is severely limited. The shoulders can be supported by slings in 45 degrees of abduction attached to a chair or to a wheelchair.

ELBOW WEAKNESS

Weakness of extension

Paralysis of the triceps can result from posterior cord lesions, poliomyelitis and myopathies; severe weakness is a common complication of fractures of the elbow, particularly the olecranon.

The operation for shortening the triceps following olecranon fractures is often undertaken to correct severe weakness of this muscle, but this in itself does not obviate the necessity for intensive redevelopment of the triceps power both before and after operation. In mild cases it may not be necessary to operate if the exercise programme has been successful, but if there is any degree of triceps weakness, surgery is advisable. Extension of the elbow is, of course, carried out by gravity as well as by the triceps. Unless this is remembered, quite severe degrees of weakness can be missed clinically. When the patient is asked to extend the elbow from full flexion with the shoulder at 90 degrees' forward flexion, it will be seen that the shoulder drops forwards so that gravity can allow the elbow to extend. If the elbow is watched carefully, it will be seen that there is no actual movement in the joint until the shoulder has dropped to less than 45 degrees. If slight resistance is given against the forearm, the trick shoulder depressor action is clearly seen.

When testing the triceps clinically, the angle of shoulder flexion at which the elbow can just be extended should be noted. To test this, the patient is asked to raise the arm above the head so that the elbow is fully flexed. The examiner supports the shoulder at gradually decreasing degrees of elevation until the patient can just extend the elbow – this angle is measured and, as the triceps increases in strength, it becomes greater. The examiner prevents trick action by his support. Appreciation of the trick action of the shoulder depressors is important for the occupational therapist and the physiotherapist.

It is easy to set up a craft and give progressive resistance exercises, the main effect of which is to build up the power of the depressors and not the triceps at all.

When the shoulder is abducted to 90 degrees and the elbow flexed, elbow extension should not be possible in the presence of complete triceps paralysis. A few patients have, however, been seen in which undoubted triceps paralysis was present, yet good extension of the elbow was possible in this position. Here the wrist extensors and brachioradialis were the muscles responsible. Re-education is therefore well worth trying in patients with triceps paralysis.

One patient has been seen who had almost total brachial plexus palsy with a very slight flicker in the biceps but no activity in the triceps or any of the other muscles acting on the elbow, and no activity in any other muscles below the elbow. He had very good action in the infraspinatus, and was able, with the arm abducted to 90 degrees, to flex and extend the elbow quite well and against slight resistance. It was noticed that extension of the elbow was obtained by depression and external rotation of the shoulder, which allowed gravity to extend the elbow.

As in all re-education programmes, resistive exercises to the muscles responsible are given in their normal range of movement; when the patient has the idea of the compensatory action, he is trained in the new range.

Compensatory or trick actions, provided that there are muscles to stabilize and fix the joints involved, can usually be taught in a co-operative patient, and can often provide adequate function.

Weakness of flexion

Apart from brachial plexus lesions, the elbow flexors can be paralysed in the rather uncommon lesion of the musculocutaneous nerve, usually due to direct violence. The brachioradialis can take over the function of elbow flexion but usually needs specific rehabilitation. The muscle works most efficiently when the forearm is in the position mid-way between pronation and supination (*Figure 3.32*). After a short period of intensive treatment, function can be indistinguishable from normal.

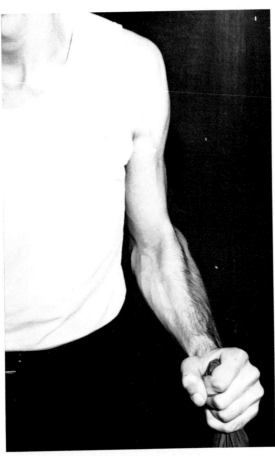

Figure 3.32 Lesion of musculocutaneous nerve. Flexion of the elbow carrying a 2.3 kg weight using brachioradialis

At the start of training the elbow is put in 90 degrees' flexion or more, the forearm into the neutral position, and the patient encouraged to bend the elbow using the brachioradialis. As soon as the patient has an idea of the movement, resistance is added, first from the physiotherapist's hand, and later using a progressive resistance technique with weights. It has been found that the most satisfactory way of retraining the brachioradialis and developing its power quickly is to give the patient a table of exercises in which he is asked to lift an increasing load an increasing number of times. On the first day of weight exercise, the patient may be able to raise 0.5 kg from the full extended position of the elbow to the maximum range of flexion, five times; thereafter the number of times the weight is lifted is increased. When the patient can raise the weight 20 times, it is increased to 1.1 kg, and when this can be lifted 20 times, it is again increased. Progression depends entirely on the rate of progress in the weight raising exercise, but the principle is to develop strength and endurance at the same time, for the elbow flexors are required not only to lift weight but also to maintain the forearm and hand against resistance over a period of time.

RECONSTRUCTIVE SURGERY

When the nerves are irreparable or recovery after suture is poor, reconstructive surgery is essential if function is to be regained. Surgical reconstruction comprises two main operative procedures – static operations to give stability, and dynamic procedures to provide movement and attempt to replace the muscle function lost by permanent paralysis. Static operations involve arthrodesis of joints. Arthrodesis of the wrist in 20 degrees' dorsiflexion will markedly improve the function of the finger flexors, if there has been permanent paralysis of all the wrist extensors and there are insufficient motors to transfer flexors to give active wrist extension.

Arthrodesis of the proximal interphalangeal joints in 30–45 degrees' flexion can be useful in high lesions of the median and ulnar nerves when there is no hope of return of active flexion and no motor available for transfer. This operation puts the fingers in the position of function for grasp and is often combined with arthrodesis of the wrist.

Dynamic procedures involve transfer of tendons of unaffected muscles to replace active movement. Such procedures can be single or multiple and may need to be combined with stabilization operations in severe lesions.

The general indications for all tendon transfer operations are as follows.

(1) The patient must have an adequate range of passive movement. Ideally no patient with paralysis should ever be allowed to develop stiff joints in the hand – regular passive movements and lively splinting should be routine. Unfortunately, these principles are not always followed and patients may present some months or years after injury for reconstructive surgery with stiff joints. It is essential that an intensive course of physiotherapy is given to restore maximum range of passive movements to stiff joints before any surgery is undertaken.

(2) Because tendon transfers lose at least one grade of power on the MRC scale, as a result of being moved, it is important to improve their power by intensive exercises, for even if not affected by the original condition, muscles are likely to have become weak through disuse. A muscle must have power 4+ to be considered for transfer.

(3) The amplitude of excursion of the transfer must be as near as possible the same as that of the paralysed tendon and it should pull in as straight a line as possible.

(4) The best function results when a transfer is expected to perform one movement only and it is therefore best to perform multiple transfers whenever possible

when several movements have been lost. This may, however, be impossible in severe cases and one must therefore concentrate on the most important movement for the particular patient's needs.

Details of surgical techniques are not considered here but a full description of current procedures can be found in *Campbell's Operative Orthopedics*.

The standard surgical procedures that have stood the test of time are widely accepted throughout the world will now be described. As the most common disorders that require such surgery are lesions of the peripheral nerves, they will be considered under each nerve lesion. Brachial plexus lesions present special problems and they are considered separately on pages 157 *et seq*. Cervical cord lesions are the third major group in which surgery can be of great value and they are discussed under a separate heading as quadriplegia.

Surgical reconstruction must be considered in the following situations.

(1)   When nerve regeneration is impossible – too great a loss of nerve for repair or grafting, inability to find one end of a nerve when explored, owing to widespread damage such as in blast injuries, burns, crush injuries, or when associated soft tissue damage militates against regrowth of the nerve.

(2)   When the lesion is at such a high level that, even if regeneration occurs, the muscles will have fibrosed and function will not return. In such cases, reconstruction can be effected immediately with minimal loss of time off work.

(3)   When there has been such a degree of coincident damage to muscles or joints that worthwhile function is impossible, even were the nerve to recover. This may occur with direct necrosis of muscle due to crush or vascular damage locally or at a distance.

Tendon transfers

The standard procedures for tendon transfers as used at the Royal National Orthopaedic Hospital under Mr Donal Brooks are as follows.

RADIAL NERVE LESIONS

To provide active wrist extension, flexor carpi ulnaris is put into extensor digitorum communis and extensor pollicis longus.

Pronator teres is put into extensor carpi radialis brevis. Palmaris longus, if present, is put into abductor pollicis longus.

Rehabilitation after radial nerve tendon transfer

The arm is kept in plaster for 3 weeks with the wrist and metacarpophalangeal joints free. The thumb is fully extended at the metacarpophalangeal joint. It is usual after the plaster has come off to provide a wrist splint to maintain wrist extension until active control is learnt.

Extension of fingers and thumb is encouraged, combined with wrist flexion and then independent of wrist movements. True long extensor action must be encouraged with interphalangeal joints flexed and movement occurring only at the metacarpophalangeal joints. Then extension of the metacarpophalangeal joints with extended fingers is allowed. Abduction of the thumb is added next and movement is usually just possible at this stage. Wrist extension is trained with pronation and then independently.

After 5–6 weeks, graduated resistance is added. Rarely, if finger extension is difficult to regain, the donor muscle is stimulated electrically.

If there is any adherence, ultrasound and massage are given over the anastomosis on the dorsum of the forearm just proximal to the wrist.

If there is any swelling at all, a sling must be worn with the hand elevated until it has disappeared. Passive movements are given to the metacarpophalangeal joints to regain flexion, the wrist being held in extension with the interphalangeal joints extended. There is no cause to treat the interphalangeal joints, as they have not been immobilized.

MEDIAN NERVE LESIONS

In lesions at the wrist, opposition needs to be restored. In isolated median nerve lesions, the adductor pollicis and often part of the flexor pollicis brevis are intact and the need is to replace the abductor pollicis brevis and opponens. The standard procedure is to transfer the flexor sublimis from the ring finger round a pulley from the flexor carpi ulnaris, divided into two slips – one inserted in the extensor pollicis longus expansion proximal to the interphalangeal joint, and the other into the abductor pollicis brevis. It is not necessary to restore the action of the first and second lumbricals.

In a high lesion of the median nerve when the long flexor action has been lost as well as intrinsic action, extensor carpi radialis longus is put into flexor pollicis longus. The profundus tendon to the ring finger is divided about 2.5 cm above the wrist joint and put into the tendons of the index and middle fingers. The distal stump of the flexor digitorum profundus to the ring finger is buttonholed into the little finger flexor. So, three profundus tendons flex four fingers.

Because no sensation is present in a high lesion, a tendon transfer for opposition is rarely indicated.

Rehabilitation after median nerve tendon transfer

The arm is immobilized in plaster or a boxing glove dressing with a plaster back slab, the wrist in flexion, the fingers semi-flexed, and the thumb flexed and abducted for 3 weeks.

Flexion of the index finger is re-educated with flexion of the other fingers. This is relatively easy to learn, but full excursion takes a few weeks to develop. Flexion of the thumb is then re-educated with wrist and thumb stabilized. If there is any adhesion formation, ultrasound and massage are used. Wrist extension is allowed to be regained in its own time. Resistance is started at 5–6 weeks, when occupational thrapy is added.

MEDIAN AND RADIAL PALSY

Here the patient has lost extension of the wrist and fingers, flexion of the index and middle fingers, and opposition of the thumb.

The wrist joint is arthrodesed. If necessary, flexor carpi ulnaris is put into extensor digitorum communis and extensor pollicis longus. A high median tendon transfer restores flexion to the index. Flexor pollicis brevis usually provides adequate pinch grip, so the paralysis of the long thumb flexor is unimportant.

ULNAR NERVE LESIONS

Here the order of opening and closing the hand is lost. The metacarpophalangeal joints should be the first to open and the last to close, and this is reversed in ulnar palsies when the interossei are paralysed. The result is that objects tend to be pushed out of the hand when gripping.

To correct the claw hand – hyperextension of the metacarpophalangeal joints – there are two possibilities: ideally to restore intrinsic function by tendon transfers or to prevent hyperextension of the metacarpophalangeal joints by tenodesis or capsulorrhaphies, for if the metacarpophalangeal joints are held slightly flexed then the long extensor of the fingers can extend the interphalangeal joints.

Tubiana (1969) has pointed out that the usual transfers for restoration of active intrinsic functions work by tenodesis effect, as one cannot reproduce the timing of the muscle interplay. He prefers the Zancolli procedure in which a triangular portion of the volar plate is removed, plicating the capsule of the metacarpophalangeal joint and holding it in slight flexion. Moreover, this operation does not require the transfer of any tendons, which are thus available for restoration of other functions. The best results are obtained if, preoperatively with the metacarpophalangeal joints held in flexion, the patient can extend the distal interphalangeal joints.

Zancolli (1979) now uses the 'lasso' operation, in which the flexor sublimis is divided distal to the pulley at the metacarpophalangeal joint, looped back and sutured to itself at the desired tension, depending on the stiffness of the joint. The procedure corrects the clawing, provides a powerful intrinsic function with initial flexion of the proximal phalanx and restores simultaneous digital flexion. To restore lateral pinch grip, the flexor sublimis extensor indicis or extensor digitorum brevis is put into the first dorsal interosseus.

COMBINED RADIAL AND ULNAR PALSY

Here the patient can flex the fingers but cannot stabilize the wrist or release finger flexion. There is weakness of flexion at the metacarpophalangeal joints, lack of abduction of the fingers and clawing of the metacarpophalangeal joints of ring and little fingers. Flexor carpi radialis longus is put into extensor digitorum communis and extensor pollicis longus to give active finger release.

The wrist is arthrodesed. The Zancolli procedure is carried out if hyperextension at the metacarpophalangeal joints is a problem (plicating the volar plate and tightening the structures anteriorly).

After all tendon transfers, immobilization is maintained for 3 weeks. Active exercises then start, resistance being allowed at 6 weeks. Graduated occupational therapy helps to restore functional patterns.

COMBINED MEDIAN AND ULNAR NERVE LESIONS

Tubiana (1969) has pointed out that the direction of tendon transfer must depend on what movement has been lost. In pure median nerve lesions, the tendon transfer is put into the abductor pollicis brevis, and in pure ulnar lesions into the adductor. In paralysis of all the intrinsics of the thumb, the transfer will be routed in the direction of the flexor pollicis brevis to attempt movement mid-way between adduction and abduction. This is combined with either a Zancolli procedure or a tenodesis to restore correct opening and closing of the hand, and transfer to provide pinch grip.

In a *high median and ulnar lesion*, the recommended procedures are:

Transfer of extensor carpi radialis longus to flexor digitorum profundus and flexor pollicis longus to provide finger flexion. Extensor carpi radialis brevis is left to extend the wrist.

Zancolli's procedure or lasso operation, or volar capsuloplasty.

The metacarpophalangeal joint of the thumb may need to be arthrodesed to provide stability.

Extensor indicis can be transferred to the first dorsal interosseus tendon of index to provide pinch grip, if necessary.

Quadriplegia

Douglas Lamb (1971) has pointed out that in cervical cord lesions if there is no activity at all 1 month after injury then no recovery can be expected, but in some cases a flicker seen at an early stage has developed into marked recovery as much as 18 months later.

Surgery, if successful, is preferable to aids and gadgets which the patient may be unable to apply himself. Contraindications include: (1) injuries above C5 or below C8; (2) marked spasticity; (3) lack of sensation. Surgery is delayed for at least 1 year after injury.

In a 10-year period 25 patients received 72 tendon transfers out of 113 cervical cord injuries in Lamb's unit. Assessment of function must be made by remaining function, not by anatomical level of the lesion.

Zancolli (1979) has reported on the results of surgery in 76 patients operated on from 12 to 18 months after injury. He agrees with Moberg (1977) that the first step should be to restore extension of the elbow by transferring the posterior part of the deltoid into the triceps. This will help the patient in his transfers, give him the ability to reach out for objects and improve his mobility in a wheelchair. It also facilitates re-education following subsequent tendon transfers. His scheme is as follows.

If only the brachioradialis is available for transfer, the metacarpophalangeal joint of the thumb is arthrodesed in 10 degrees' flexion, and tenodesis of the extensor pollicis longus is carried out at Lister's tubercle so that passive flexion of the wrist will produce extension of the thumb at the carpometacarpal and interphalangeal joints. Tenodesis of the abductor pollicis longus is then carried out to maintain the first metacarpal in slight abduction and antepulsion. The brachioradialis is transferred into the extensor carpi radialis brevis. Tenodesis of the flexor pollicis longus is carried out so that lateral pinch of the thumb is provided as the wrist is extended.

Zancolli points out that one must always attempt to reproduce lateral pinch grip and not a pulp pinch. He chooses the dominant hand first, and the one with most sensibility.

If weak wrist extension is present, he tenodeses the extensor digitorum communis and extensor pollicis longus, fusing the metacarpophalangeal joint of the thumb, tenodesing the abductor pollicis longus and performing the lasso operation on the flexor sublimis digitorum to stabilize the metacarpophalangeal joint, some movement being provided by the viscoelastic properties of the muscle. If there is strong wrist extension, the brachioradialis is transferred to the extensor digitorum communis and extensor pollicis longus, and the other procedures listed above are carried out as for weak wrist extension. It may be possible to transfer the extensor carpi radialis longus or pronator teres to the finger flexors. Clearly, the more muscles available, the greater the possibility of tendon transfers increasing function.

In all these procedures the hand is immobilized for 4 weeks; thereafter, passive flexion of the fingers and wrist is carried out to prevent intrinsic plus deformity.

APPENDIX: MANUFACTURE OF LIVELY SPLINTS

Splint for dropped wrist

The object of this splint is to maintain the wrist in moderate dorsiflexion and to allow active flexion and extension of the wrist. It may be useful in radial nerve palsies and any other situation in which there is paralysis of the wrist extensors.

The splint consists of a wire framework with a palmar pad fitting into the cup of the palm. The position of this pad is critical and must not interfere with the full range of metacarpophalangeal movement. Wire supports are provided coming under the wrist, then out and round to form a coil each side of the wrist. The wire then passes back each side of the forearm and terminates by curving around the volar aspect of the forearm about 10 cm below the elbow. In addition, there is a padded support under and just proximal to the wrist, from which a leather strap passes over and around the wrist, and is secured with Velcro. Two 16 s.w.g. wire stiffeners are soldered under the wrist support.

Thus the palmar pad supports the wrist in dorsiflexion, with the strap over the wrist and the forearm support forming the other two points of leverage.

As each splint is made to fit the patient, no set sizes can be given, but the wrist support is approximately 3.8 cm wide and the forearm support approximately 0.6 cm wide. Both these are padded with Dalzafoam and covered with leather. The outer covering of the wrist support is made of tanned leather and is long enough to go round the wrist and back under itself to fasten with Velcro.

The palmar pad is reinforced with tin and padded with Molefoam 0.6 cm thick, then covered with leather; 16 s.w.g. wire has been found adequate for this type of splint (*Figure 3.33*).

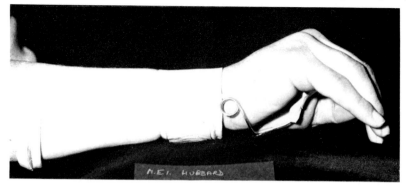

Figure 3.33   Lively splint for wrist drop, side view

The method of construction is as follows.

(1)   Select a length (approximately 90 cm) of 16 s.w.g. wire.
(2)   Starting approximately at the centre of the wire, make the forearm support to fit the patient. Allow sufficient room for the tin strap and padding. The wire is then a long-sided U.
(3)   Bend each side of the U distally to fit along the midline of the forearm.
(4)   At the level of the wrist joint form the coils around a suitable jig (approximately 9.5 mm diam.), making two and a quarter complete turns on each side.
(5)   Bend each side inwards around the wrist.
(6)   Under the centre of the wrist, bend the sides forwards.
(7)   Form the outline of the palmar pad, binding and soldering the two ends together where shown, after cutting off surplus wire.
(8)   When the shape and fit are satisfactory, bind and solder the ends of the wires where they meet under the wrist.
(9)   Cut a tin palm plate to shape, then bend and solder in position.
(10) Cut and bend the forearm and wrist supports to fit, then solder in position. Bend and solder the stiffeners in place.
(11) Fit padding and cover.
(12) Fit Velcro to the strap and to the volar surface of the wrist support.

Splint for claw hand

Here the requirement is for a splint to prevent the long extensors hyperextending the metacarpophalangeal joints, but to allow flexion at these joints. This may be used in ulnar nerve lesions or any situation where there is paralysis of muscles supplied by the first thoracic root. The principle of the 'knuckle duster' is used. The splint provides support over the back of the metacarpals, support over the dorsal surface of the proximal phalanges, with coils forming hinges at the metacarpophalangeal joints and a palmar pad providing the fulcrum.

It is important to keep the bulk of the splint to a minimum in the palm, so as not to interfere with function. Tin and piano wire (19 s.w.g) are used with Dalzafoam padding on the back pad and Molefoam wrapped round the palmar grip. The finger cups are shaped to fit the fingers and are covered with unpadded leather (*Figure 3.34*).

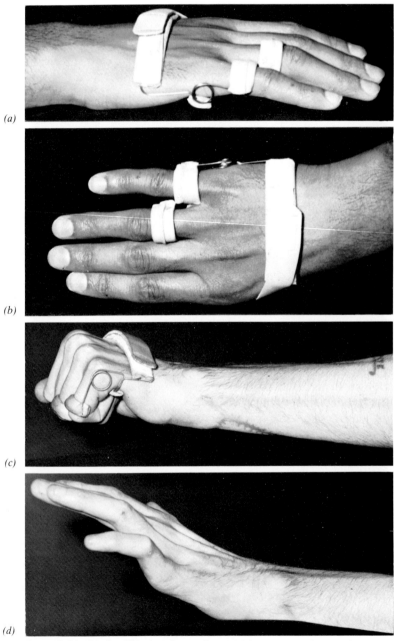

(a)

(b)

(c)

(d)

Figure 3.34   Lively splint for ulnar palsy. (a) Ulnar aspect. (b) Aerial view. (c) Flexion. (d) Hyperextension deformity without splint

The method of construction is as follows.

(1)   Select a 45 cm length of 19 or 20 s.w.g. piano wire (whichever is available).
(2)   Form a hairpin bend at the centre without closing the bend too tightly. This loop forms the palmar grip.
(3)   Measuring against the patient, bend one end back alongside the edge of the hand, then up and over the back of the hand to form the back pad.
(4)   Curve the end of the wire back on itself to hold the tin securely. Cut off surplus wire.
(5)   Bend the other end forwards in line with the little finger.
(6)   With the palmar pad in the cup of the palm, form a coil to lie on the axis of the metacarpophalangeal joint, making two and a half complete turns. The wire should not lie along the outer side of the little finger.

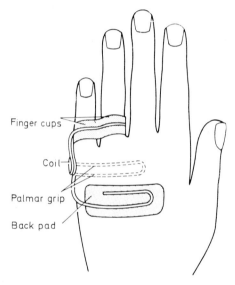

Figure 3.35   Diagram of splint for claw hand

(7)   Approximately two-thirds distal to the metacarpophalangeal joint, bend the wire up and over the back of the little finger, modelling closely to its contour, and likewise over the ring finger.
(8)   Cut off surplus wire.
(9)   Form the strips for the finger cups 1.3 cm wide approximately) and back pad (1.9 cm wide).
(10) Solder tin in position, ensuring fit is correct. NB: it is almost impossible to bend the wire and the tin when they are soldered together without breaking the soldered joint.
(11) Cut the strap to size and attach it to the loop of the palmar grip with several turns of strong thread sewn through the leather.
(12) Fit padding to palmar grip and back pad. Cover all necessary parts with matching soft leather. Fit Velcro to strap and back pad.

It is important to note that all fittings to the patient must be made with the hand in the *corrected* position.

Splint for intrinsic paralysis

Splints are necessary when there is a combination of claw hand and a flattened thenar eminence following nerve lesions due to trauma or neuropathies (e.g. leprosy) (*Figure 3.36*).

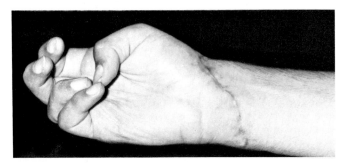

Figure 3.36   Attempted opposition in patient with median and ulnar nerve palsy

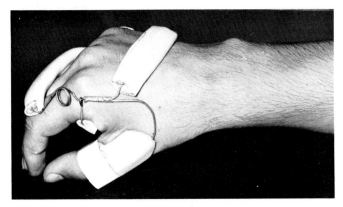

Figure 3.37   Opposition with lively splint

A not uncommon injury is severance of both median and ulnar nerves and multiple tendons at the wrist. The splint provides support at the metacarpophalangeal joints to prevent hyperextension and keeps the thumb in palmar abduction. The spring wire construction allows active movements at all joints (*Figures 3.37* and *3.38*).

Splint for combined median and ulnar paralysis

(1)   The main portion of the splint is formed from one piece of 19 or 20 s.w.g. wire approximately 60 cm long.

(2)   Starting at the centre of the dorsum of the hand, mould the wire round towards the thumb and carry it distally to the metacarpophalangeal joint of the index finger.

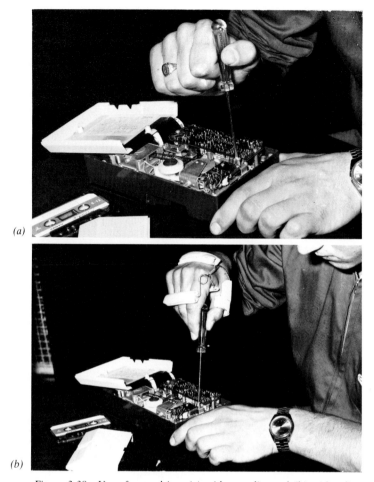

Figure 3.38   Use of screwdriver (a) without splint and (b) with splint

(3)   Form a coil in line on the axis of the metacarpophalangeal joint, making two complete turns. Approximately two-thirds of the way along the proximal phalanx of the index, bend up the wire and form it over the dorsum of the fingers. Bend back along the side of the little finger.

(4)   Form a coil in the axis of the metacarpophalangeal joint, making two complete turns.

(5)   Make a 'kink' in the wire in line with the distal palmar crease to locate the palmar bar.

(6)   Finally, bend it up and curve over the dorsum of the hand to meet the other end. Cut off surplus wire and solder ends together.

The method of construction of palmar bar and thumb spring is now given.

(1)   Select a piece of 18 s.w.g. wire approximately 30 cm long and, allowing sufficient length for the palmar bar, make a right-angle bend.

(2)   Lay the wire in position alongside the main splint and shape the palmar bar to follow the contour of the distal palmar crease and hook over the kink in the side bar. Cut off surplus wire.

(3)   Allowing sufficient length for a pivot tube (see 5), make a slight kink in the thumb spring to prevent any axial movement along the pivot tube.

(4)   Form the thumb spring as shown in *Figure 3.39*, adjusting to hold thumb in corrected position. The short bend at the end provides a solid location for a thumb cup.

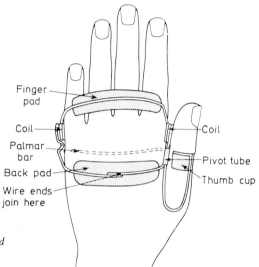

Figure 3.39   Diagram of splint for combined median and ulnar palsy

(5)   Now make the pivot tube by rolling a piece of tin around both wires. Solder the seam overlap and then solder the tube to the side bar of the main assembly. Ensure that the palmar bar/thumb spring is free to rotate, and is also located correctly in relation to the coil. This should be in line with the metacarpophalangeal joint with the palmar bar lying in the distal palmar crease.

(6)   Cut and form the thumb cup, 1.3 cm wide, halfway round thumb. Solder in position.

(7)   Cut and form the finger pad (1.3 cm wide) and back pad (1.9 cm wide) and solder in position, ensuring a close fit.

(8)   Pad the palmar bar with 0.5 cm Molefoam, the finger and back pad with Dalzafoam and cover with soft leather.

(9)   Cover the thumb cup with the outer covering long enough to strap around the thumb and fasten with Velcro.

Splint for thenar paralysis

Splintage is required in any condition causing paralysis of the intrinsic muscles of the thumb and in particular in median nerve lesions. It is relatively easy to provide a splint which holds the thumb in palmar abduction, but the key problem is to provide rotation of the metacarpal to allow opposition by the long flexor of the thumb, as this muscle is spared in lesions at the wrist. As yet we have not been able to provide an adequate base for opposition without bringing the dorsal bar across to the ulnar fingers.

Our previous splint for thenar paralysis is bulky (*Figure 3.40*), but patients do find the pull of the rubber more effective for opposition than the push of the spring wire in the combined splint. However, some patients prefer the latter and we try both.

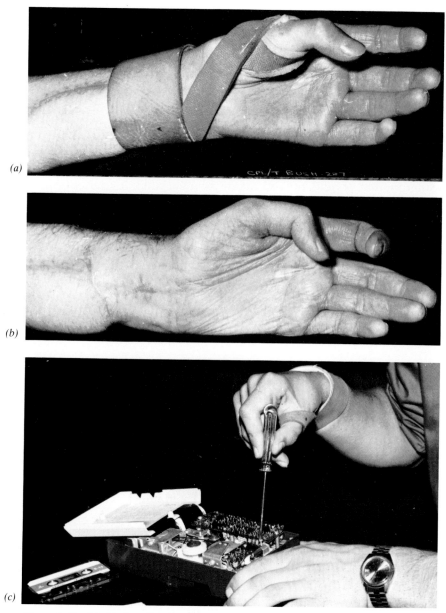

Figure 3.40   (a) Lively splint for thenar paralysis. (b) Deformity in median nerve lesion without lively splint. (c) Splint in use

The cost of materials is at present less than 50 pence a splint. The splints can be made by workshop technicians or occupational therapists.

All the patients who have worn them are pleased with the appearance of the splints and find them more acceptable and useful than previous models.

Materials necessary for these splints are as follows.

PIANO WIRE

This is the general name for spring steel wire, the material used in the splints described above. The following points should be noted.

(1)   It is supplied in standard wire gauge (s.w.g.) thicknesses.
(2)   A simple guide to the diameter of any wire can be taken as follows:
        10 s.w.g. = 3.2 mm ($^1/_8$ in) approx.
        14 s.w.g. = 2.4 mm ($^3/_{32}$ in) approx.
        16 s.w.g. = 1.6 mm ($^1/_{16}$ in) approx.
        20 s.w.g. = 0.8 mm ($^1/_{32}$ in) approx.
(3)   The s.w.g. of the wires mentioned in the text are all as used at the MRU, Chessington, but should not be taken as invariable. Experience will indicate when different sizes should be used for a particular patient.
(4)   Bulk supplies are usually delivered in coils, but it has been found that shops dealing with model aircraft supplies sell straight 1-metre lengths of a wide range of thickness at quite reasonable prices (about 10 pence per length).

TIN

Rectangular one-gallon cans have provided excellent material for the 'tins'; also plaster of Paris containers, bandage tins, bean tins and Coke cans.

Earlier type of lively splint for thenar paralysis (*Figure 3.40*)

AIM

The aim is to lift the thumb metacarpal into palmar abduction, rotation and opposition so that the thumb is held in a position of function.

INDICATIONS

Any condition with weakness or paralysis of thenar muscles will benefit from the use of a lively splint.

MATERIALS

The materials required are: calf hide, 5 cm wide × patient's wrist measurement plus 7.5 cm; rubber sheeting, 0.3 cm thick; non-slip foam liming; 10 cm Velcro fastening; adhesive and linen thread.

METHOD OF CONSTRUCTION

(1) Cut a strip of rubber sheeting approximately 2.5 × 20 cm.
(2) Mark one end A, the other B.
(3) Draw a line across the rubber 7.5 cm from A.
(4) With the patient holding the thumb in palmar abduction, place the marked line over the web of the thumb, with A over the palm and B at the dorsal surface.
(5) Bring both ends round the metacarpophalangeal joint in a downward movement, folding end B round and over end A opposite the base of the thumb nail, in a moulding movement. (They should then form a V.)
(6) Mark on the edge of B where the wrist meets B, and vice versa. Allow A to wrap underneath it until it reaches the wrist border, B (*Figure 3.41*). This prevents the short, cut end of A being pressed on to the skin over the metacarpal by B, thus causing discomfort.

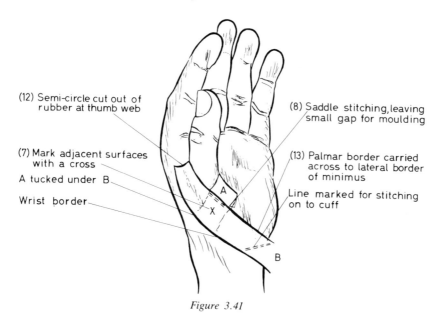

(12) Semi-circle cut out of rubber at thumb web

(7) Mark adjacent surfaces with a cross

A tucked under B

Wrist border

(8) Saddle stitching, leaving small gap for moulding

(13) Palmar border carried across to lateral border of minimus

Line marked for stitching on to cuff

Figure 3.41

(7) Mark an X on each of the two adjacent surfaces to facilitate stitching when removed from the patient's thumb. It is sometimes difficult to pick up the exact markings if the splint has had to be put down for some reason or other and then picked up at a later date, when stitching can so easily be done on the wrong side of the rubber, thus making it for the wrong thumb.
(8) Using the linen thread, stitch B to A with three or four large running stitches. (Small stitches will perforate the rubber.) Make sure that the knot is between the two surfaces to avoid skin friction. Stitch three-quarters of the way only so that a small gap will be left to allow for moulding the rubber.
(9) Now prepare the wrist cuff. Take the width of the patient's wrist plus an extra 7.5 cm (5 cm for overlap, 2.5 cm for lining). Cut a piece of calf hide 5 cm in width to the above measurements.

(10)   Stick the Velcro fastening on to one end of the upper surface of the leather, and the other half to the opposite end of the cuff on the under surface. To ensure that contact is firm it is advisable to apply the adhesive to both surfaces and wait until they are 'tacky' before pressing them together. Provided this is properly done, there should be no need to stitch the Velcro to the leather.

(11)   Attaching the thumb piece to the cuff is the most important stage and can make the splint quite useless and ineffective if incorrectly applied. The patient must be told how to apply the splint correctly: (*a*) the V of the rubber under the thumb nail; (*b*) the rubber band moulded round the palmar aspect of the thumb and wrist until the lateral border of minimus is reached (*Figure 3.41*). The paper-backed foam lining is now placed inside the cuff, and on the patient's wrist. The opening should be on the ulnar side of the dorsal aspect. It is then fastened securely.

(12)   Place the thumb piece over the metacarpophalangeal joint and as far down the metacarpal as possible. Cut out a small semi-circle of rubber over the thumb web area to permit this.

(13)   Lift and rotate the metacarpal, stretching and moulding the wrist border of the rubber until the palmar border of the rubber is in line with the lateral border of minimus, and the thumb is in a good position of function. There should be sufficient pull on the rubber to enable the patient fully to extend his thumb against it. Mark the angle made on the rubber along the edge of the leather and mark on the leather the two ends of the angle line. Remove the two parts.

(14)   Saddle stitch the rubber on to the leather where marked, and trim off the surplus.

(15)   Remove paper backing from non-slip lining and stitch on to cuff, except on the overlap.

(16)   Apply the splint to the patient, stressing once more the important points of application, and then ask him to put it on himself to make sure that he is well aware how to avoid faulty positioning. Review in a few days' time in case of any stretch that may have occurred in either the calf or the rubber; adjust if necessary.

PRECAUTIONS

(1)   Make sure that the patient knows how to apply the splint to achieve maximum function of the thumb.

(2)   If the thumb piece does not have sufficient rubber cut over the thumb web, the rubber will not reach far enough down the metacarpal, probably resulting in lateral angulation of the proximal phalanx. The splint will then become useless.

(3)   If the attachment of the rubber to the wrist cuff has too much tension, the wrist will be pulled into flexion.

(4)   The wrist cuff must be lined with non-slip material.

(5)   If the stitching on the V section of the thumb piece is too tight, there will be impairment of circulation. The patient should be warned about any colour change in his skin, and should remove the splint for a short time if this happens. It may become necessary to 'break in' the thumb to the splint by applying it for short spells each day and gradually increasing the time until it can be worn all day.

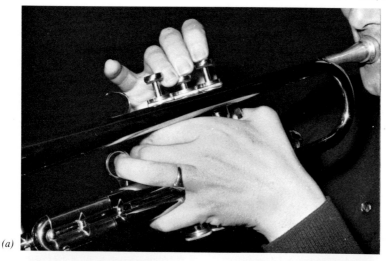

(a)

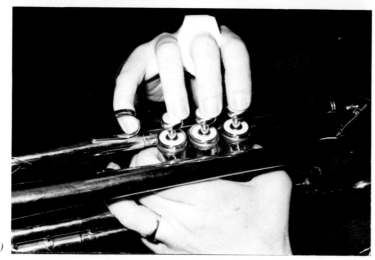

(b)

Figure 3.42   This shows the difficulty experienced by a professional trumpeter with a complete ulnar nerve lesion, in controlling the valves due to loss of metacarpophalangeal joint stability. A Plastazote wedge gave him the necessary support and the extensors were able therefore to act as abductors

(6) Occasionally, there may be hypersensitivity due to nerve regeneration, and pressure from the cuff will be uncomfortable. This can be relieved by placing two strips of 1.3 cm sponge rubber on the top of the non-slip lining, bounding the hypersensitive area, so that a small channel is made for it, and pressure is thus lessened over that area.

(7) The patient must be able to extend his thumb fully against the pull of the rubber, and the tension should just be sufficient to return him to a position of function.

(8) Occasionally, one finds a patient whose skin cannot tolerate the rubber sheeting used on the median splint in cases of peripheral nerve injury. In such a case that part of the sheeting which is in direct contact with the metacarpal can be

replaced with an identical piece in fibreglass. This is attached to the part of the splint which passes across the palmar aspect of the hand to be attached on the ulnar side of the hand; the rubber sheeting is then stitched on to the fibreglass. It is important to take an accurate cast of the thumb in its position of function, since the fibreglass is an exact reproduction of the part and, if faulty, another cast would have to be made. The inside of the splint must be rubbed down very smoothly to avoid small wrinkles which would be uncomfortable to the patient during movement of the thumb.

REFERENCES AND BIBLIOGRAPHY

Adams, S. J. E. (1976). Naloxone reversal of analgesia produced by brain stimulation in the human. *Pain* **2,** 161

Akil, H. and Richardson, D. E. (1974). Electrical, surgical and pharmacological management of pain. Proceedings of the Neurolectric Society 7th Annual Meeting, New Orleans, 20–23 November, p. 50

Almquist, E. E. (1970). Conduction velocity and two-point discrimination in sutured nerves. *Journal of Bone and Joint Surgery* **52A,** 791–794

Anderson, L. S., Black, R. G., Abraham, J. and Ward, A. A. (1971). Neuronal hyperactivity in experimental trigeminal deafferentation. *Journal of Neurosurgery* **35,** 444

Andres, K. H. and von During, M. (1967). Morphology of cutaneous receptors. *Handbook of Sensory Physiology* pp. 3–20

Barnes, R. (1949). Traction injuries of the brachial plexus in adults. *Journal of Bone and Joint Surgery* **31B,** 10–16

Barnes, R. (1954). In *Peripheral Nerve Injuries*, p. 156. Ed. by H. J. Seddon. (Medical Research Council Special Report Series, No. 282) London: HMSO

Bonica, J. J. (1977). Neurophysiologic and pathologic aspects of acute and chronic pain. *Archives of Surgery* **112**(6), 750–761

Bonney, G. (1954). The value of axon responses in determining the site of lesion in traction injuries of brachial plexus. *Brain* **77,** 588–609

Bowden, R. E. M. and Napier, J. R. (1961). The assessment of hand function after peripheral nerve injuries. *Journal of Bone and Joint Surgery* **43B,** 481–492

Bratton, B. R., Hudson, A. R. and Kline, D. G. (1979). Experimental interfascicular nerve grafting. *Journal of Neurosurgery* **51,** 323–332

Brewerton, D. A. and Daniel, J. W. (1969). Return to work after injury. *The Hand* **1,** 125–128

Brooks, D. M. (1949). Open wounds of the brachial plexus. *Journal of Bone and Joint Surgery* **31B,** 17–33

Brooks, D. M. (1952). Nerve compression by simple ganglia. *Journal of Bone and Joint Surgery* **34B,** 391–400

Brooks, D. M. (1954). Nerve injuries and fractures. In *Peripheral Nerve Injuries*, p. 82. Ed. by H. J. Seddon. (Medical Research Council Special Report Series, No. 282) London: HMSO

Burgess, P. R. and Perl, E. R. (1973). Cutaneous mechanoreceptors and nociceptors. *Handbook of Sensory Physiology* pp. 29–78.

Cabaud, H. E., Rodkey, D. V. M., McCarrol, R., Mutz, H. and Niebauer, J. S. (1976). Epineural and perineurial fascicular nerve repairs – a clinical comparison. *Journal of Hand Surgery* **4,** 131–137

Campbell, W. C. (1971). *Operative Orthopedics,* 5th edn. Rev. by A. H. Crenshaw. St Louis, Mo: C.V. Mosby

Capener, N. (1949). The use of orthopaedic appliances in the treatment of anterior poliomyelitis. *Journal of Bone and Joint Surgery* **37B,** 591

Cervero, F., Iggo, A. and Ogawa, H. (1976). Nociceptor driven dorsal horn neurones in the lumbar spinal cord of the cat. *Pain* **2,** 5–24

Clarkson, P. W. and Pelly, A. (1962). *The General and Plastic Surgery of the Hand.* Oxford: Blackwell

Cochrane, R. G. and Davey, T. F. (1964). *Leprosy in Theory and Practice,* 2nd edn. Bristol: John Wright

Copeland, S. and Landi, A. (1979). Value of the Tinel sign in brachial plexus lesions. *Annals of the Royal College of Surgeons* **61,** 470–471

Dellon, A. L. (1976). Reinnervation of denervated Meissner's corpuscles. A sequential histologic study in the monkey following fascicular nerve repair. *Journal of Hand Surgery* **1,** 98–109

Dellon, A. L., Curtis, R. M. and Edgerton, M. R. (1974). Reeducation of sensation in the hand after nerve injury and repair. *Plastic and Reconstructive Surgery* **53,** 297–302

Dickhaus, H., Zimmerman, M. and Zotterman, Y. (1976). The development in regenerating cutaneous nerve of C fibre receptors responding to noxious heating of skin. In *Sensory Function of Skin in Primates*, pp. 415–425. Ed. by Y. Zotterman. Oxford: Pergamon Press

Dickson, R. A., Dinten, J., Rushworth, G. and Colwin, A. (1977). Delayed (degenerate) interfascicular nerve grafting – a new concept in peripheral nerve repair. *British Journal of Surgery* **64**, 698–671

Drake, C. G. (1964). Diagnosis and treatment of lesions of the brachial plexus and adjacent structures. *Clinical Neurosurgery* **11**, 110–127

Duport, C., Cloutier, G. E., Prevoisk, Y. and Dion, M. A. (1965). Ulnar tunnel syndrome at the wrist. *Journal of Bone and Joint Surgery* **47B**, 757–761

Edshage, S. (1964). Peripheral nerve suture. A technique for improved intraneural topography. Evaluation of some suture materials. *Acta Chirurgica Scandinavica* Suppl. 331

Foreman, R. D., Beall, J. E., Applebaum, A. E., Coulter, J. D. and Willis, N. D. (1976). Effect of dorsal column stimulation on primate spinothalamic tract neurons. *Journal of Neurophysiology* **39**, 534

Francis, J. B. (1858). Extracting teeth by galvanism. *Dental Report* **1**, 65–69

Greene, M. H. (1969). Use of biceps for digital function. *Journal of Bone and Joint Surgery* **51A**, 789

Gwathney, J. T. (1914). *Anesthesiology*, pp. 628–643. New York: Appleton

Hallin, R. G. and Torebjork, H. E. (1974). Activity in unmyelinated nerve fibres in man. In *Advances in Neurology*, pp. 19–27. Ed. by J. J. Bonica. New York: Raven Press

Hannington-Kiff, J. G. (1974). Intravenous regional sympathetic block with guanethidine. *Lancet* **i**, 1019–1020

Heath, R. G. (1963). Electrical self-stimulation of the brain in man. *American Journal of Psychiatry* **120**, 517–577

Henderson, W. R. (1948). Clinical assessment of peripheral nerve injuries: Tinel's test. *Lancet* **ii**, 801

Highet, W. B. (1954). Grading of motor and sensory recovery in nerve injuries. In *Peripheral Nerve Injuries*, p. 356. Ed. by H. J. Seddon. (Medical Research Council Report Series, No. 282) London: HMSO

Hughes, J. (1975). Isolation of an endogenous compound from the brain with pharmacological properties similar to morphine. *Brain Research* **88**(2), 295–308

Iggo, A. (1977). Cutaneous and subcutaneous sense organs. *British Medical Bulletin* **33**, 97–102

Inouye, Y. and Buchthal, F. (1977). Segmental sensory innervation determined by potentials recorded from cervical spinal nerves. *Brain* **100**, 731–737

Jabeley, M. E., Burns, J. E., Orcutt, B. S. and Bryant, W. M. (1976). Comparison of histologic and functional recovery after peripheral nerve repair. *Journal of Hand Surgery* **1**, 119–130

Jones, S. (1979). Investigation of brachial plexus traction lesions by peripheral and spinal somatosensory evoked potentials. *Journal of Neurology, Neurosurgery and Psychiatry* **42**, 107–116

Kabat, H. (1961). Proprioceptive facilitation in therapeutic exercise. In *Therapeutic Exercise*. New Haven, Conn: E. Licht

Lain, T. M. (1969). The military brace syndrome. A report of sixteen cases of Erb's palsy occurring in military cadets. *Journal of Bone and Joint Surgery* **51A**, 557–560

Lamb, D. W. (1971). The hand in quadriplegia. *The Hand* **3**, 31–37

Lamb, H. (1971). Ulnar nerve compression lesions at the wrist and hand. *The Hand* **2**, 17–18

Landi, A., Copeland, S., Jones, S. and Wynn Parry, C. B. (1980). The role of somatosensory-evoked potentials and nerve conduction studies in the surgical management of brachial plexus injuries. *Journal of Bone and Joint Surgery*, **68**, 492–496

Lang, S. M. and Goldner, J. L. (1969). Transfers of biceps brachii tendon into digital flexor tendons. *Journal of Bone and Joint Surgery* **51A**, 789

Littler, S. W. (1959). Neurovascular skin island transfer in reconstructive hand surgery. *Transactions of the International Society of Plastic Surgeons 2nd Congress*, p. 175. Edinburgh: Livingstone

Loeser, J. D. and Ward, A. A. (1967). Some effects of deafferentiation on neurons of the cat spinal cord. *Archives of Neurology, Chicago* **17**, 629–636

Loeser, J. D., Ward, A. A. and White, L. E. (1968). Chronic deafferentation of the human spinal cord neurons. *Journal of Neurosurgery* **29**, 48–50

Loh, L. and Nathan, P. W. (1978). Painful peripheral states and sympathetic blocks. *Journal of Neurology, Neurosurgery and Psychiatry* **41**, 664–671

Long, D. M. and Hagfors, N. (1975). Electrical stimulation in the nervous system. The current status of electrical stimulation of the nervous system for relief of pain. *Pain* **1**, 109

Lotem, M. (1971). Radial palsy following muscular effort. A nerve compression syndrome possibly relating to a fibrous arch of the lateral head of the triceps. *Journal of Bone and Joint Surgery* **53B**, 500–506

Mazars, G. J. (1976). Contribution of thalamic stimulation to the physiopathology of pain. In *Advances in Pain Research and Therapy*, vol. 1, pp. 483–485. Ed. by J. J. Bonica and D. Albe-Fessard. New York: Raven Press

Melzack, R. (1975a). The McGill pain questionnaire – major properties and scoring methods. *Pain* **1**, 277–299

Melzack, R. (1975b). Prolonged relief of pain by brief intense transcutaneous somatic stimulation. *Pain* **1**, 357–373

Melzack, R. (1977). *The Puzzle of Pain*. Harmondsworth: Penguin

Melzack, R. and Loeser, J. D. (1978). Phantom body pain in paraplegics. Evidence for a central pattern generating mechanism for pain. *Pain* **4**, 195–210

Melzack, R. and Wall, P. D. (1962). On the nature of cutaneous sensory mechanisms. *Brain* **85**, 331–356

Melzack, R. and Wall, P. D. (1965). Pain mechanisms. A new theory. *Science* **150**, 971–979

Millesi, H., Meissl, G. and Berger, A. (1972). The interfascicular nerve grafting of the median and ulnar nerves. *Journal of Bone and Joint Surgery* **54A**, 727–750

Millesi, H., Meissl, G. and Berger, A. (1976). Further experience with interfascicular grafts. *Journal of Bone and Joint Surgery* **58A**, 209–218

Moberg, E. (1958). Objective methods in determining the functional value of sensibility in the hand. *Journal of Bone and Joint Surgery* **40B**, 454–476

Moberg, E. (1977). Surgical treatment for absent single hand grip and elbow extension in quadriplegia. *Journal of Bone and Joint Surgery* **57A**, 196–206

Mountcastle, V. B. (1968). *Medical Physiology*, vol. 2, 12th edition, p. 285. St Louis, Mo: C. V. Mosby (14th edn, 1979)

Narakas, A. (1977). Indications et resultats du traitement chirurgical direct dans les lesions par elongation du plexus brachial. Les indications du traitement chirurgical direct. *Revue Chirurgical Orthopedie* **63**, 88–106

Nashold, B. S., Urban, B. and Zorub, D. S. (1976). Phantom pain relief by focal destruction of the substantia gelatinosa of Rolando. *Advances in Pain Research and Therapy*, vol. 1, pp. 959–963. Ed. by J. J. Bonica and D. Albe-Fessard. New York: Raven Press

Nathan, P. W. (1962). In *The Assessment of Pain in Man and Animals*, pp. 129–134. Ed. by C. A. Keele and R. Smith. Edinburgh: Livingstone

Nathan, P. W. (1972). Pain. *British Medical Bulletin* **33**, 249

Nicholson, O. R. and Seddon, H. J. (1957). Nerve repair in civil practice. Results of treatment of median and ulnar lesions. *British Medical Journal* **2**, 1065–1071

Olds, J. and Milner, P. (1954). Positive reinforcement produced by electrical stimulation of septal area and other regions of rat brain. *Journal of Comparative Physiology and Psychology* **47**, 419–427

Omer, G. E. (1968). Evaluation and reconstruction of the forearm and the hand after acute traumatic peripheral nerve injuries. *Journal of Bone and Joint Surgery* **50A**, 1454–1478

Onne, L. (1962). Recovery of sensibility and sudomotor activity in the hand after nerve suture. *Acta Chirurgica Scandinavica* Suppl. 300

Osborne, G. (1970). Compression neuritis of the ulnar nerve at the elbow. *The Hand* **2**, 10–13

Owen, E. (1976). Editorial. *Journal of Bone and Joint Surgery* **58B**, 397–398

Paul, R. L., Goodman, H. and Merzimch, M. (1972). Alterations in mechanoreceptor input to Brodman's areas one and three in the postcentral hand area of *Macaca mulatta* after nerve section and regeneration. *Brain Research Reports* **39**, 1–19

Payan, J. (1970). Anterior transposition of the ulnar nerve; an electrophysiological study. *Journal of Neurology, Neurosurgery and Psychiatry* **33**, 157–165

Pulvertaft, R. G. and Campbell Reid, D. A. (1963). Surgery of the hand in Great Britain. *British Journal of Surgery* **50**, 673–688

Randsford, A. O. and Hughes, P. F. (1977). Complete brachial plexus lesions. *Journal of Bone and Joint Surgery* **59B**, 417–442

Reynolds, D. V. (1969). Surgery in the rat during electrical analgesia induced by focal brain stimulation. *Science, New York* **164**, 444

Robins, R. H. C. (1961). *Injuries and Infections of the Hand*. London: Edward Arnold

Russel, W. R. and Harrington, A. B. (1944). Early diagnosis of peripheral nerve injuries in battle casualties. *British Medical Journal* **2**, 4

Santini, M. (1976). Towards a theory of sympathetic sensory coupling. In *Sensory Function of the Skin in Primates*, pp. 15–37. Ed. by Y. Zotterman. Oxford: Pergamon Press

Scott, P. J. and Huskisson, E. C. (1977). Measurement of functional capacity with visual analogue scales. *Rheumatology and Rehabilitation* **16**, 257–259

Seddon, H. J. (1952). Carpal ganglion as a cause of paralysis of the deep branch of the ulnar nerve. *Journal of Bone and Joint Surgery* **34B**, 386–390

Seddon, H. J. and Brooks, D. M. (1954). Open wounds of the brachial plexus. In *Peripheral Nerve Injuries*, p. 418. Ed. by H. J. Seddon. (Medical Research Council Special Reports Series, No. 282) London: HMSO

Shea, J. D. and McClain, E. J. (1969). Ulnar nerve compression syndrome at and below the wrist. *Journal of Bone and Joint Surgery* **51A**, 1095–1103

Sinclair, D. C. (1955). Cutaneous sensation and the doctrine of specific energy. *Brain* **78**, 584–614

Stevens, J. H. (1934). Brachial plexus paralysis. In *The Shoulder*, pp. 332–399. Ed. by E. A. Codman. Boston, Mass

Sunderland, S. (1944). Voluntary movements and the deceptive action of muscles in peripheral nerve lesions. *Australian and New Zealand Journal of Surgery* **13**, 160

Sunderland, S. (1975). The pros and cons of funicular nerve repair. *Journal of Hand Surgery* **3**, 201–211

Trojaborg, W. (1976). Motor and sensory conduction in the musculocutaneous nerve. *Journal of Neurology, Neurosurgery and Psychiatry* **39**, 890–899

Tubiana, R. (1969). Reconstruction of the thumb. *Journal of Bone and Joint Surgery* **51A**, 643–660

Tubiana, R. and Duparc, J. (1960). Restoration of sensibility in the hand by neurovascular skin island transfer. *Journal of Bone and Joint Surgery* **43B**, 474–480

Vallbo, A. B. and Hagbarth, K. E. (1968). Activity from skin mechanoreceptors recorded percutaneously in awake subjects. *Experimental Neurology* **21**, 270–289

Wall, P. D. (1961). Two transmission systems for skin sensations. In *Sensory Communication*, pp. 475–496. Ed. by W. A. Rosenblith. Cambridge, Mass: MIT Press

Wall, P. D. (1967). The laminar organisation of dorsal horn and effects of descending impulses. *Journal of Physiology* **188**, 403–423

Wall, P. D. and Gutnik, M. (1974). Properties of afferent nerve impulses originating from a neuroma. *Nature, London* **248**, 740–743

Wallin, G., Torebjork, E. and Hallin, R. (1976). Preliminary observations on the pathophysiology of hyperalgesia in the causalgic pain syndrome. In *Sensory Function of the Skin in Primates*, pp. 489–502. Ed. by Y. Zotterman. Oxford: Pergamon Press

Weddell, G. (1961). Receptors for somatic sensation. In *Brain and Behavior*, vol. 1, pp. 13–48. Ed. by M. A. R. Brazier. Washington DC: American Institute of Biological Sciences

White, J. C. (1954). Conduction of pain in man: observations on its afferent pathways within spinal cord and visceral nerves. *American Medical Association Archives of Neurology and Psychiatry* **71**, 1–23

White, J. C. and Sweet, W. H. (1969). *Pain and the Neurosurgeon*. Springfield, Ill: Charles C. Thomas

Wynn Parry, C. B. (1970). New types of lively splints for peripheral nerve lesions affecting the hand. *The Hand* **2**, 31–38

Wynn Parry, C. B. (1974). The management of injuries to the brachial plexus. *Proceedings of the Royal Society of Medicine* **67**, 488–490

Wynn Parry, C. B. and Salter, M. (1976). Sensory re-education after median nerve lesions. *The Hand* **8**, 250–256

Yeoman, P. M. and Seddon, H. J. (1961). Brachial plexus injuries: treatment of flail arm. *Journal of Bone and Joint Surgery* **43B**, 493–500

Zancolli, E. and Mitre, H. J. (1972). Elbow flexoroplasty by a bipolar transposition of the latissimus dorsi. Reported to 27th Annual Meeting of American Society for Surgery of the Hand

Electrodiagnosis   4

Traditional methods of electrodiagnosis, using strength duration curves to detect the proportion of innervated to denervated muscle fibres, have been largely superseded by nerve conduction studies and electromyographic records of muscle activity which offer an accurate means of localizing the level of a lesion in the peripheral nerve, and demonstrate whether the lesion is in the anterior horn cell, peripheral nerve or muscle itself.

However, there is still a limited place for plotting strength duration curves for they provide a simple, quick, reliable and cheap method of determining whether denervation is present; if so, approximately how much, and, by serial studies, if reinnervation is proceeding satisfactorily.

The conduction of the nerve impulse and the subsequent contraction of muscle are associated with changes in membrane polarity which can be measured accurately by electrical methods. The use of stimulation techniques to study the state of innervation of the lower motor neuron dates back to the late nineteenth century, when Erb (1883) described the faradic-galvanic test.

In this test a short-duration current (originally using the output of an induction coil and hence called the faradic current) is passed through the muscle under test and it is noted if the muscle contracts or not, and if so, what amount of current is required. When using a faradic coil this value cannot be accurately measured and only a rough estimate can be made.

Next, a long-duration current, conventionally from a galvanic battery, is passed through the muscle and the type of muscle contraction obtained is noted – whether brisk or sluggish.

A normal innervated muscle contracts briskly with a low output from the faradic coil, and briskly also with a low output of the galvanic battery. A denervated muscle will not usually respond to the faradic current, though, if a high output is used, some denervated muscles will show a contraction. The contraction with the galvanic current is sluggish due to direct conduction of the current along the muscle fibres instead of via the intramuscular nerve fibres.

A sluggish response indicates only that some fibres are denervated, and partially denervated muscles can show a sluggish response in the presence of voluntary contraction.

Normal muscle, when cold, tends to contract sluggishly, as do muscles in myxoedema; in contrast, the response of denervated muscle when warm can become quite brisk. The clinical value of the sluggish response is therefore limited, merely drawing attention to the possibility of some denervation in the muscle under test. During reinnervation the muscle which has hitherto failed to respond to a faradic current now contracts weakly with a very high output. This so-called 'weak faradic response' has been widely misrepresented, for many who use the test have wrongly assumed that a denervated muscle will never contract with the faradic current, whereas Erb (1883) himself pointed out that denervated muscle would occasionally contract provided sufficient current was used. During World War II Ritchie (1954) had the opportunity of studying a large number of patients in whom the findings of the faradic-galvanic test were known and in whom the actual state of the lower motor neuron was also known. He found that the test was accurate in only 50 per cent of cases. Moreover, the better the physiotherapist carrying out the test, the more likely she was to be wrong in her assessment of the case. The more efficient physiotherapist kept her faradic coil in better condition and encouraged patients to tolerate higher outputs than her more timid colleagues. Thus she would obtain a higher proportion of positive responses in denervated muscles and often concluded wrongly that this meant recovery or lack of degeneration. Frequently, too, it was observed that muscles would not show a faradic response when some voluntary movement was clearly present. Moreover, using an electronic stimulator, Wynn Parry (1953) has shown that 76 per cent of denervated muscles will respond to the 1 ms output. The test will, if interpreted thus, be still more inaccurate using modern equipment with its higher output and more comfortable stimulus. The test is qualitative only; it will not allow serial expression of the state of the lower motor neuron, and in view of the fallacies described above it is entirely unsuitable for clinical use. With the established use of strength duration curves and their sound basis in routine practice, there is no longer any place for the faradic-galvanic test; requests to physiotherapists for its perform-ance should cease and the term reaction of degeneration (RD) should be dropped.

STRENGTH DURATION CURVES

Rationale

This method allows the expression of the characteristic excitability-response of the tissue under test, in graphical form. A long-duration square wave electrical impulse is applied to the muscle under test and the amount of current required to elicit minimal contraction (rheobase) is measured and expressed in milliamps or volts. The duration of the impulse is progressively shortened and the intensity of current required to produce minimal contraction is measured for each duration. A curve relating strength of current and duration of impulse can now be drawn. In normally innervated muscle the intensity of current for minimal contraction is the same over a wide range of pulse durations and has only to be increased when very short pulse durations are used. This is due to the much lower excitability of muscle compared with that of the nerve (chronaxie 3 ms or greater). In partially innervated muscle, the curve is broken, showing elements of both excitable tissues – muscle and nerve. This break is known as a kink or a discontinuity; *Figure 4.1* shows the three curves of normal, denervated and partially innervated muscle.

It can be seen from *Figure 4.1* that the excitability curve of muscle is the same shape as that of nerve but is shifted to the right. If the muscle curve were prolonged to the right it would be horizontal, as the point obtained by using a pulse of 100 ms duration is by definition the rheobase and represents the threshold of the tissue.

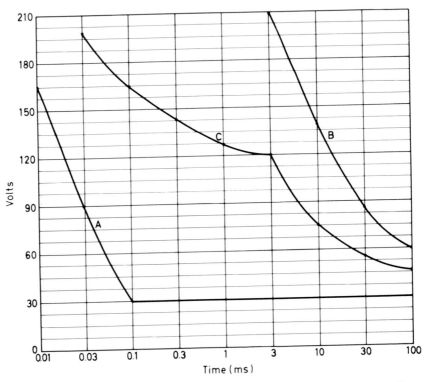

Figure 4.1 Strength duration curves on normal (A), denervated (B), and partially innervated (C) muscle. The top left-hand portion of curve C represents the activity of reinnervated fibres (compare with A); the bottom right-hand portion represents the activity of still denervated fibres (compare with B)

The earliest signs of reinnervation after degeneration on the strength duration curve are the appearances of discontinuities, the presence of more points on the curve and a shift of the curve to the left (*Figure 4.2*).

Should recovery be halted, the curve will reflect this by showing no change at repeated intervals. In the same way, in progressive denervation the curve will show gradually increasing abnormality with the appearance of kinks, a rise in slope and a shift to the right. Abbreviated tests such as the 100/1 ms ratio are open to the same objections as chronaxie and are not recommended. Plotting a strength duration (SD) curve offers the full facts of the excitability of the tissue, and is easily and rapidly accomplished. The SD curve will show only the state of innervation of the fibres stimulated by the current but in small muscles (such as the intrinsic muscles of the hand) the curve is likely to give a true picture of the state of the whole muscle, although in a very large muscle (such as the quadriceps) it may be that the superficial fibres which are most easy to stimulate are in a different state of innervation from the deeper ones and that the SD curve will not, therefore, give a true picture of the activity of the whole muscle.

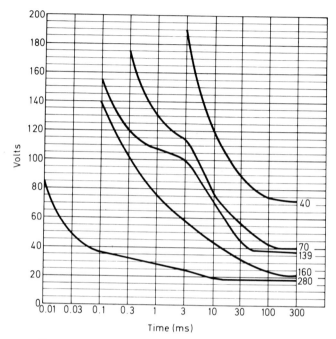

Figure 4.2   Strength duration curves on the abductor digiti minimi in a recovering ulnar nerve lesion. From above down the curves are 40, 70, 139, 160 and 280 days, respectively, after secondary nerve suture. All the signs of progressive reinnervation are seen on the curve — shift to the left, lowering of slope and development of kinks

It is well known that in motor neuron disease a muscle may be severely wasted and weak, yet the strength duration curve can be surprisingly normal and the electromyogram may show little or no fibrillation. In states of chronic denervation, denervated fibres are incorporated into a surviving motor unit, by sprouts from normal axons. Thus, there are few denervated muscle fibres left to give their characteristic electrical response in the SD curve.

Rheobase

The rheobase of a tissue is defined as the amount of current passing for an infinite duration required to cause minimal detectable response. For practical purposes, infinite duration is taken to be any value of 100 ms or greater. In denervated muscle the rheobase represents the excitability threshold of muscle tissue, while in normally innervated muscle the rheobase represents the excitability threshold of the intra-muscular nerve fibres. The rheobase varies for different muscles. Facial muscles have a very low rheobase (1–2 V) while in proximal limb muscles the average is 15–30 V, and in small hand muscles 40–60 V. A sudden rise in the value of rheobase is often regarded as evidence of recovery but Wynn Parry (1953) found no change in the rheobase with reinnervation in 60 per cent of a series of 101 cases of peripheral nerve injury.

Chronaxie

This is a measure of excitability and is defined as the minimum time required to excite the tissue with a stimulus of twice the rheobase. Special instruments known as chronaximeters were once used to determine chronaxie. A range of condensers of different capacities were charged to a potential of twice the rheobase and then discharged. The capacity required to produce minimal muscular contraction was then found and the chronaxie was calculated by multiplying by a constant which depended upon the particular instrument. The chronaxie can easily be obtained from the SD curve by finding the point where the curve cuts the abscissa at twice the rheobase (see *Figure 4.1*).

Chronaxie, like rheobase, is subject to the same variations in temperature, blood supply, skin resistance and oedema. The value of chronaxie in a partial lesion will depend on the shape of the s.d. curve. If the curve has a high slope in the right-hand portion with a kink to the left, the chronaxie will be long and will suggest total denervation. Similarly, if the curve has a low slope with the kink to the right, the chronaxie will be short and will suggest normal innervation. Thus there is a real source of error in relying on chronaxie as the sole index of the state of innervation. The tendency will be for it to be long in the early stages of reinnervation when the SD curve shows undoubted recovery, and to be short in the early stages of denervation when the SD curve will show a marked kink (*Figure 4.2*). Harris (1962) exhaustively reviewed the value of chronaxie and came to the same conclusion as Ritchie (1954) and Wynn Parry (1953), that chronaxie is of little value in diagnosis and dangerously misleading in prognosis or in the serial assessment of reinnervation or denervation.

Technique of strength duration curves

The muscle under examination must be well lit and warm. The skin should be clean but elaborate precautions in an attempt to lower skin resistance are not needed. Although skin resistance is theoretically more likely to be of importance when using a constant voltage stimulator, in practice it can be ignored. Experiments on various methods of lowering skin resistance have been carried out by the author (Wynn Parry, 1971), which show that the shape of the curve is exactly the same whether or not it is lowered to its minimum. As the maximum difference between the threshold of curves before and after lowering skin resistance was 10 V, this question need cause no concern.

Two techniques are available – the unipolar and bipolar methods. In the unipolar method a large dispersive electrode is placed behind the neck and upper back when testing the arm muscles, and a small active electrode is used to stimulate this muscle. In the bipolar technique, two similar electrodes are used and are placed on either side of and equidistant from the 'motor point' of the muscle to be tested. In both techniques the active electrodes must be kept moist throughout the test. With the unipolar technique the active electrode should be placed over the motor point. A convenient diameter for active electrodes is 1 cm.

Using the 100 ms pulses the voltage at which the minimum response occurs is measured – this is the rheobase.

As soon as the rheobase has been determined, the pulse selector switch is turned to the next shortest pulse duration and the amount of current required for minimal contraction is again determined. This is repeated for each pulse duration down to the 0.01 ms pulse or as far as a response can be obtained. Should the operator be inexperienced, or if the charting of the curve presents peculiar difficulty, the electrode should be frequently moistened because the rheobase will become much higher if the electrode is dry. An audible signal is most useful to indicate to the operator when the stimulus arrives.

The SD curve is a reliable method of detecting slight signs of denervation, by the presence of a kink or discontinuity in the curve. Trojaborg (1962) showed a good correlation between abnormalities in SD curves and reduced conduction velocity in neuropathies. The SD curves were normal in over two-thirds of 44 patients in whom conduction velocity was normal. He pointed out that in some partial traumatic lesions the fast-conducting motor fibres may survive, giving a normal conduction latency, yet the SD curve is clearly abnormal. Moody (1965), in a study of carcinomatous neuromyopathy, stated, 'In the present study an abnormal SD curve was always associated with slowed motor conduction in the nerve to the muscle and in every case in which motor conduction was reduced, there was an abnormality in the SD curve; this correlation suggests that all the large diameter fast-conducting fibres of the nerve are affected early in the disorder.'

The time lag between the appearance of nascent polyphasic ('recovery') units in the electromyogram and a kink in an SD curve previously typical of total denervation is usually only 10–14 days, and unless there is urgent need of electromyography to settle the issue, either for medicolegal reasons or because surgical treatment is proposed, EMG is not usually necessary in the routine follow-up of peripheral nerve injuries. The SD curve allows a fairly accurate and quick means of assessing the proportion of denervated to innervated fibres and can be used as a guide to the severity of denervation; it may also be helpful in following the progress of a case when serial curves are plotted at regular intervals. This is particularly valuable when a rapid survey of many muscles is required, as for instance in a brachial plexus palsy with multiple root or cord involvement.

Clinical applications

It must be emphasized that SD curves only offer information on the presence or absence of denervation and an approximate index of its extent. They give no guide to the localization of the lesion in the anterior horn cell, peripheral nerve or muscle. This can be obtained only from a study of the type and amount of motor unit activity observed in the electromyogram and from a consideration of conduction velocities in the peripheral nerves at various levels. It may therefore be unnecessary to plot SD curves in a case where there is obvious wasting and weakness, and the problem is to determine the level of the lesion in the lower motor neuron or the site of compression of a peripheral nerve. In young children, it is better to study the electromyogram first and only subsequently to plot an SD curve, as the procedure may be distressing and general anaesthesia may be necessary in the very young.

Direct nerve stimulation

In this technique nerves are stimulated with a short-duration (1 ms) current at accessible points and the muscle is observed to see if it contracts and, if so, at what threshold, the threshold to stimulation between the two sides being measured when appropriate. Thus at Erb's point (at the root of the neck) the C5, 6, 7 roots and sometimes in thin subjects C8, T1 roots can be stimulated; in the axilla all three nerves are excitable. The radial nerve can be stimulated in the spiral groove and just above the elbow and the median and ulnar nerves at the elbow and wrist. One must observe if muscles normally supplied by that nerve respond or if there are anomalies of innervation, which occur in some 20 per cent of normal subjects.

The most common anomaly is for the ulnar nerve to supply all the flexor pollicis brevis, the opponens or the second lumbrical, the median nerve to supply the third lumbrical or all the flexor pollicis brevis. Cases of complete ulnar or median supply to all the intrinsics are not excessively rare – although the median supply to abductor pollicis brevis is sufficiently constant for it to be chosen for conduction studies in suspected median nerve lesions. Anomalies of sensory supply are also common and there is no correlation between motor and sensory anomalies, nor are they symmetrical; subjects can have a markedly anomalous nerve supply in one hand and a 'textbook' supply in the other. It is common, too, for fibres from the median nerve to cross over to the ulnar at some point in the forearm and this can furnish puzzling situations in the diagnosis of neuropathies. It is therefore essential that every electrodiagnostic examination of the hand musculature starts with percutaneous stimulation of the median and ulnar nerves at the elbow and wrist, and by carefully observing which muscles respond. If stimulation of the ulnar nerve at the wrist demonstrates activity in muscles conventionally supplied by the median nerve, quantitative studies should be undertaken – surface electrodes are placed over the abductor pollicis brevis and abductor digiti minimi, and the amplitudes to supramaximal stimulation measured on stimulation of both median and ulnar nerves at wrist and elbow; this will reveal any significant degree of cross-over in the forearm.

When a hysterical palsy is suspected, the demonstration of strong contractions of the paralysed muscles on nerve stimulation, the normal SD curves and normal amplitudes to supramaximal stimulation, will exclude an organic lesion of the peripheral nerve.

In a neurapraxia a response below the level of block indicates that there is little or no degeneration. Occasionally with a high output one can get a response above the block and if the SD curve is also normal one can thus give a good prognosis. The electromyogram will be no help because there will be no signs of denervation until 21 days and, if there is a block only, no motor units will be under voluntary control. This test is particularly valuable in patients with a dropped wrist due to a pressure palsy.

ELECTROMYOGRAPHY

Rationale

In this technique a surface or needle electrode picks up electrical activity in muscle which is displayed on a cathode ray oscilloscope and the sound recorded on a loudspeaker. The apparatus has facilities for stimulating nerve and triggering the time base so that the response to a stimulus is related in time. The normal motor subunit comprises the anterior horn cell, its axons and 20–50 muscle fibres. These subunits are scattered about in three dimensions in muscle so that subunits of different anterior horn cells lie close together.

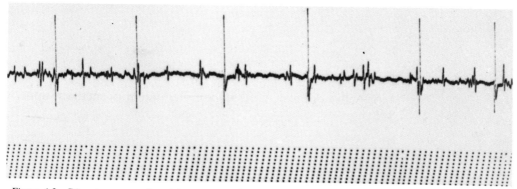

Figure 4.3   Discrete motor unit activity on minimal effort in a normal subject. Time scale 10 ms; amplitude 200 μV

Minimal contraction comprises the discharge of one motor subunit (*Figure 4.3*) and increasing demand involves an increase in the number of units and their frequency of discharge, until on maximum effort the whole trace on the cathode ray oscilloscope is obliterated, giving the so-called full interference pattern (*Figure 4.4*).

The normal motor subunit has an amplitude of 300 μV to 5 mV – according to the type of muscle. The small muscles of the hand may have units up to 5 mV. If many anterior horn cells are lost or axons have degenerated there is a reduction in the interference pattern.

In chronic partial denervation, degenerated muscle fibres secrete a neurotrophic substance which attracts collateral sprouts from neighbouring intact axons; thus the motor unit has many more muscle fibres than normal, and so the motor unit is much enlarged on the screen. This is seen as the so-called 'giant' unit and may be up to 10 mV in amplitude (*Figure 4.5*).

In the embryo, before being innervated by the nerve at the sixth week, muscle fibres are in a state of constant activity, each fibre contracting regularly and

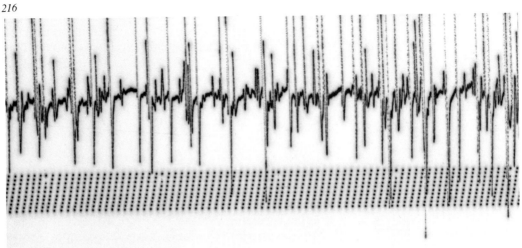

Figure 4.4 Full interference pattern of normal motor unit activity. Time scale 10 ms; amplitude 200 μV

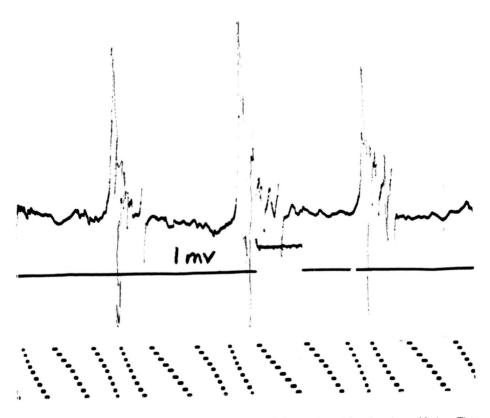

Figure 4.5 Giant units in the first dorsal interosseus muscle in a patient with a chronic cord lesion. Time scale 10 ms; amplitude 1 mV

spontaneously – so-called fibrillation. After the muscle is innervated, this activity ceases and the muscle fibre only contracts with the others in the subunit to give a motor unit discharge under voluntary control. Some 18–21 days after denervation, muscle fibres revert to their embryonic behaviour and start to discharge spontaneously and rhythmically. This is seen on the electromyogram as fibrillation. These potentials have an amplitude of 100–200 μV and a duration of 0.5–1 ms (*Figure 4.6*).

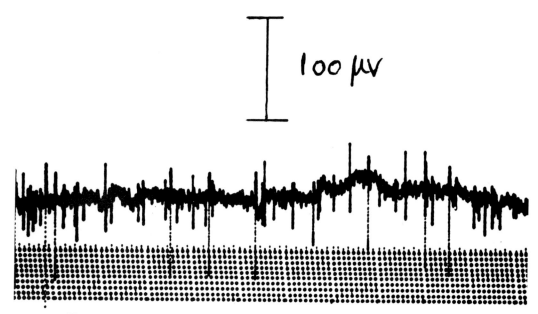

Figure 4.6   Spontaneous fibrillation. Time scale 10 ms; actual amplitude of unit 80 μV

The amount of fibrillation is some guide to the amount of surviving muscle tissue; healthy denervated muscle should fibrillate freely. If the nerve does not reinnervate the muscle, fibrillation will gradually decrease as the muscle becomes fibrotic – starting after 18–24 months. As reinnervation starts, fibrillation stops suddenly. At the beginning of reinnervation the motor unit comprises only a few muscle fibres, as reinnervation of fibres takes place gradually. Moreover, the myelin sheath takes a long time to mature and so the speed of conduction along the preterminal axons is slow. This causes a temporal dispersion in the motor unit which has a longer duration than normal and is polyphasic, while the amplitude is lower because there are fewer fibres within the unit. In degeneration, similar potentials will be seen as the motor unit disintegrates (*Figure 4.7*).

In myopathies, where the lesion may be primarily one of muscle fibres, motor units are much smaller than normal because individual fibres are lost within the unit; however, whole units are not lost and thus the interference pattern is not reduced. So a full interference pattern of short-duration low-amplitude units, which on the loudspeaker give characteristic harsh sounds, is typical of muscle disease (*Figure 4.8*). In pure degenerative myopathies spontaneous fibrillation is not usually seen, but in inflammatory diseases of muscles (e.g. polymyositis) the nerve terminals may be involved and spontaneous fibrillation may be quite a prominent feature.

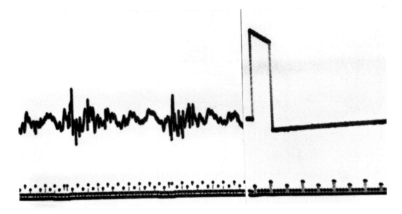

Figure 4.7   Polyphasic units in recovering nerve lesion. Time scale 5 and 10 ms; amplification 1 mV

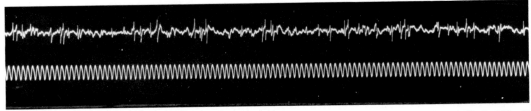

Figure 4.8   Motor units in heredofamilial muscular dystrophy. Time scale 2 ms peak to peak; amplitude 100 μV

So far we have been considering the shape, amplitude, duration and amounts of fibres as seen on the screen or measured from film. This will help to establish denervation and reinnervation, but in order to distinguish lesions of the axon from the anterior horn cell and to localize the level of a pressure lesion it is necessary to measure the conduction velocity at various levels of the nerve in the limb.

Technique of measuring motor conduction velocity

A needle or surface electrode is placed in or on muscle and a stimulus applied to the nerve at various levels, such as the axilla, elbow and wrist, and, using supramaximal stimulation, the latency is measured. This is the time from stimulation to first deflection of the motor unit action potential (*Figure 4.9*).

The distance between the points of stimulation is measured and velocities are calculated.

If it is necessary to detect spontaneous fibrillation, the motor conduction velocity is measured using concentric needle electrodes, taking care that the same unit is responding at each level by observing that the shape is the same at each level. It is useful in some instances to measure the total activity of muscle in response to nerve stimulation using a surface electrode and supramaximal stimuli measuring the amplitude from the 'isoelectric line' to peak. This allows the estimate of the amount of activity and, therefore, the number of fibres responding. If the faster fibres are spared (as may happen) velocities will be normal but amplitudes may be lower than normal, indicating fibre loss. This was elegantly shown by Fullerton (1966) in a group of patients with lead poisoning who retained their fast conducting fibres but lost the slower fibres.

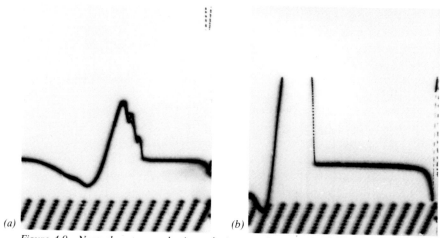

Figure 4.9   Normal motor conduction velocity recording with needle electrode in abductor pollicis brevis and stimulating (a) at wrist and (b) at elbow. Time scale 1 ms

Gombault in 1880 described myelin disappearing from part or the whole of an internodal segment without distal generation in guinea-pigs who had been poisoned with lead. In 1957 Waksman, Adams and Mansmann showed that experimental diphtheritic neuropathy in guinea-pigs and rabbits was associated with severe segmental demyelination, starting close to the nodes of Ranvier. Kaiser and Lambert (1962) then studied conduction velocity in such guinea-pigs and showed marked slowing down to 20 m/s with temporal dispersion. McDonald (1962) showed that this was due to segmental demyelination, not to drop-out of fast fibres. On recording in the nerve roots with single fibres he was able to show that conduction in the peripheral nerve was normal and that the velocity decreased only when different impulses reached the roots where segmental demyelination had occurred. It is known that guinea-pigs kept in wire mesh cages develop a neuropathy of the plantar nerves of the hind foot and histological examination shows localized demyelination with slowing of conduction in the leg but very marked slowing in the foot, suggesting that the toxin made the nerve abnormally vulnerable to pressure. Hopkins and Morgan Hughes (1969) have kept guinea-pigs in slings and shown that they do not develop distal slowing.

In poisoning with triorthocresyl phosphate, isoniazid or nitrofurantoin, the neuropathy is due to primary neuronal damage with scanty segmental demyelination – the primary disorder is in the axis cylinder. The amplitude to supramaximal response falls rapidly, indicating loss of fibres, but the conduction velocity remains normal.

Fullerton and Barnes (1966) studied acrylamide neuropathy in rats (a poison in man) and showed only slight reduction in conduction velocity; this was confirmed in baboons, and fibre counts showed that the slight slowing was due to loss of large-diameter fibres, which conduct at the faster rates. It is now believed that there are two types of neuropathy: those in which the disease process affects the myelin and is therefore associated with marked slowing of conduction, and those affecting the axis cylinders direct, causing drop-out of fibres in a random fashion.

In neuropathies due to segmental demyelination very low values for conduction velocity can be found – down to 5 or 10 m/s, for the mechanism of saltatory conduction is lost and values approaching pure cable conduction are found. In neuropathies due to axis cylinder drop-out the velocity is 30–40 per cent below the maximum conduction velocity (i.e. 35–40 m/s). As drop-out occurs in a random fashion, some nerves will conduct normally, since the fastest conducting fibres may be spared while others, in whom the fastest fibres are affected first, will show velocities of 40 m/s (i.e. the speed of the smallest diameter fibres). It is therefore important in electromyography to study the motor conduction velocity in several nerves.

The mechanism of pressure lesions of peripheral nerves is believed now to be due to derangement of the myelin at the level of the lesion by mechanical compression. Conduction is slowed over the compressed segment but will be normal above and below. Thus, measuring conduction velocities at various levels in the limb will help determine the level of the lesion.

For example, in a case of ulnar neuritis caused by compression of the nerve at the elbow, the latency to abductor digiti minimi stimulating the ulnar nerve at the wrist will be normal, and normal also when stimulating below the elbow. However, when the electrode is moved above the elbow, the latency will be prolonged. Sometimes the latencies may be normal in a case of ulnar neuritis at the elbow if the fastest fibres have been spared. In such a case measurement of the amplitude, using surface electrodes, to supramaximal stimulation may show reduction of the amplitude between stimulation above the elbow and at the wrist, indicating that some fibres are not responding (*Figure 4.10*). Reduction of more than 20 per cent between elbow and wrist is taken as significant.

A well recognized clinical disorder of the ulnar nerve is compression of the deep branch in the palm, following repeated pressure, due to occupational causes such as despatch riders or drivers of heavy lorries using powerful gears.

The deep branch supplies all the interossei, medial two lumbricals, adductor and flexor pollicis brevis, and these muscles will be weak or paralysed.

The superficial branch supplies sensation and the abductor digiti minimi, and will be spared in lesions of the deep branch.

Thus, stimulation of the nerve at the wrist and recording with a needle electrode in the abductor digiti minimi will produce a response of normal latency and normal compact shape. When recording in the first dorsal interosseus the response will be delayed and dispersed due to derangement of the myelin (see *Figure 4.13c*).

In the carpal tunnel syndrome, pressure on the median nerve at the wrist causes localized demyelination and, thus, slowing of conduction across this segment. The normal latency from the wrist to the abductor pollicis brevis should be less than 5 ms. Values greater than 6 ms but less than 7 ms indicate a moderate degree of compression.

Goodman and Gilliatt (1961) showed that if the latency is greater than 7 ms, conservative treatment using splints or steroid injections will not be successful and surgery is required.

Thus, electromyography is useful not only in diagnosing the condition but also in indicating the severity and, so, suggesting the appropriate course of treatment. Occasionally latencies may be normal despite an obvious clinical picture of the carpal tunnel syndrome. In such cases, if the difference between the latencies for median and ulnar nerves is more than 1.5 ms, despite the median latency being within the usually accepted normal limits, then there is a lesion of the nerve at the wrist.

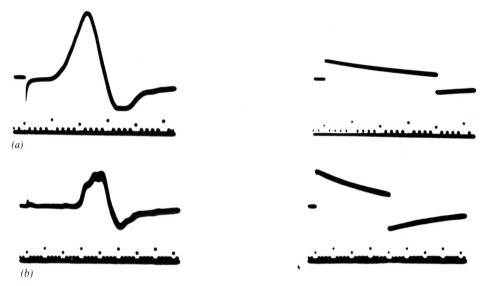

(a)

(b)

Figure 4.10   Stimulation of ulnar nerve (a) just below the elbow and (b) just above the elbow in a patient with ulnar neuritis due to compression of the nerve at the elbow by a tight band. Recording using surface electrodes over abductor digiti minimi; amplitude 1 mV; time scale 1 ms. Note prolonged latency and grossly diminished amplitude above elbow

Sometimes a delayed response to threshold stimulation (i.e. very weak shocks) is seen. This is called a late unit and indicates compression of the nerve which is pathologically excitable. This may be the only sign of nerve damage and it is therefore important to look for the response to such minimal shocks and not only to look for the response to supramaximal stimuli which may be normal (Preswick, 1963).

Sensory studies

The refinement of apparatus and technique has allowed measurement of conduction in sensory fibres (Gilliatt and Thomas, 1960). In this technique ring electrodes are placed round the index or little finger, or indeed any digit, and the sensory action potential is recorded over the nerves at the wrist with surface electrodes. If good amplifiers are used with a low noise level, and if there is no interference and the patient relaxes well, the technique is easy. The normal median sensory action potential has an amplitude of 10 μV or more and a latency of 3 ms or less, the ulnar sensory potential 9 μV or more and a latency of 3 ms or less (*Figure 4.11*).

The radial sensory action potential can be measured using an antidromic technique, stimulating in mid-forearm and recording with surface electrodes over the first dorsal interosseus space – amplitudes are 30 μV or more and latencies 4 ms or less. The demonstration of a normal radial sensory action potential in the presence of weakness of C7 muscles or paraesthesiae in C7 distribution will be helpful confirmation of a root lesion, not a nerve lesion. Sensation is affected earlier in some polyneuropathies and although objective signs of sensory disturbance may not be present, sensory action potentials are lost. This is particularly evident in the early stages of the Guillain–Barré syndrome. Sensory potentials are lost early in the carpal tunnel syndrome, often before motor latencies are prolonged, and should be routinely studied in all suspected cases; they are also a good guide to recovery after surgery (*Figure 4.12*).

Sometimes the localization of a lesion can be difficult, for motor conduction velocity may be normal and amplitudes to supramaximal stimulation at various levels may also be normal. In such cases stimulation of the nerve at the wrist and recording over the nerve with surface electrodes at the elbow will give a mixed motor and sensory response and may show a difference between the two sides. The demonstration of a normal mixed potential stimulating above the elbow and recording in the axilla, when abnormalities have been demonstrated in finger to wrist or wrist to elbow studies, will firmly localize the lesion to the elbow.

Sensory action potentials are valuable in distinguishing pre- and postganglionic lesions of the brachial plexus. The presence of normal sensory action potential in the anaesthetic hand indicates a preganglionic lesion and a bad prognosis. Its absence may indicate a postganglionic lesion.

In axis cylinder disease, as already mentioned, slowing of conduction is mild; thus in motor neuron disease conduction velocities in median and ulnar nerves may be 40 m/s. The sensory action potentials are normal because the sensory system is not affected. The electromyogram shows a reduced pattern of giant units. This picture is not diagnostic of motor neuron disease or myelopathy; any condition of chronic partial denervation will lead to this phenomenon and is therefore seen in poliomyelitis, syringomyelia and the rare chronic motor neuropathies, but in practice motor neuron disease is the most common cause. If denervation can be demonstrated in the legs this will clearly point to a motor system disease and distinguishes cervical spondylosis causing lower motor neuron signs in the arms and upper motor neuron signs in the legs.

Symptoms of paraesthesiae in the median distribution, so typical of a carpal tunnel syndrome, may be the first indication of a widespread polyneuropathy (e.g. alcoholism, diabetes and collagen disease) and it is therefore always advisable to look at one other nerve as well as the contralateral median nerve. A recommended routine in a case of suspected carpal tunnel syndrome is as follows.

(1)   Response to percutaneous nerve stimulation at elbow and wrist to detect any anomalous nerve supply.

(2)   Insertion of a concentric needle electrode in abductor pollicis brevis to detect spontaneous fibrillation and to study the number, shape and amount of motor units on volition; e.g. polyphasic or giant units.

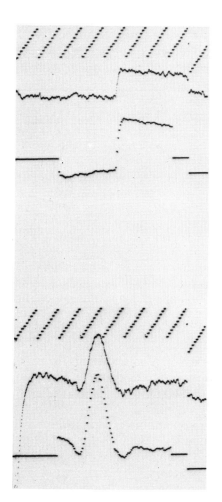

Figure 4.11 *Normal sensory action potential. Stimulating index with ring electrodes and recording with surface electrodes over the median nerve at the wrist. Time scale 1 ms; amplitude 10 μV*

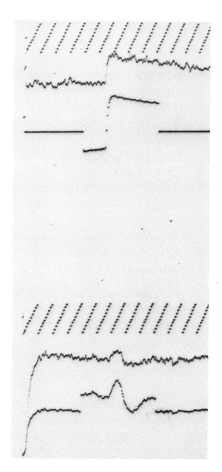

Figure 4.12 *Diminished amplitude and prolonged latency of sensory action potential in a patient with the carpal tunnel syndrome. Index finger stimulated with ring electrodes and recording made with surface electrodes over the wrist. Time scale 1 ms; amplitude 10 μV. Lower tracing average of 30 responses*

(3) Stimulation of the median nerve at the wrist with threshold shocks to demonstrate any late units and then supramaximal shocks to obtain the latency of the fastest conducting fibres at the wrist and elbow, thus measuring conduction velocity in the forearm.

(4) Measurement of amplitude and latency of the sensory action potential stimulating index and recording over median nerve at the wrist.

(5) Measurement of amplitude and latency to peak of the sensory action potential stimulating the little finger and recording over the ulnar nerve at the wrist.

(6) Repeat steps (1) to (5) on the other side.

(7) If an abnormality is also seen in the ulnar nerve, then study motor conduction velocity and sensory conduction in legs. By this means one will avoid missing generalized disease.

A recommended routine in suspected ulnar nerve lesions is given below.

(1) Percutaneous stimulation of the ulnar and median nerves at wrist and elbow on both sides, observing muscles that respond to exclude any anomalous supply.

(2) Insertion of concentric needle electrode in abductor digiti minimi – look for spontaneous fibrillation, and numbers and types of units on volition. Stimulation of ulnar nerve at wrist and elbow and measurement of motor conduction velocity in forearm.

(3) Insertion of concentric needle electrode in the first dorsal interosseus – look for spontaneous fibrillation, and the numbers and types of units on volition. Measure latency to supramaximal stimulation to exclude a lesion of the deep branch of the ulnar nerve.

(4) With surface electrodes over the abductor digiti minimi, stimulate with supramaximal shocks at the wrist above and below the elbow and measure the amplitude to see if a decrement exists between above and below elbow.

(5) Measure amplitude and latency to peak of sensory action potential, stimulating little finger and recording over ulnar nerve at the wrist.

(6) Study sensory potential in median nerve to exclude a generalized neuropathy.

(7) Stimulate the ulnar nerve at the wrist, record above the elbow to measure amplitude and latency of the mixed action potential, and compare with result on the other arm.

(8) Stimulate the ulnar nerve above the elbow and record over axilla, measuring amplitude and latency.

The extent and order in which these tests are done will vary with clinical examination. If, for example, the clinical picture suggests a root lesion with paraesthesiae in ulnar distribution, it may only be necessary to demonstrate a normal sensory action potential from finger to wrist. Payan (1969) has shown how accurately ulnar nerve lesions can be localized by a rigorous and painstaking examination using needle electrodes to pick up the response of nerve at various levels. This may well take up to 3 hours but is well worth while if the above procedure does not give a clear answer – it must be realized that even the basic examination just described takes up to an hour. But the more experience one has in this field the more one realizes that a really thorough electrophysiological examination of many nerves will amply repay the time spent.

Rheumatoid arthritis

This systemic disease illustrates well how valuable EMG studies can be in elucidating the exact cause of neurological symptoms. The peripheral nervous system can be involved in several ways in rheumatoid disease. The most common is one of the entrapment neuropathies – pressure of rheumatoid synovitis on the median nerve in the carpal tunnel, effusion in the elbow joint pressing on the ulnar nerve, effusion in the knee joint compressing the lateral popliteal nerve. Indeed, symptoms of carpal tunnel syndrome may be the first indication of rheumatoid disease, and all patients who present with such symptoms must be carefully examined to see if there is any soft tissue swelling in the carpal tunnel and followed up carefully to see if they develop manifestations of the disease later. However, many patients with established rheumatoid arthritis develop symptoms of median nerve compression due to rheumatoid synovitis or wrist effusion and these symptoms may merge in the general picture of pain and limitation of joint movement. It is therefore most important to examine patients with rheumatoid arthritis at regular intervals with the possibility in mind that they may be developing a superimposed carpal tunnel syndrome. If there is any such suspicion they should be referred for electrodiagnosis, for timely decompression will relieve their symptoms due to mechanical causes – too often such cases are missed and the drug regimen is increased not only without benefit to the patient but with the attendant dangers of the drugs and increasing damage to the median nerve.

Pallis and Scott (1965) have described a type of sensory neuropathy in rheumatoid disease which affects the digital nerves in a patchy fashion and is not confined to the territory of one nerve. Measurements of sensory action potentials for each digit will clearly demonstrate the random involvement of sensory nerves in such cases.

Patients with severe rheumatoid arthritis may develop generalized polyneuritis; this is often associated with other systemic manifestations such as arteritis, lung involvement and high titres of rheumatoid factor. The demonstration of slowing of motor and sensory conduction in several nerves throughout their length will confirm the clinical diagnosis and exclude localized pressure lesions. Finally, rheumatoid arthritis affecting the cervical spine is being increasingly recognized and involvement of the atlantoaxial joint may cause cord compression with sensory symptoms in the hands and long tract signs in the legs. The signs in the legs may not be obvious either because the patient is bedridden by her disease or because the acutely painful joints in the lower limbs mask central nervous symptoms, and the paraesthesiae in the hand may be diagnosed as median nerve compression or generalized neuropathy. There, the demonstration of normal motor and sensory conduction in the nerves of the upper limbs will suggest a central cause for the symptoms and appropriate investigations and treatment of the cervical spine.

Brachial plexus palsies

As emphasized in Chapter 3, it is vital to determine as early as possible after an injury to the brachial plexus whether the lesion is preganglionic or postganglionic. EMG has several contributions to make in brachial plexus lesions. Sensory studies will distinguish pre- and postganglionic lesions. In the presence of an anaesthetic hand, the detection of normal sensory action potentials (SAPs) for the median and ulnar nerves must indicate that C8 and T1 roots are affected proximal to the posterior root ganglion. Absent SAPs, however, may mean a postganglionic lesion – they certainly indicate that there has been wallerian degeneration distal to the ganglion, although in some injuries there may be damage both proximal and distal to the ganglion; myelography may clarify the issue. The spinogram (page 164) is a more refined means of establishing the level of the lesion.

Sampling representative muscles supplied by each root will indicate if some, at any rate, of the nerve fibres are in continuity. Suggested sampling procedures are:

C5   Infraspinatus, deltoid
C6   Biceps
C7   Triceps, extensor carpi radialis longus
C8   Flexor digitorum sublimis or flexor carpi ulnaris
T1   Interossei or thenar group

In the early stages before fibrillation can be expected to develop (i.e. within the first 18 days after injury) EMG will be no help; not only will spontaneous fibrillation not be found but inhibition due to pain may make voluntary movement impossible. It is here that percutaneous nerve stimulation at Erb's point at the root of the neck may show a response in muscles supplied by C5, 6 roots and stimulation of the radial nerve, at the spiral groove and just above the elbow and the median and ulnar nerves at the elbow, may show responses in muscles supplied by C7, C8 and T1, respectively. Detection of spontaneous fibrillation in posterior cervical muscles will also show that the lesion is preganglionic, as their supply comes off the posterior primary ramus proximal to the ganglion. However, there is so much overlap of innervation that failure to detect spontaneous fibrillation does *not* mean that there has been no lesion of the lower motor neuron.

Electromyography now has a most important part to play in the operating theatre (page 167).

Peripheral nerve lesions

Electromyography can be most valuable in determining the extent of a traumatic lesion of a peripheral nerve. The detection of even one or two motor units under voluntary control, which will not be clinically detectable, will indicate that part at least of the nerve is in continuity and may profoundly affect the surgeon's attitude to surgery. The demonstration of profuse spontaneous fibrillation and absence of any units on volition will show that the lesion is complete, but will not of course decide if it is an axonotmesis or neurotmesis. This can only be determined on clinical grounds or at operation. Electromyography will help the surgeon determine the extent of a lesion by showing which muscles are denervated and which are not, and thus localize the level of damage. The first signs of reinnervation – the presence of low-amplitude polyphasic units – precede clinical signs of a flicker of voluntary movement by many weeks, and therefore EMG can be of value if performed at about the time after suture or damage that recovery would be expected, according to the usual rate of nerve regeneration. After a fracture of the mid-shaft of the humerus involving a complete radial nerve lesion, the first evidence of reinnervation of brachioradialis should occur about 100 days after injury and at this time sampling with concentric needle electrodes can be expected to show early recovery units. The absence of EMG signs of recovery at a time when they should be expected, if nerve regeneration were occurring, can be most valuable in helping the surgeon to decide on. exploration. As peripheral nerves regenerate, so the number of motor units under voluntary control increase, the amplitude to supramaximal stimulation increases, the motor conduction velocity increases and spontaneous fibrillation becomes increasingly difficult to detect. Sensory action potentials rarely return to normal – indeed with conventional surface recording techniques SAPs may never be elicited – for with sutured nerves there is always a degree of scarring at the wrist which effectively prevents the recording of a signal from the underlying nerve.

Electrical investigations at open operation (Kline and De Jonge, 1968) may be able to distinguish a recoverable lesion from one requiring suture. The nerve is stimulated above the lesion and recording made below. The presence of an action potential indicates that the lesion is in continuity.

It is important that EMG should not be regarded only as a means of confirming a lesion that is fairly obvious clinically. Certainly it is a wise precaution to ask for the electrical investigations before operating on a suspected compression lesion, for root pressure on C8 in cervical spondylosis can mimic the carpal tunnel syndrome remarkably faithfully, and the demonstration of normal motor and sensory latencies in a clinical setting of paraesthesiae in the median distribution – particularly if there is no more than 1 ms difference between the latency for median and ulnar nerves – may save the patient from an unnecessary operation and direct attention to treatment of the lesion in the neck. But even if the electrical tests do show a local compression lesion, it is always wise to examine at least one other nerve to ensure that one is not dealing with a generalized subclinical neuropathy. The nerves which commonly exhibit symptoms early in generalized neuropathies are often those that are most vulnerable to pressure – the median nerve in the carpal tunnel, the ulnar nerve at the elbow and the lateral popliteal nerve at the knee. Rheumatoid arthritis and myxoedema can both present at onset with symptoms of carpal tunnel compression, and ulnar neuritis may be the first manifestation of diabetic neuropathy. Thus, as a routine in the investigation of a carpal tunnel syndrome, we always record the ulnar sensory potential, and the contralateral median motor and sensory studies are also carried out. Philosophically speaking, EMG can be used as a means of trying to disprove what seems to be an obvious clinical diagnosis.

Normal results in patients with symptoms suggestive of peripheral nerve disorders can be of equal importance. We have referred already to the value of normal studies in differentiating carpal tunnel syndrome from cervical spondylosis; demonstration of normal ulnar motor and sensory conduction in patients with paraesthesiae in the ulnar distribution will suggest a proximal lesion such as a cervical rib or thoracic outlet syndrome.

Case 4.1. This patient had complained for several years of paraesthesiae in the median distribution of both hands. The symptoms were suggestive of carpal tunnel syndrome, being nocturnal and relieved by shaking the hands. Decompression was carried out without preoperative EMG studies, but symptoms were not relieved.

Subsequently the paraesthesiae became localized in the ulnar distribution of both hands and, again without EMG studies preoperatively, ulnar nerve transposition was carried out with no relief of symptoms. She was referred for EMG studies, her symptoms being worse than ever – with pins and needles in all fingers, some clumsiness in fine movements, but no true weakness and no wasting. Sensory conduction studies on both median and ulnar nerves were entirely normal.

Motor latencies from wrist to abductor pollicis brevis and abductor digiti minimi on both sides were normal and motor conduction velocity was normal for all nerves in the forearm. However, denervation was demonstrated in the interossei on both sides and in right abductor pollicis brevis. At first sight this suggested either a root or a cord lesion involving C8 and T1. Had only the interossei been denervated one could have postulated bilateral T1 compression lesions, but the involvement of abductor pollicis brevis implied a more sinister prognosis.

However, routine nerve stimulation of both nerves at elbow and wrist had demonstrated that on the right the thenar muscles were all supplied by the ulnar nerve, but were supplied by the median nerve on the left. It was thus likely that the patient had a bilateral T1 root lesion with an anomalous nerve supply. Subsequently, rudimentary cervical ribs were demonstrated which responded to treatment.

Several morals emerged from this case history. The importance of preoperative electrical studies to confirm the presence of nerve compression – four operations could have been avoided in this case – the importance of full investigation including sampling for denervation despite normal conduction studies, and the need to exclude or demonstrate an anomalous nerve supply.

Case 4.2. A labourer reported with sensory loss over the whole of the forearm and hand on both sides. There was no wasting of muscle. Sensory conduction tests for both median and ulnar nerves, and ulnar nerve on the right, were normal but that for the right median was absent. The normal conduction studies in the presence of absent sensation indicated a preganglionic lesion and were consistent with syringomyelia. The explanation for the absent sensory action potential for the median nerve became apparent when the conduction latency across the wrist was found to be 7 ms with normal motor conduction velocity in the forearm. There was thus a coexisting carpal tunnel syndrome.

Case 4.3. This patient presented with pain in the right shoulder, radiating down the right arm into the hand for 15 months. This had gradually become worse and began latterly to be associated with blanching of the hand and paraesthesiae in the ulnar two fingers. No muscle wasting or loss of power were noted but sensation was dull to pin-prick and cotton wool in the ulnar distribution. Both radial pulses were diminished with shoulder elevation. X-rays showed a large transverse process of C7 on the right and there was tenderness to deep pressure on the root of the neck.

EMG studies revealed normal sensory action potential of 10 μV amplitude and latency to peak 3 ms for the ulnar nerve stimulating the little finger and recording over the ulnar nerve at the wrist. Motor conduction velocity was 55 m/s in the forearm and there was no decrement in the amplitude to supramaximal shocks stimulating at the wrist and above the elbow, recording over the abductor digiti minimi with surface electrodes.

A diagnosis of root compression by a cervical rib or tight band was made and shoulder raising exercises were prescribed. These were ineffective and surgery was undertaken. A fibrous band deep to the scalenus anterior was found which compressed the plexus on shoulder depression. This was divided, with complete relief of symptoms. EMG had been useful in excluding a lesion at the elbow and confirmed the clinical impression of a thoracic inlet syndrome.

Case 4.4. A housewife complained of paraesthesiae, clumsiness and weakness in the median distribution of both hands. On examination she had blunting of sensation in the tips of the index and middle fingers of both hands and wasting of abductor pollicis brevis on both sides. She also had some wasting of the interossei on the muscles of the left hand but no sensory loss in the ulnar distribution. The question arose as to whether she was suffering from a generalized systemic peripheral neuropathy. SAPs were absent for both median nerves but normal for both ulnar nerves, stimulating index and little fingers and recording over the appropriate nerves at the wrist. Distal latencies were grossly abnormal, stimulating the median nerve at the wrist and recording with needle electrodes in abductor pollicis brevis on both sides (*Figure 4.13*). Distal latencies were normal, stimulating the ulnar nerves on both sides and recording with needle electrodes in abductor digiti minimi; however, the latency stimulating the ulnar nerve at the wrist and recording in the first dorsal interosseus was 3 ms on the right but 7 ms on the left, with marked dispersion of action potential (*Figure 4.13c*).

Motor conduction velocities in the lateral popliteal nerves were normal. Close questioning revealed that the patient had recently acquired a new washing machine which required a vigorous application of the palm of the left hand to a knob to make it work. The diagnosis of bilateral carpal tunnel syndrome and lesion of the deep branch of the ulnar nerve on the left was consequently made. Bilateral median nerve decompression and change of technique with the washing machine completely relieved her symptoms.

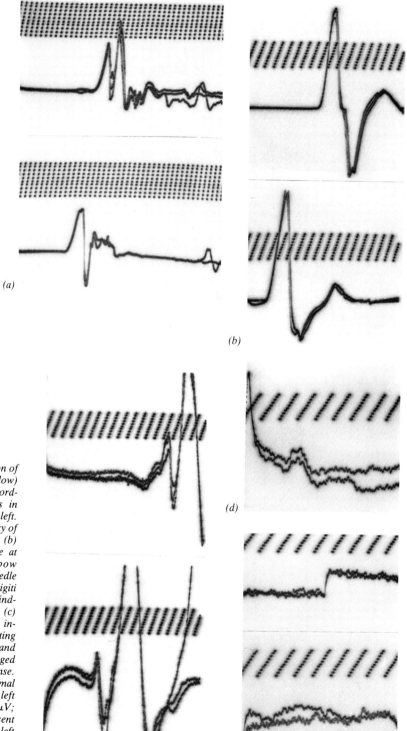

Figure 4.13 (a) Stimulation of median nerve at wrist (below) and at elbow (above), recording with needle electrodes in abductor pollicis brevis on left. Note prolonged distal latency of 9 ms. Time scale 1 ms. (b) Stimulation of ulnar nerve at wrist (below) and elbow (above), recording with needle electrodes in abductor digiti minimi on left — normal findings. Time scale 1 ms. (c) Recording in first dorsal interosseus on left, stimulating ulnar nerve at wrist (below) and elbow (above). Note prolonged latency and dispersed response. Time scale 1 ms. (d) Normal sensory action potential, left ulnar nerve. Amplitude 10 μV; time scale 1 ms. (e) Absent sensory action potential, left median nerve

Case 4.5. This patient presented with symptoms, which had been present for some months, of tingling in the ulnar two fingers of the right hand. There was mild subjective sensory disturbance, but no wasting and only slight weakness. The conduction studies listed in *Table 4.1* show the preoperative findings and the improvement in nerve action potential, motor unit action potential and conduction velocity 3 months after transposition of the ulnar nerve at the elbow. The sensory action potential finger to wrist may take many months or years to reappear.

Case 4.6. This patient had had her ulnar nerve transposed at the elbow in February 1975 for symptoms typical of ulnar neuritis, which were relieved temporarily. In November 1976 the question was raised as to whether the nerve needed reoperation, for the symptoms had recurred. Serial studies showed (*Table 4.2*) that the electrical findings were improving and it was subsequently shown that her symptoms were due to a cervical rib. Serial studies can be most helpful in deciding whether the condition is progressing, recovering or remaining static.

Table 4.3 shows how long the sensory conduction takes to recover after decompression. The antidromic technique was used in which an amplitude of 13 μV is well below normal.

Table 4.1 Transposition of right ulnar nerve, 3 September 1976

	2 Sep. 76	*9 Dec. 76*
Sensory action potential	Absent	Absent
Nerve action potential (μV)	10 (R = 30)	16
Motor unit action potential, elbow (mV)	1 (R = 5)	2.5
Motor conduction velocity (m/s)	27	44

Table 4.2 Transposition of ulnar nerve, February 1975 (Case 4.6); presented with pain and paraesthesiae, October 1976

	11 Nov. 76	*20 Jan. 76*
Sensory action potential (μV)	3	3
Nerve action potential (μV)	7	9
Motor unit action potential:		
Wrist (mV)	2	7
Elbow (mV)	3	5

Table 4.3 Left carpal tunnel syndrome; operation 24 May 1976

	1 Apr. 76	*21 June 76*	*22 July 76*
Right			
Amplitude (μV)	13	13	25
Latency (ms)	4.3	3.5	3.5
Left			
Amplitude (μV)	33	NS	33
Latency (ms)	3.2	NS	3.2

NS, not studied

Guillain–Barré syndrome

The hands are frequently involved in this condition. In the early stages there is clinical paralysis of the intrinsic muscles of the hand.

Electromyographic studies show highly typical findings. Distal latencies may be remarkably prolonged up to 10, 15 or 20 ms, but the amplitude to supramaximal stimulation at the wrist is usually within normal limits, while that at the elbow is grossly diminished, indicating a block to conduction, reflected pathologically in segmental demyelination in the nerve. Motor conduction velocities are usually slowed and become progressively slower as the disease continues; paradoxically, there are some cases in which the motor conduction velocity is relatively normal early in the disease, becoming slow as the patient begins to recover. This is compatible with segmental demyelination starting in the roots and progressing distally, for with segmental demyelination at root level motor conduction velocity is not affected distally.

Sensory studies can be very helpful, for sensory action potentials are often absent at an early stage when, clinically, sensation is normal. This is most valuable in the differential diagnosis, for it shows that one is dealing with a mixed sensorimotor neuropathy and not a purely motor disorder. Serial records of motor and sensory conduction are useful as an index of recovery, although distal latencies often remain prolonged for many months, even when the patient is clinically normal.

SUMMARY OF ELECTRODIAGNOSTIC FINDINGS IN LESIONS OF THE LOWER MOTOR NEURON

Myelopathy

This term is used to describe lesions of the anterior horn cell; for example, motor neuron disease (amyotrophic lateral sclerosis, progressive muscular atrophy), syringomyelia, poliomyelitis, transverse myelitis.

In the early stages spontaneous fibrillation may be readily found. Spontaneous fasciculation is common, motor units of large amplitude – 6 mV or more and polyphasic in shape – occurring irregularly and at a rate not usually exceeding 1 every 3 or 4 seconds. On volition, interference patterns will be moderately reduced with normal and giant units. Motor conduction velocity is normal or slowed to 40 per cent of maximum values but, as there is random drop-out of axons in this disease, some affected nerves will show normal motor conduction velocity. Amplitudes to supramaximal stimulation recording over the small muscles of the hand will be reduced in proportion to the loss of axons. Sensory conduction is normal. In the later stages spontaneous fibrillation is increasingly difficult to detect, as denervated fibres are mopped up by collateral sprouts from neighbouring normal axons. The number of motor units decreases until only discrete giant units are seen on volition.

Neuropathy

Spontaneous fibrillation is readily found on volition, interference patterns are reduced in proportion as motor units are lost, and the units themselves are broken up and polyphasic due to slowing of conduction in the preterminal axons. Motor conduction velocity is slowed – the extent of slowing depends on the underlying pathology. If segmental demyelination is the underlying disorder, slowing will be marked, in severe cases reaching 5–10 m/s. If the lesion is due to axis cylinder drop-out, slowing will be slight and values of 40 m/s are usual. Amplitudes to supramaximal stimulation will be reduced according to the extent of neuronal loss. Common neuropathies affecting the hand include Guillain–Barré, polyneuritis, leprosy, diabetes, carcinomatous neuropathies, rheumatoid disease, collagenoses, triorthocresyl phosphate poisoning. Charcot–Marie–Tooth disease and Déjérine–Sottas' heredofamilial disorder. Sensory action potentials are almost always lost even if, clinically, sensation appears normal, for sensory conduction is a highly sensitive index of sensory nerve function. There are rare cases of pure motor neuropathies in which sensory conduction remains normal. The distinction between such cases and myelopathies depends, apart from the clinical picture, on finding slow motor conduction velocity in some nerves.

PRESSURE NEUROPATHIES

If the peripheral nerve lesion is due to localized pressure, the findings depend on whether the pressure has caused only local demyelination (neurapraxia) or has been sufficiently severe to cause some wallerian degeneration. In a pure neurapraxia there will be no signs of denervation; if degeneration has occurred then spontaneous fibrillation will be found at rest and polyphasic units on volition, provided the block is not so severe as to preclude any conduction of the impulse along the nerve. Classically a response should be detected in the muscle when stimulating the nerve below the block, but not when stimulating above it – when no response is found or a response at very high thresholds. The amplitude to supramaximal response recorded over a distal muscle (e.g. the abductor digiti minimi in a suspected lesion of the ulnar nerve at the elbow) will be low when stimulating above the block and normal when stimulating below the suspected block. Similarly, SAPs will be abnormal below the block if sensory fibres have degenerated and normal above the block. The retention of normal SAPs in a pressure neuropathy is clearly a favourable prognostic sign. Thus the retention of the radial sensory action potential in a wrist drop indicates a temporary neurapraxia only.

In a distal compression lesion (e.g. carpal tunnel syndrome) distal latencies will be prolonged in both motor and sensory fibres, while motor and sensory conduction velocities will be normal above the site of compression.

Myopathy

The traditional view of the pathology of myopathies has been that the disease process affects the muscle fibres direct. As fibres are lost from the motor unit, the motor unit on the electromyograph screen is seen to be shorter in duration and lower in amplitude. The interference pattern remains normal until a late stage because axons are not lost, only muscle fibres. Thus the characteristic picture of a myopathy is a full interference pattern of short-duration low-amplitude units. Motor and sensory conduction velocities are, of course, normal, and spontaneous fibrillation is not seen. In inflammatory myopathies (e.g. polymyositis) an element of denervation may be present and fibrillation can be detected. In polymyositis also the disease tends to affect the muscle in a patchy fashion so in many areas the EMG picture is normal. In the heredofamilial myopathies, however, it is usual for the whole muscle to show a myopathic pattern and for fibrillation to be absent. Myopathies affecting the hand muscles are rare – dystrophia myotonica and the Scandinavian distal familial myopathy are the only distal myopathies seen in practice, but it is in just such cases that EMG can be so useful.

REFERENCES AND BIBLIOGRAPHY

Erb, W. (1883). *Handbook of Electrotherapeutics.* Translated by L. Putzel. New York: Williams Wood

Fullerton, P. M. and Barnes, J. M. (1966). Chronic peripheral neuropathy produced by lead poisoning in guinea pigs. *Journal of Neuropathology and Experimental Neurology* **25**, 214–236

Fullerton, P. M. and Barnes, J. M. (1966). Peripheral neuropathy in rats produced by acrylamide. *British Journal of Industrial Medicine* **23**, 210–221

Gilliatt, R. W. (1966). Nerve conduction in human and experimental neuropathies. *Proceedings of the Royal Society of Medicine* **59**, 989–998

Gilliatt, R. W. and Thomas, P. K. (1960). Sensory nerve action potentials in patients with peripheral nerve lesions. *Journal of Neurology, Neurosurgery and Psychiatry* **23**, 312–320

Gombault, A. (1880). Contribution a l'etude anatomique de la nevrile parenchymateuse subaique et chronique ne-vrile segmentaire peri-axile. *Archives de Neurologie* **1**, 11

Goodman, H. V. and Gilliatt, R. W. (1961). The effect of treatment on median nerve conduction in patients with the carpal tunnel syndrome. *Annals of Physical Medicine* **6**, 137–155

Harris, R. (1962). Chronaxie. In *Electrodiagnosis and Electromyography.* Ed. by Sidney Licht. New Haven, Conn: E. Licht. (3rd edn, 1971)

Hopkins, A. P. and Morgan Hughes, J. A. (1969). The effect of local pressure in diphtheritic neuropathy. *Journal of Neurology, Neurosurgery and Psychiatry* **32**, 614–623

Kaiser, H. E. and Lambert, E. H. (1962). Nerve function studies in experimental polyneuritis. *Electroencephalography and Clinical Neurophysiology* Suppl. **22**, 29

Kline, D. G. and De Jonge, B. R. (1968). Evoked potentials to evaluate peripheral nerve injuries. *Surgery, Gynecology and Obstetrics* **127**, 1239–1248

McDonald, W. I. (1962). Conduction in muscle afferent fibres during experimental demyelination in cat nerve. *Acta Neuropathologica* **1**, 425–432

Moody, J. (1965). Electrophysiological investigations into the neurological complications of carcinoma. *Brain* **88**, 1023–1036

Pallis, C. A. and Scott, J. T. (1965). Peripheral neuropathy in rheumatoid arthritis. *British Medical Journal* **1**, 1141–1147

Payan, J. (1969). Electrophysiological localisation of ulnar nerve lesions. *Journal of Neurology, Neurosurgery and Psychiatry* **32**, 208–220

Preswick, G. (1963). The effect of stimulus intensity on motor latency in the carpal tunnel syndrome. *Journal of Neurology, Neurosurgery and Psychiatry* **26**, 398–401

Ritchie, A. E. (1954). In *Peripheral Nerve Injuries.* Medical Research Council Report Series, No. 282. Ed. by H. J. Seddon. London: HMSO

Trojaborg, W. (1962). Correlation between motor nerve conduction velocity electromyography and strength duration curves. *Danish Medical Bulletin* **9**, 23–25

Waksman, B. H., Adams, R. D. and Mansmann, J. (1957). Experimental studies of diphtheritic polyneuritis in the rabbit and guinea pig. Immunologic and histopathologic observations. *Journal of Experimental Medicine* **105**, 591

Wynn Parry, C. B. (1953). Strength duration curves. In *Electrodiagnosis.* Ed. by Sidney Licht. New Haven, Conn: E. Licht

Wynn Parry, C. B. (1971). Strength duration curves. In *Electrodiagnosis and Electromyography,* 3rd edn. Ed. by Sidney Licht. New Haven, Conn: E. Licht.

The Stiff Hand   5

This chapter is concerned with the treatment of stiffness of the fingers whether due to fractures, soft-tissue contracture, burns, joint disease or generalized conditions affecting the hand. All the conditions discussed present basically the same problems; that is, restoration of joint function, muscle power and the co-ordinated functions of the hand.

FRACTURES

Fractures of the metacarpals and phalanges rarely result in non-union but are a frequent cause of stiffness in neighbouring joints. When it is realized that it is the immobilization of the fracture which causes the stiffness of the joints it will be appreciated how important it is to immobilize fractures of the hand for the minimum period of time necessary and to institute early movements. It is most important not to immobilize more fingers than is absolutely essential. Mobility of the metacarpophalangeal and interphalangeal joints is vital to the normal function of the hand, and it is disastrous when the radiological result of a fracture of the hand is perfect, but the patient is left with a stiff frozen hand.

The commonest fractures in the hand are, in order of frequency: fractures of the base of the metacarpals; second, fractures of the shaft of the phalanges; third, fractures of the neck of the metacarpals; and, fourth, Bennett's fracture-dislocation of the thumb. Our series comprised 426 fractures serious enough to warrant intensive rehabilitation, fractures of the metacarpals being three times as common as all other types.

Fractures of the metacarpals

Fractures of the metacarpals can be divided into those involving the shaft and those involving the neck.

METACARPAL SHAFT

Following reduction the patient is immobilized in a dorsal slab for a maximum of 3 weeks and free use of the unsplinted fingers is encouraged from the start. Following removal of the plaster or splintage, active movements are instituted and full function should be obtained in 4 weeks. Provided the patient will use his hand as much as possible following removal of the plaster, full-time intensive rehabilitation is not necessary.

When fractures of the metacarpal shaft show much displacement, and in the presence of multiple fractures, it is more satisfactory to treat the fractures by intramedullary nails. This allows for accurate reduction and early movements.

METACARPAL NECK

The common fractures of the metacarpal neck involve the index and little fingers, and are commonly found in boxing. It is important to obtain accurate reduction in this type of fracture; otherwise, angulation may occur, thus encroaching on the palmar arch and causing marked stiffness of the metacarpophalangeal joint. Immobilization is required for 3 weeks, followed by active exercise. Unless there have been any complications, full-time treatment is not necessary and the patient is encouraged to use his hand. An effort should be made to discourage boxers from continuing their sport for some time, if not for ever.

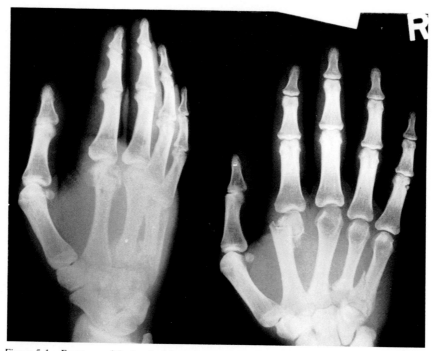

Figure 5.1   Fractures of the head of the index metacarpal and bases of metacarpals of ring and little fingers (Case 5.1)

In the presence of multiple fractures with soft-tissue damage and subsequent weakening of the hand, and where a patient requires very skilled and fine function to perform his job, it may be necessary to institute full-time intensive treatment to obtain the best result.

The following case histories illustrate these points.

Case 5.1.   This patient sustained fractures of the neck of the index metacarpal and bases of the ring and little metacarpals in a motor cycle accident in Novement 1962. The radiograph shows the fractures (*Figure 5.1*). He was in plaster for 2 weeks and was admitted to the MRU on 4 December 1962. At this stage there was full extension of the metacarpophalangeal joints and flexion only to 130 degrees. Grip was half that of the normal side. It was necessary to institute intensive treatment here in view of the patient's job as an armament mechanic. He was under treatment for 6 weeks, at the end of which time there was a full range of joint movement.

Power was 5 kg as compared with 6.3 kg on the normal side, and function as assessed at his job was normal.

Case 5.2.   This patient sustained fractures of the mid-shaft of the metacarpals of the index, middle and ring fingers in a motor cycle accident on 29 October 1958. He was in a plaster back slab for 2 weeks and then started active exercise. At this stage there was only 45 degrees' flexion at the metacarpophalangeal joints and 30 degrees' limitation of movement at both terminal and proximal interphalangeal joints. After 2 weeks of intensive treatment, full range of movement at all joints was obtained and the patient was returned to his trade as an armament mechanic. The fractures are shown in *Figure 5.2.*

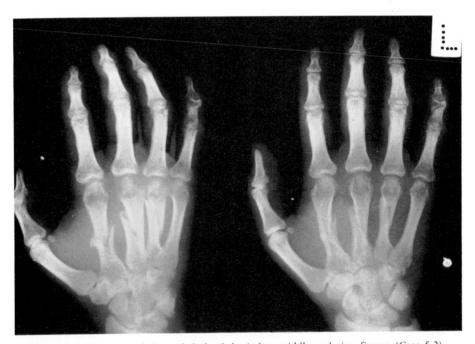

Figure 5.2   Fractures of the mid-shaft of the index, middle and ring fingers (Case 5.2)

Case 5.3.   This patient suffered a severe head injury following a motor cycle accident on 20 October 1962, fracturing the skull and developing a left-sided hemiparesis. He also fractured the necks of the four metacarpals of the left hand. He was unconscious for 3 weeks, and when treatment was started there was virtually no movement of the metacarpophalangeal joints of the left hand either actively or passively. He was first seen for intensive rehabilitation some 5 months after the accident. His maximum active flexion of the metacarpophalangeal joints measured 15 degrees index, 16 degrees middle, 16 degrees ring and 16 degrees little. He had a marked stereognostic deficit of the left hand. *Figure 5.3a* shows the condition of the hand at the beginning of treatment. Apart from the usual exercises in the occupational therapy department, intensive sensory re-education was given to cope with the stereognostic defect; also, passive movements, oil massage and plaster stretches were carried out twice a day for

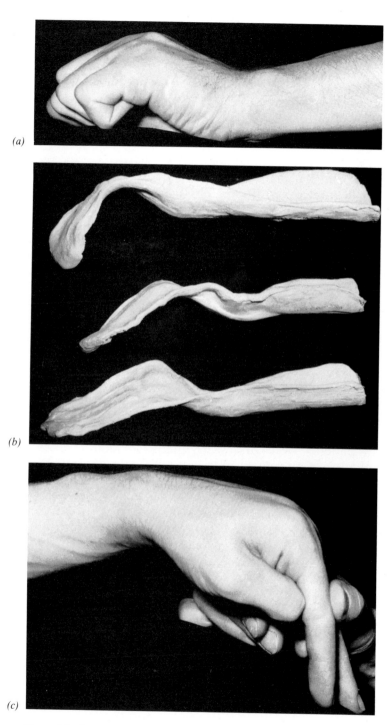

(a)

(b)

(c)

Figure 5.3   Fractures of necks of index, middle, ring and little finger metacarpals and hemiplegia. (a) Maximum flexion possible at beginning of treatment. (b) Serial plasters used in the same case. (c) Maximum passive flexion at end of treatment in Case 5.3

some weeks (*Figure 5.3b*). An excellent result was obtained and the patient was discharged 2 months later with a range of movement of index 70 degrees, middle 50 degrees, ring 60 degrees and little 45 degrees (*Figure 5.3c*). He could make a full fist and the grip was the same on the two sides. An important factor in the rehabilitation of this patient was that he was a member of the Magic Circle, and was formerly an expert conjurer. On discharge from treatment he was able to perform all the tricks to the satisfaction of the professionals as well as of the doctors.

Fractures of the phalanges

Fractures of the shaft of the proximal and middle phalanx are the most common. In fractures of the proximal phalanx the proximal fragment is pulled dorsally by the extensor tendon. In fractures of the middle phalanx the proximal fragment will be extended if proximal to the insertion of flexor sublimis digitorum and flexed if distal to it. Fractures are immobilized with the wrist in 20 degrees' dorsiflexion, 40 degrees' flexion of metacarpophalangeal joints, proximal interphalangeal joint 40 degrees, and a few degrees' flexion of the interphalangeal joint. If displacement is present, stability is maintained by a nail. Kirschner wiring is usually essential in distal phalangeal fractures.

Simple fractures of the phalanges require immobilization for approximately 2 weeks for pain and swelling to disappear; full function should be obtained within 2–3 weeks after mobilization.

Dislocations of the interphalangeal joints also require about 3 weeks' immobilization. Full function is restored after a few weeks. If for any reason active rehabilitation is delayed, some loss of movement inevitably results. Except when a patient needs a full range of movement in his job, the function usually returns without treatment. Wherever possible, plaster immobilization should be avoided by substituting such devices as strapping two fingers together.

A number of patients were first seen some 2–3 months after fracture, with considerable limitation of movement of the interphalangeal joints. Despite this delay before rehabilitation, function returned very rapidly once intensive treatment was started. In several patients as much as 6 months had elapsed since fracture, and there was limitation of movement of 45–60 degrees. After 3 weeks of full-time treatment, a full range of movement was restored. The average rate of return of movement was found to be 15 degrees a week.

COMPLICATIONS

Angulation of the fracture site

This inevitably leads to loss of movement. In such a case intensive treatment is advisable. Full range of movement cannot be expected, but without treatment poor function is the rule.

Case 5.4. This patient sustained closed fractures of the shafts of the proximal phalanges of the ring and little fingers and, as will be seen from *Figure 5.4*, there was marked angulation at the site of the fracture of the little finger. This was immobilized in plaster for 18 days, following which the patient was transferred for full-time rehabilitation. After treatment for 18 days, grip was 7.2 kg on the normal hand, and 6.3 kg on the affected hand. He could make a full fist but the little finger lacked the palm by 1.5 cm.

He was assessed in the workshops as an engine fitter and was found to be able to carry out all the duties of his highly skilled trade without any disability.

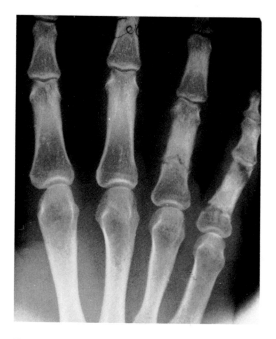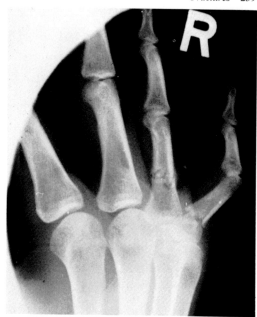

Figure 5.4   Fractures of the proximal phalanges of ring and little fingers with angulation of the little finger fracture (Case 5.4)

Adherence of extensor tendons

It is not uncommon for the extensor tendon to become adherent to the callus. Mild cases respond well to conservative treatment, which should include oil massage to free the tendon from the callus, and progressive resistance exercises to build up the power of extension. Mild degrees of adherence do not limit function and, provided there is a good range of metacarpophalangeal joint movement, no further treatment is required.

With severe degrees of adherence, however, conservative treatment will not offer a good result. It is important to free the tendon from the bone surgically as soon as possible when the adherence is severe. If delayed too long, inveterate stiffness of the metacarpophalangeal joints develops and there are few more difficult joints to restore to a full range of movement. After operation, 1 or 2 weeks' treatment to restore function of the grip and to re-educate the extensor tendon is all that is required.

Sudeck's atrophy

The development of Sudeck's atrophy is more common with metacarpal fractures than with fractures of the phalanges. The principles of early intensive treatment in Sudeck's atrophy have now been accepted. When associated with fractures of the metacarpal, it is important that intensive work should not be started until sound union has occurred. Should mobilization start too soon, pain will result and this will perpetuate the vicious circle of vasomotor instability.

Non-union

Non-union is a rare complication. Following bone grafting, the patient may need many weeks in plaster before union is satisfactory. If the patient uses the arm throughout the period in plaster, full function should be obtained within 3–4 weeks after removal of the plaster. Full-time treatment is only needed should there be an undue stiffness of the joints, or if the patient's job demands particularly fine function.

Delayed union

Should plaster immobilization be required for longer than 6 weeks, some degree of metacarpophalangeal stiffness is likely. If the patient is not using the hand vigorously throughout immobilization, stretch splints, resistance exercises and occupational therapy will be needed. Once enough movement has been obtained for the patient to carry out his job, further progress can be expected with use.

The critical angle of metacarpophalangeal flexion is, in our experience, 45 degrees. Once this has been achieved, further improvement can be expected with normal use, and this amount of flexion is adequate for most tasks.

Incorrect positioning in the plaster

Bad positioning, lack of use of the hand during immobilization and immobilizing more than one finger, all lead to avoidable stiffness of the interphalangeal and metacarpophalangeal joints.

Limitation of flexion follows invariably after immobilizing the fingers in extension. The capsule shortens, adhesions form in the extensor hood, and there is retraction of the collateral ligaments whose insertions are closer together in extension than in flexion, and fixation of the volar plate, preventing it gliding in flexion. Because the volar plates are connected by the transverse metacarpal ligament, stiffness of one metacarpophalangeal joint is often followed by stiffness of the other metacarpophalangeal joints. Finally, the interossei will act as extensors of the metacarpophalangeal joint if it is extended, as their insertion is dorsal to the axis of movement in flexion and extension. Prevention is of paramount importance because stiffness in extension makes the hand useless. This is achieved by minimal time of immobilization, elevation to prevent oedema and accurate reduction of fractures, particularly if there has been dislocation of the joint or articular involvement. The position of immobilization is critical – 45 degrees of flexion of metacarpophalangeal joints and the proximal interphalangeal joints held at 30 degrees.

However severe the stiffness, it is always worth attempting intensive rehabilitation. This will include oil massage several times a day to loosen scarring, slow gentle sustained passive stretches, application of serial plasters, active exercises, occupational therapy, games, and possibly wearing a 'lively' stretch splint (page 292). When the stiffness is so severe that these measures fail, despite at least 3 weeks' continued treatment with no measurable increase in range, surgery is indicated if function is inadequate.

In the operative treatment of joint stiffness, there must be a viable motor to make surgery worth while. Resection of collateral ligaments, taking care not to damage the interosseus, may be sufficient – if not, a major part of the capsule may need to be excised.

Curtis (1970) described a procedure in which he dissects out the proximal and distal margins of the transverse retinacular ligaments on each side of the proximal interphalangeal joint. The collateral ligament is totally resected and the transverse retinacular ligaments retained for lateral stabilization. Next, a tiny dental probe is passed dorsally beneath the extensor mechanism and also over the dorsal surface of the interphalangeal joints, thus freeing all adhesions. This instrument is slipped through the proximal interphalangeal joint and the volar plate freed of adhesions. Finally, the lumbrical canal is opened in the distal palmar area and the lumbrical freed from adhesions.

At the end of the operation, steroid is injected into the joint to minimize adhesions and postoperative pain. Active exercises start immediately.

There may be an indication for arthroplasty and Silastic prostheses of Swanson in severe stiffness of the metacarpophalangeal joints, provided there is good motor power and the soft tissues are healthy.

The following case history illustrates some of the problems associated with multiple complicated injuries of the upper limb which may result in severe disability of the hand although the hand itself has not been involved in the injury.

Case 5.5. This patient was driving his car with his elbow out of the window when a passing lorry hit it. He sustained an open dislocation of the elbow with multiple fractures (*Figure 5.5*), including loss of the capitellum, loss of the extensor muscles of the forearm, and damage to the radial and ulnar nerves (Mr Geoffrey Osborne's case).

The injuries necessitated prolonged immobilization, and eventually a pseudarthrosis developed which required bone grafting. One of the major disabilities in this patient was gross stiffness of the metacarpophalangeal joints for which capsulotomy had been carried out on two occasions but with little success.

Mr Osborne was kind enough to refer the patient for intensive treatment in an attempt to obtain increased range in these joints.

On starting treatment on 6 July 1961 the movements at the metacarpophalangeal joints were index 10–30 degrees, middle 0–20 degrees, ring and little fingers fixed in full extension. A lively splint to assist elbow flexion was supplied to compensate for the considerable weakness of the elbow muscles and joint instability. This had a cock-up and spring for the wrist in view of the loss of wrist extensors. Stretching of the stiff metacarpophalangeal joints six times a day was carried out and stretch plasters were applied between treatments and at night.

So resistant were the joints in this patient that a posterior plaster was used with the distal end projecting over the dorsal surface of the fingers and pressing on them.

Figure 5.5b shows the range at start of treatment; *Figure 5.6* shows some of the serial plasters used and *Figure 5.7* the range of passive movement that could be obtained by the patient 10 weeks after starting treatment. The increased range allowed further reconstructive procedures to be carried out.

Fractures involving the interphalangeal joints

When a fracture of the phalanx involves the interphalangeal joint, it must be accepted that full function can never return. There is inevitably stiffness of the joint and ultimately some degree of arthritis. Under these circumstances, treatment should be directed towards obtaining maximum movement by active exercise and maximum power by building up the grip. On no account should plaster stretches or passive movement be given to the joint. These will not improve the range of movement but will certainly increase pain and stiffness. Two or three steroid injections at two-weekly intervals are well worth trying, as increased range and diminished pain often follow.

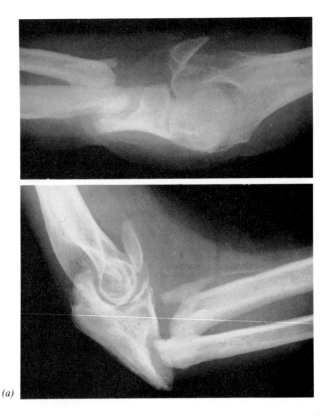

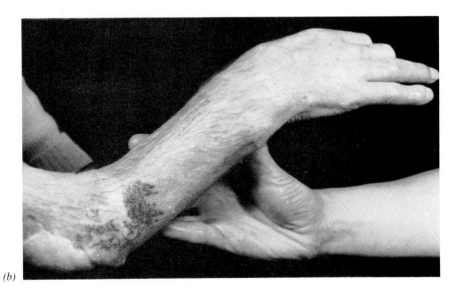

(a)

(b)

Figure 5.5 (a) Fractures of the elbow sustained when the patient rested it out of his car window, to be struck by an oncoming lorry. (b) Maximum flexion of the metacarpophalangeal joints on starting rehabilitation. (Case 5.5)

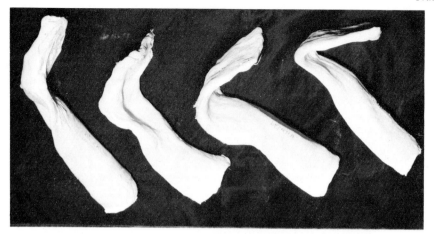

Figure 5.6 Serial plasters used in Case 5.5

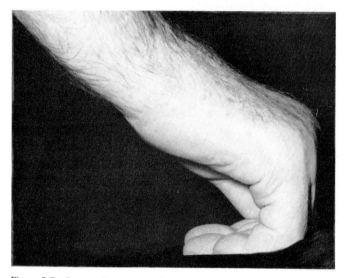

Figure 5.7 Range of metacarpophalangeal joints on discharge (Case 5.5)

MALLET FINGER

This is defined as a flexion deformity of the terminal interphalangeal joint following a lesion of the extensor mechanism. Flexion of the terminal interphalangeal joint is carried out by the retinacular ligaments of Landsmeer from 90 to 45 degrees, and by the lateral slips of the common extensor tendon from 45 to 0 degrees; Landsmeer's ligaments are unable to extend the joint beyond 45 degrees as they cross the joint volar to its axis. Thus when the extensor tendon is cut, the finger is held at 45 degrees, for the retinacular ligaments become tense when the extensor action is lost. Only in severe crush injuries are the retinacular ligaments also damaged and then there is a 90 degree deformity. The lesion usually occurs with a flexion force applied to the terminal phalanx when it is under tension in pushing movements. It is not uncommon after blows from a cricket ball (or baseball) on the tip of the finger.

The treatment of choice is immobilization for 6 weeks in a special metal mallet finger splint (*Figure 5.8a*) which holds the finger in extension and allows the proximal interphalangeal joint a full range of movement. The patient is given a card explaining the rationale of the splint (*Figure 5.8b*). Successful restoration of tendon and joint function can be achieved even 6 months after injury; if seen later than 6 months, however, surgical treatment is necessary.

Bennett's fracture-dislocation

Many cases of Bennett's fracture-dislocation will achieve a perfect result if treatment is provided early, but some may develop osteoarthritis, and this condition is particularly disabling and painful. The fracture is conventionally treated by skin traction in extension, and immobilization may be required for 5–8 weeks.

In this injury the dorsal ulnar oblique ligament is torn and, unless this heals properly, the thumb will be unstable. The ligament can be either repaired at open operation or treated conservatively by manipulation and plaster; if this fails, it must be repaired operatively. With fractures involving the joint, wiring may be necessary to avoid angulation and subsequent stiffness. Most cases of fracture will not require

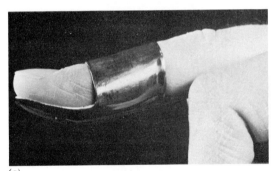

(a)

Figure 5.8   Metal splint for mallet finger: (a) in use; (b) explanatory card for the patient

MALLET FINGER SPLINT

The aim of the splint is to keep the tip of the finger straight for 6 weeks.

The splint is made of stainless steel so that it can be worn whilst washing. When the splint is removed to dry the finger the affected finger tip should be kept straight by pressure with the thumb. (See Diagram)

Dry the finger with surgical spirit before replacing the splint to prevent soreness.

The splint must be worn continuously for 6 weeks and then at nights for a further 2 weeks.

(b)

functional rehabilitation, and full range of movement and normal power can be expected 4 weeks after removal of the plaster. Occasionally, however, it may be necessary to institute intensive treatment, particularly if the patient has bilateral fractures and has an arduous skilled job. The following case history illustrates this point.

Case 5.6. This patient was boxing for the RAF when he sustained bilateral Bennett's fracture-dislocation on 8 February 1962. He was in a plaster for 3 weeks and was sent to the MRU following this for intensive treatment. At this stage his grip measured 0.45 kg on the right and 1.6 kg on the left, and there was considerable pain in the wrists (*Figure 5.9*).

After treatment for 3 weeks his grip was 6.8 kg on each side and movements were normal.

He was fully assessed at his work and found able to complete the test jobs given to him as a general fitter perfectly satisfactorily, except that he found he had considerable fatigue in the hands at the end of work. He was supplied with a light fibreglass support for the right thumb, which was the most painful, to use when he developed any severity of pain after work. This he wore for a few weeks but was able to discard it and has remained pain-free with full function ever since.

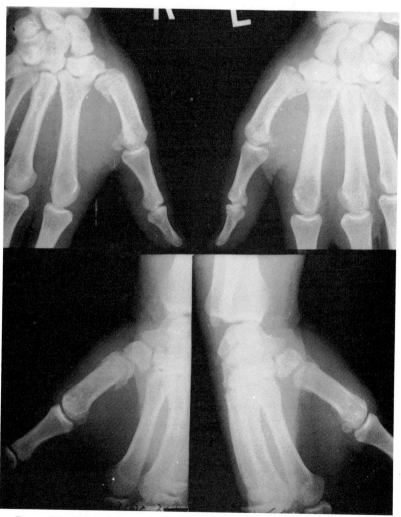

Figure 5.9 Bilateral Bennett's fracture-dislocations due to boxing (Case 5.6)

When osteoarthritis develops, careful supervised treatment is necessary. The patient's first complaints are usually of pain on extremes of movement of the thumb, on grip and when holding tools for long periods. Next, the hand becomes generally weak so that the patient may drop things and be quite incapable of guiding or manipulating tools. Many patients complain of deep-seated grinding which is particularly uncomfortable. Once pain has been present for any length of time, a vicious circle sets in of pain – increasing weakness resulting in exposure to further damage of the joint – and more pain.

The patient feels acute pain over the joint, the grip will be extremely poor and the circulation of the hand may be impaired. There is often subjective numbness of the thumb, and the skin over the thumb is felt to be colder than the fingers. *Figure 5.10* shows the radiological appearance of a typical case.

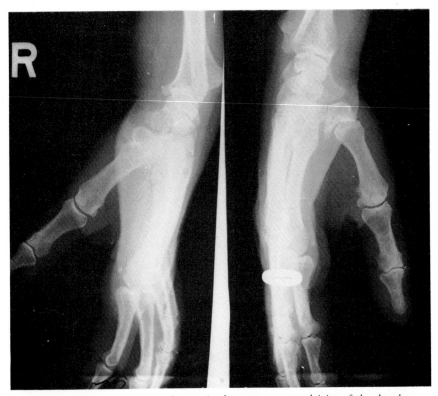

Figure 5.10   Osteoarthritic changes in the carpometacarpal joint of the thumb

Conservative treatment should be tried first. It is always worth while injecting hydrocortisone, 0.5 ml (12.5 mg), or an equivalent dose of soluble steroid into the joint as a preliminary measure, and this may be repeated three times at weekly intervals. In the early stages this may relieve the pain sufficiently for the patient to resume his occupation and thus redevelop the power of the thumb muscles. It may be necessary, if the patient's job does not involve gripping and turning movements of the thumb, to prescribe occupational therapy; conversely, if the patient's job is too hard, a lighter form of work must be prescribed or, again, suitable occupational therapy. If this treatment does not succeed and the patient continues to complain of increasing pain and weakness of the thumb, some form of splintage is applied. The rationale of splinting is to prevent or limit movement in the joint for a few weeks so that the patient can build up the power of the thumb muscles, thus breaking the vicious circle of pain – weakness – pain.

If the condition is severe it is advisable to immobilize the thumb completely so that all movement is prevented.

In milder cases or in severe cases where complete immobility prevents the patient doing his job, modified immobilization can be used by providing a leather splint, with or without Perspex reinforcement on the extensor aspect. Within a few days the pain will be materially reduced, certainly enough to allow the patient to use the hand in moderately hard activities. It is important not to stop immobilization too soon. It has been found that if immobilization is removed before the grip by measurement is over one-half that of the normal side, the patient will certainly relapse. The test as to whether the patient is ready for mobility is the power of the stabilizing muscles.

Where pain is an outstanding feature, a combination of intra-articular hydrocortisone injections and splintage is worthwhile. Additional measures can be used to help relieve the pain; heat to the patient's hand before occupational therapy is of value not only in relieving the pain, but also for its beneficial effect on the impaired circulation. In severe cases the splintage may be worn for 3–4 months before the pain is completely relieved. Patients often find it useful to keep their splint for many months, or even years, wearing it while undertaking heavy work. Should this treatment fail, then operative measures are the only ones likely to offer permanent relief of the pain; this will mean arthrodesis or excision of the trapezium.

Those patients who are constantly using their hand for heavy tasks will benefit more by arthrodesis. When immobilization is stopped after this operation, most patients will require formal rehabilitation because they will have had, in almost all cases, many months of severe pain and weakness of the hand; therefore, they will require re-education in activities of the hand as well as improvement in gross muscle power. The average time for restoring maximum function after removal of the plaster following arthrodesis is 6 weeks. The length of time bears a direct relation to the time in plaster as well as to how long the patient had symptoms before operation.

Excision of the trapezium

After simple excision of the trapezium or implantation of a space-filling prosthesis, the hand is elevated for 48 hours and then active exercises begin.

There is a good deal of discomfort after operation. Patients subconsciously try to use the thumb, so important a part of the hand is it, and this may last up to 6 or 8 weeks.

As normal use of the thumb involves only its middle range, one has to prescribe intensive exercises using the whole range of movement.

The scar may become adherent over the tendons of extensor and abductor pollicis longus. This must be mobilized with oil massage and ultrasound.

It is usually 3 months before full function returns after operation.

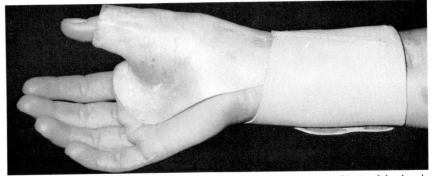

Figure 5.11   Fibreglass splint used in osteoarthritis of the carpometacarpal joint of the thumb

Figure 5.11 shows the splint used for partial immobilization of the carpometacarpal joint in osteoarthritis. The manufacture of the splint is described in Appendix D of this chapter.

Fracture of the sesamoid bone of the thumb

This must be a rare condition. *Figure 5.12* shows a radiograph of a patient who sustained such an injury when he slipped and fell on the thumb.

    Case 5.7.   This patient was immobilized for 3 weeks in plaster. Following its removal he was admitted to the rehabilitation centre. At this stage the thumb was very tender and stiff. Grip was 3.2 kg compared with 5.9 kg on the normal side.
    The fracture had not united; intensive rehabilitation by exercises and occupational therapy was therefore prescribed to restore full function.
    He was discharged with no pain, and full power and function 1 month later.

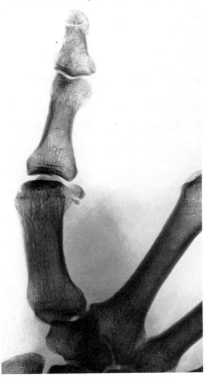

Figure 5.12   Fracture of sesamoid bone of thumb

SPRAINS AND DISLOCATIONS

Sprains

Sprains of the metacarpophalangeal and interphalangeal joints should be treated with early movements; in the case of metacarpophalangeal joints, localized tenderness to one spot in the collateral ligaments will often respond dramatically to an injection of 0.5 ml lignocaine and 0.5 ml steroid. Sprains of the thumb are sometimes associated with a tear of the ulnar collateral ligaments and these require repair at open operation or, if too severe for repair, arthrodesis.

It is essential to rule out damage to the ligaments in any traumatic lesion of the hand. If a full range of active movement is not possible, there may be damage to the volar plate. If there is any doubt as to the integrity of the ligaments, a local block should be given and lateral stress imposed, as muscle spasm due to pain may cause impaction of the joint surfaces, wrongly suggesting stability. Unstable fingers should be rested for 21 days, instead of the normal 10 days for uncomplicated sprains. The patient must be warned that it is common for such fingers to be swollen and stiff for many months.

Case 5.8.   This patient knocked his right middle finger against an aircraft; no bony injury was sustained but the joint swelled and became very painful. When seen 2 weeks later the joint lacked 45 degree extension and had 50 degrees' active flexion. Steroid and local anaesthetic was injected into the joint and a lively Capener splint provided. Twelve days later movements were 20/110 and all pain had been abolished. He was fit to return to work as a pilot.

Dislocations

The interphalangeal joints, the metacarpophalangeal joints and the carpometacarpal joints can all become dislocated with concomitant fractures. These injuries must always be immobilized in a position of function for sufficient time to allow healing of the ligaments and subsidence of the joint effusion. Quite often following removal of the plaster or splintage it is some time before a reasonable range of movement and function is obtained. This is because the injury is more severe than one would imagine and soft-tissue damage can be quite extensive. It is wise to give 2 or 3 weeks' intensive treatment if the patient does not regain a full range of movement speedily after the immobilization is removed. The following two case histories illustrate these points.

Case 5.9.   This patient dislocated the metacarpophalangeal joint of the right thumb on 29 May 1959. He was in plaster for 1 month and in a splint for a further 3 weeks. On removal of the immobilization the joint was found to be painful. There was a good range of passive movement but a very limited range of active movement and good power. It was still necessary, however, to wear a light fibreglass splint because after a long period of work as wireless operator he would develop pain and tiredness in the muscles.

Case 5.10.   This patient sustained a fracture of the radial styloid and dislocation of the carpometacarpal joints of the index and middle fingers in a road traffic accident on 26 November 1961. He was manipulated under anaesthesia and put in plaster for 7 weeks. When he came out of plaster there was a 0.9 kg grip on the left, 5.9 kg on the right, and virtually no movement in the hand. The major disability was the almost complete absence of passive movements in the thumb web. The stiffness of the thumb as well as of the index and middle fingers was due not only to the long period of immobilization and the soft-tissue damage sustained at the time of injury, but also to damage of the radial lateral ligaments attached to the styloid process of the radius, which could be felt to be tight. Intensive treatment comprising oil massage, stretching and exercises was given and, over a period of 3 months, good function was obtained.

On discharge he had a 4.5 kg grip on the left, 7.7 kg grip on the right, and the workshop assessment showed that he was fully fit for his duty as an air frame mechanic.

SCAPHOID FRACTURES

These are the most common fractures of the carpus; 90 per cent unite but prolonged immobilization may be necessary (in 45 degrees' dorsiflexion and some radial flexion). The patient can usually rehabilitate himself after removal of plaster.

It is surprising how symptom-free non-union can be. Fisk (1971) has shown that we have been wrong to regard scaphoid fractures as isolated injuries to the wrist, for the scaphoid braces the mid-carpal joint and the mid-carpal joint supports the scaphoid. Movement about the scaphoid occurs vertically at its proximal pole, horizontally at its distal pole and coronally at its articulation with the capitate. Thus, scaphoid fractures seriously upset wrist movements. It is not only the bony damage that is relevant in scaphoid fractures, it is also the damaged ligaments and capsules. Fisk showed that it was the volar carpal ligament which was the major factor in maintaining the stability of the carpus, and to a lesser extent the joint capsule, between the capitate, scaphoid and lunate.

Damage usually occurs in hyperextension injuries when the patient falls on the outstretched hand – the position of maximum instability of the carpus. Falls on the hand in ulnar deviation do the most damage, for in radial deviation the scaphoid is protected and subject only to stress along its long axis.

When avascular necrosis of the scaphoid develops, and in cases of complicated perilunate and trans-scaphoid fracture-dislocations, all the proximal rows of carpals can be excised. This operation allows return of some wrist movement. If unsuccessful, arthrodesis can always be performed later.

Of 11 cases treated by us, 7 regained almost full range of movement and good power, 2 regained 50 per cent of range and movement, and 2 had poor results with continuing pain and weakness who required arthrodesis.

The rehabilitation of such patients may need to be prolonged, particularly if symptoms have been present for many months before operation. A supportive splint can be useful in the early stages to immobilize the wrist while muscle power is built up. It is important not to put too heavy a demand on the wrist in the first few weeks and certainly until muscle power is adequate. Carpentry, gardening and hand games are particularly valuable, including gymnasium activities and games with padded rackets such as table tennis, badminton and tennis.

If non-union is established, the proximal fragment moves with the proximal row of carpal bones and the distal fragment with the distal row. The scaphoid tuberosity becomes impacted against the radial styloid, leading to arthritis. If the carpus is stable the wrist should be immobilized in plaster until revascularization occurs. If there is instability of the carpus then there is a flexion deformity at the scaphoid, persistent pain and the fracture will not unite. Styloidectomy should be performed and the scaphoid grafted. If arthritis has developed, arthrodesis is indicated.

DUPUYTREN'S CONTRACTURE

Description

Skoog (1948) gave the incidence of Dupuytren's contracture as 1.5 per cent. In his series, 18 per cent had involvement of the plantar fascia as well as the hands. The feet, however, only require treatment if the condition is causing pain.

Conversely, there are very few patients who, once Dupuytren's contracture with deformity is established in the hand, do not require surgical treatment. The length of time the patient has suffered from the onset of symptoms before seeking advice depends on the disability it causes him and its rate of development. Furthermore, the intelligence of the patient is a considerable factor. One is constantly amazed to see how patients will put up with appalling degrees of disability before they come for advice; in several cases the only treatment that could be offered was amputation of the little finger which was flexed completely into the palm and beyond any aid.

In our series the time from onset of contracture to operation varied from 2 months to 10 years, with an average of 4 years. In only 7 per cent was there a family history. In 20 per cent only there was a history of some trauma, common precipitating factors being blows sustained in football games, constant digging and crush injuries of the hand. Very few patients were seen who had had the condition following repeated trauma in the palm from a tool, such as a drill or a screwdriver.

In 50 per cent the left hand alone was affected, in 20 per cent the right hand alone and in 30 per cent both hands were affected.

Treatment

If the disability is slight and the condition progressing only very slowly, surgery is not indicated. Hydrocortisone has been used by some workers, notably Baxter and his colleagues (1952), but they were unable to arrive at any definite conclusions except to point out that this treatment does not replace surgery. It is important to advise the patient who presents with a very early Dupuytren's contracture to report back if and when the disability increases, and for this reason it is advisable to follow up such patients at regular intervals.

Bassot (1965) described a technique for correcting flexion deformity by conservative means. Trypsin, together with local anaesthetic and hyaluronidase, is injected at various points along the length of the thickened band and nodule. Fifteen minutes later a forced extension is given to rupture the thickened band; this procedure is repeated several times at intervals of a few days until maximum correction is achieved. Hueston (1971) confirmed these findings and has shown marked increase in extension after this procedure. The rationale is to use proteolytic and inflammatory enzymes to depolymerize and spread the ground substance. Hueston has suggested that it is worth considering in patients unfit for general anaesthesia, where extensive surgery is best avoided and in a severe case to provide correction of the metacarpophalangeal deformity before fasciectomy.

In the early stages of this condition, it may be possible to restore full extension of a flexed proximal interphalangeal joint by oil massage and serial plaster finger splints –

particularly valuable in patients in whom surgery is contraindicated. The patients most likely to respond are those in whom the fibrosis is relatively superficial, one finger only is involved and the deformity is less than 45 degrees.

Healing of the operative scar may be slow due to poor circulation after months or years of fibrosis, and the disability when active rehabilitation starts may not be much less than it was before correction. However, even with skin grafting, when the patient will have had the condition for a long time, permanent contraction of the fingers must be overcome and the deep fibrosis resolved by physiotherapy. The average time from operation to the commencement of intensive rehabilitation is 5 weeks. In some patients, who have had the condition for many years and in whom the skin is of poor quality, the surgical scar may not heal fully for 4 or 5 weeks. During this stage saline solution soaks should be given and the patient encouraged in active exercise both in the saline bath and with the physiotherapist. The object of these saline baths is to reduce the scaling, clean the skin, relieve pain and thus encourage the patient to exercise the hand. Under no circumstances must heat be used, as the recently and thinly dissected skin of the palm is liable to be necrosed by heat. The physiotherapist must encourage active flexion at the metacarpophalangeal and interphalangeal joints, each joint being supported in turn. Between treatment sessions a tulle gras dressing is worn. Light occupational therapy is essential but the patient must wear his dressing. It may be advisable in the early stages for the patient to have the arm elevated in a sling if there is the slightest sign of oedema which, if allowed to persist for even 2 days, will result in further fibrosis. The deformity of the hand at this stage is normally 45 degrees' flexion of the proximal interphalangeal joint, and a slight – maybe 10 degrees' – flexion deformity at the terminal interphalangeal joint. In a very severe case the metacarpophalangeal joint may also be held in flexion, sometimes as much as 55 degrees (at 125 degrees). There is unlikely to be any movement in the terminal interphalangeal joint or proximal interphalangeal joint. In those patients where flexor sheaths are extensively affected, little or no active flexion can be expected to return. Full-time intensive treatment is required for a period, on average, of 6 weeks after operation, except in the severe cases which may need up to 5 months' treatment.

In about 25 per cent of patients the little finger remains solid and in 45 degrees of flexion (135 degrees) at the proximal interphalangeal joint, no active movement returning. This deformity is particularly liable to be seen in patients with a long history in whom there has been some complication at operation, such as haematoma. Provided the flexion deformity is not severe, function can be excellent. If it interferes with any of the patient's activities, amputation is the best treatment.

The stiff little finger so often seen in severe cases is due to diffusion of the affection from digital fasciculi of the palmar aponeurosis invading the anterior capsule where the fasciculi fuse with it around the free tendons.

The principles of treatment, once the scarring has healed, are to tackle the fibrosis by increasing the vigorous oil massage, to stretch the contracted soft tissue by graduated plaster stretch splints, to restore, where possible, the function of the remaining flexors and the extensors, and to redevelop the grip and general function of the hand.

For the first few days after the scar has healed, oil massage is given only twice a day, and only lightly. By the end of the first week, the massage can become vigorous and be given four times a day. In those cases where the flexion deformity is not being rapidly overcome by this means, serial stretch splints should be started. The stretch is increased as the deformity responds and the patient must wear the splint at night. Re-education of the long flexor action and long extensor action is given at every treatment session as described in Chapter 2; all the various exercises and games described there are appropriate to these patients.

The fingers must be stretched not only in flexion but also in abduction, adduction and rotation of the metacarpal heads where so much tightness exists. It should not be forgotten that, as the fingers may have been flexed for months or even years, the extensors are involved and require re-education. It must not be expected, though, that more than a few degrees' controlled extension at each joint will return, but this need be no bar to good function.

The underlying principle of all treatment in patients with Dupuytren's contracture is to maintain the correction of the soft-tissue deformity obtained at each treatment session by the stretch splint. The physiotherapist will be able to judge, by the amount of correction being obtained each day, whether or not progress can be speeded up. The careful measurement at weekly intervals of flexion deformity will also indicate whether treatment needs to be intensified. An improvement in extension of 5 degrees or more each week is satisfactory progress.

The regimen for a Dupuytren's contracture, then, comprises first oil massage to soften the skin, promote circulation and reduce pain, which is bound to result from the subsequent stretches. Next, passive movements at all joints; then stretches, the scarred tissue being rolled, stretched and pulled, followed by re-education of tendon function at each joint; finally, group action of flexors, extensors and grip.

During the exercise session the physiotherapist grips the hand, with her own hand moulding round the metacarpophalangeal and interphalangeal joints. With the patient's palm down, the physiotherapist puts her fingers under the proximal phalanges, her hand on the dorsum of the patient's hand, and stretches the whole hand up. Then, with the wrist down on the table, a full active and passive stretch is attempted with the wrist and fingers being stretched.

Patients are encouraged to carry tennis balls to improve grip during the day.

Physiotherapy must be repeated as often as possible, preferably four times a day. Patients who have an hour's treatment two or three times a week do not do well. There is no hope of mastering the deformity and retaining progress at each session if patients come so seldom.

Hueston (1963) carried out some interesting work on the results of operation in Dupuytren's contracture. He examined two aspects of surgical treatment. First, the postoperative morbidity in 96 fasciectomies, limited to the macroscopically involved region, and, second, the recurrence rate in 35 limited and 35 total fasciectomies more than 5 years after investigation. No difference in the long-term recurrence rate was found after limited or radical fasciectomy. The most important factor in determining the rate of recurrence or extension of the disease was found to be the constitutional make-up of the patient. He found that in the presence of knuckle pads, plantar lesions or a strong family history it can be assumed that a strong diathesis of the production of Dupuytren's tissue can be presumed, and, particularly in a young man, recurrence is likely regardless of the operation carried out, whether limited or radical fasciectomy. Hueston concluded, therefore, that the operation for Dupuytren's contracture should aim simply at the correction of the disabling deformity rather than attempting to cure the general diathesis, and he formed the opinion that limited fasciectomy was the logical procedure to be adopted.

Clarkson and Pelly (1962) are also against radical fasciectomy. They pointed out that damage to nerves, necrosis of skin and haematoma formation are more common, and even then there are recurrences although less commonly than after limited fasciectomy.

When, after intensive physiotherapy for 4–6 weeks, it is clear (by measurement of the deformity and inspection of the stretch plaster) that further progress is not being obtained, the patient should be returned to work since further intensive treatment may, in fact, produce recurrence rather than improvement. Time must be allowed for the condition to settle down.

The following case histories illustrate the points described above.

Case 5.11. This patient had a recurrence of Dupuytren's contracture in the right hand 4 years after operation. This was removed, as was the recurrent contracture of the palmar fascia. Three weeks after operation the patient presented with a very thick scar 2.5 cm proximal to the metacarpophalangeal joint of the little finger and 5 cm across. It was 10 days more before the scar healed fully. At this stage treatment comprised intensive oil massage four times a day for 30 minutes at each session combined with stretch splints, active exercises and games. Three weeks after commencement of rehabilitation he returned to work with a full range of movement and function at all joints.

Case 5.12. This patient developed Dupuytren's contracture following a long period of digging as a prisoner of war. He had a 10-year history, both hands and both feet being affected. Two months after operation he presented with an unhealed very adherent scar; the metacarpophalangeal joint of the index finger was held in 60 degrees of flexion while the middle, the ring and the little fingers were held in 55 degrees of flexion.

There was no active flexion in any joint of the ring or little fingers and there was no grip.

Saline solution soaks were given until the scar healed, when a full programme of oil massage four times a day, stretch splinting, exercises and games was carried out.

After 3 months the flexion deformity at the metacarpophalangeal joints was completely overcome. The grip was excellent but there was no return of flexor action in the interphalangeal joints of the ring or little fingers. The rate of return of metacarpophalangeal extension was 8 degrees a week. *Figure 5.13* illustrates the progress of this patient.

Case 5.13. This patient had a 3½-year history before operation, the first symptom being the development of knuckle pads. There was no family history and no history of trauma. The palmar fascia and the ring finger were affected in both hands. Six weeks after operation the scar had healed and intensive rehabilitation was started. The little fingers were held in 45 degrees of flexion at the proximal interphalangeal joints, and the ring fingers in 50 degrees of flexion. There was a deep thick scar 3.1 cm proximal to the metacarpophalangeal joints. After 3 weeks' intensive treatment, full function and full movement were restored to all joints.

Case 5.14. This patient sought advice 10 years after being hit by a cricket ball in the palm of his hand. There had been one operation which resulted in a complete cure, but in the months before the second operation he noticed gradually increasing flexion of the little finger until it was almost completely bent into the palm. One month after operation the patient started active rehabilitation. There was a thick scar along the whole of the ulnar aspect of the palm, measurements of the ring and little fingers were at the terminal interphalangeal joint 50–55 degrees, proximal interphalangeal joint 30–28 degrees, and metacarpophalangeal joint 5 degrees of hyperextension to 30 degrees of flexion; the grip was non-existent. After 1 month's intensive treatment, full movement and full flexion were restored.

BURNS

Principles of surgery

When skin loss is not associated with damage to bone, joint or tendons, free grafts are used, particularly on the dorsum of the hand and fingers, being taken from the forearm, inner aspect of upper arm or, for large grafts, the thigh. To cover small areas

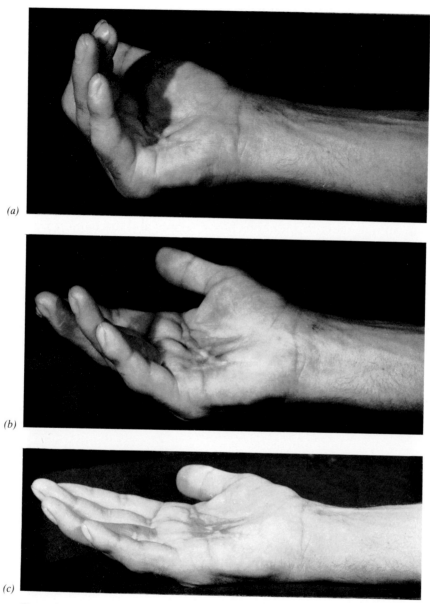

(a)

(b)

(c)

Figure 5.13 Progress in a patient with Dupuytren's contracture. (a) Two months after surgery. (b) Six weeks after commencing rehabilitation. (c) On discharge after 3 months rehabilitation. (Case 5.12)

when bone or tendon has been exposed, local flaps are used – giving bulk and sensory protection over the flexor surfaces of the middle and proximal phalanges and on the palm. These flaps may be from the dorsum of the hand, or adjoining finger flaps can be taken from other parts of the body – from the other arm, the abdomen or the chest. They are used when multiple flaps are needed or where there is a large area of skin to cover. Cross-arm flaps are used for finger tips. Finally, tube pedicles are used to cover a completely degloved thumb or finger. Further details of techniques are well described in the British Association of Surgery of the Hand's Symposium on the Burnt Hand (1970).

Rehabilitation

One of the major problems in the rehabilitation of the burnt hand is the distortion of the normal anatomy, due to severe soft-tissue damage which leads to contractures. A typical example is seen in *Figure 5.14*, with flexion of the interphalangeal joints and hyperextension of the metacarpophalangeal joints.

Often the skin is tethered to bone with either little soft tissue between or a layer of solid fibrosis, so that there is a tenuous blood supply and the hand is easily infected and vulnerable to trauma.

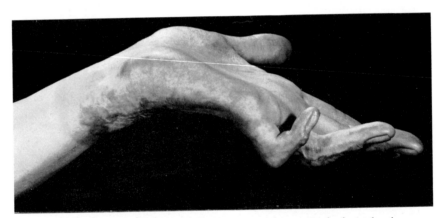

Figure 5.14   Hyperextension deformity commonly seen in the burnt hand

Gross stiffness of the metacarpophalangeal and interphalangeal joints is common, but the major problem is restoration of metacarpophalangeal range, as the proximal interphalangeal joints are often fixed in an acceptable position of flexion.

With severe burns, one can only aim at limited objectives – restoration of either power or pinch grip, depending on damage to the thumb web.

There are certain special difficulties in the early rehabilitation of the burnt hand – wounds are often still unhealed at a stage when restoration of the range of movement is essential and urgent. Active movements must therefore be started in warm water and wounds dressed as lightly as possible to allow simple functional activities.

Elevation of the limb is essential if there is the slightest sign of oedema, and in the early stages the patient should wear a sling (see *Figure 2.17*).

Patients have difficulty with the activities of daily living – their morale is often low, and they may need nursing and some help with toilet, feeding and dressing for some time.

There may often be associated joint disorders, such as stiff elbows and shoulders which inevitably complicate treatment (*Figure 5.15a*), and in very severe cases

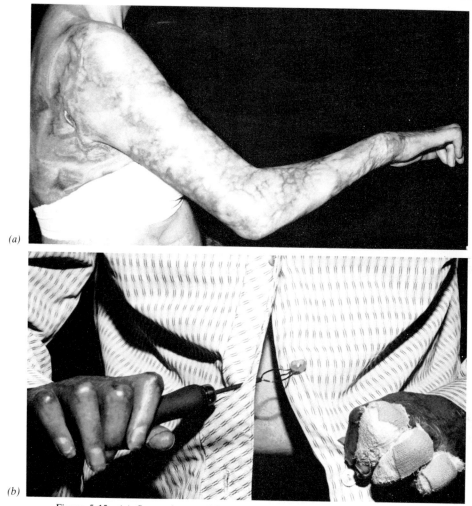

Figure 5.15 (a) Severe burns of hand and upper limb. (b) Use of button hook

periarticular calcification and ossification occur round the elbow joint, causing permanent stiffness if infection occurs and rehabilitation is delayed (Kolar and Vrabec, 1959).

In the early stages gentleness is vital. Too much stretching and too vigorous exercise are liable to flare up a soft-tissue reaction, causing breakdown of wounds. Further immobilization is therefore necessary, leading to further restriction of joint movement.

Heat must be avoided at all costs. Skin cover is sensitive and heat will cause sloughing.

Friction or trauma of any sort can undo weeks of devoted plastic surgery – when not under treatment patients must therefore be protected in slings or gloves and must constantly be educated in precautions against damage until there is complete healing. Plaster stretches, such as one uses for traumatic stiffness, are contraindicated in the early stages because the skin is too delicate.

Physiotherapy

Skin massage with hydrous ointment (Nivea Creme) is very useful in the early stages of rehabilitation to improve the texture of the skin. Later, when all wounds have healed, massage gradually becomes deeper to loosen contracted soft tissues and resolve fibrosis. This must start gently and slowly become more vigorous. It should be given at least twice a day, and preferably four times a day, in order to gain the best results quickly.

Following oil massage, gentle passive stretches are given to restore flexion to the metacarpophalangeal joints and to open out the thumb web. These passive stretches must be very gentle, slow and sustained, and should never be painful. Under no circumstances is anything remotely approaching a manipulation or forced movement used. Following a session of stretching, active exercises are given to build up power and maintain the passive range of movement. Proprioceptive neuromuscular facilitation techniques, particularly relaxation, are excellent for tight muscles. In order to maintain the correction obtained by these techniques, a light polyethylene foam (Plastazote) splint or wedges, fashioned exactly to the shape of the deformity, are worn between treatments and a resting night splint is worn (*Figure 5.16*). These are changed frequently in the early stages – even as often as twice a day, later daily,

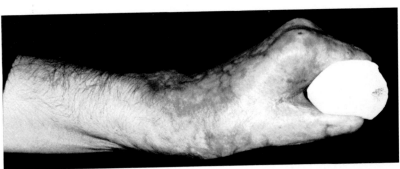

Figure 5.16   Plastazote wedge to correct deformity in the thumb web

then, as the deformity yields, two or three times a week. It is useful to keep one splint each week and label it with the date. This shows in a dramatic manner how correction is proceeding – encouraging for both patient and staff, and is much more satisfactory than attempting to record angles with a goniometer since the anatomy is often so distorted that measurements are difficult, if not impossible.

The physiotherapist can also remove dead pieces of skin and apply dry dressings to any exposed area. She must also warn the patient continually about the need to avoid rubbing the skin, putting hands on radiators or near fires, always wearing gloves in cold weather when outdoors, and avoiding getting them exposed to strong sunlight as burnt skin is highly susceptible to sunburn. Care of the nails is vital and the physiotherapist should cut the patient's nails frequently so as to prevent sharp nails digging into the skin.

Later, plaster stretches with cotton wool lining can be used, but only when all open wounds have soundly healed, the circulation is good and maximum benefit has accrued from the Plastazote techniques.

Again, serial plasters can be used and dated to show progress.

Both polyethylene foam (Plastazote) and plaster are versatile media and can be moulded to fit any deformity, however complex, and we prefer this to any type of splint with elastic bands and pulleys which, in our experience, usually produce more deformity than they correct.

Very occasionally a lively splint can be useful for a particular deformity at a particular stage; for example, to encourage wrist movement if there has been stiffness of the wrist joint or a lively 'ulnar' splint to help in correction of hyperextension deformities.

Occupational therapy

Either the physiotherapist or the occupational therapist can help the patient with activities of daily living and, as in so many fields of modern therapy, their functions overlap.

Great attention has to be paid to personal toilet (i.e. washing, feeding, dressing, toilet, etc.). Velcro fastening can be sewn in places normally requiring a button or zip fastening (*Figure 5.15b* and *5.17*).

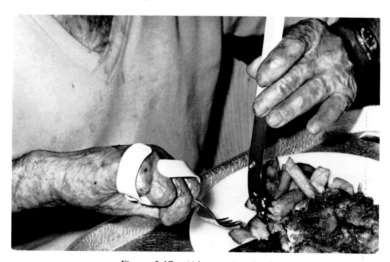

Figure 5.17 Aid to eating for burns

Handle adaptations for cutlery have to be specially designed to the individual, depending on finger contractures.

The occupational therapist can be a great help in managing personal appearance such as hair styling and make-up, and making aids to hold a comb, lipstick, powder puff or toilet paper.

Patients dislike small, intricate mechanisms or bag fastenings and these can be made easier to manipulate.

Once the patient has been taught independence, remedial occupational therapy can be introduced to provide increased joint range and power. Printing is helpful to stretch contractures and the idea of printing their own writing paper usually appeals to patients. Rug-hooking with a padded handle also provides a useful exercise and a welcome addition to the home. All the remedial hand games already described are appropriate. Carpentry should not be attempted unless the skin is thoroughly well healed. Polishing table tops with a padded block is popular and polyethylene gloves are useful to protect the skin from dust.

Case 5.15. This patient suffered extensive burns when the tent in which he was sleeping caught fire. He sustained 40 per cent total body surface burns, mainly full or deep partial thickness and affecting the head and neck, both arms and hands, the left foot and most of the back. The forearm and hands of both arms were skin grafted using the left thigh as donor area. The left hand was more deeply burned than the right but neither palm was affected. Both upper arms were Thiersch grafted using the right thigh as the donor site. He was transferred 10 weeks later to the MRU. By this time the grafted areas were healed, but there was marked webbing of the posterior axillary folds and gross limitation of movement at both elbows. There was reasonable function in the right hand but gross limitation of movement at the left metacarpophalangeal joints and a tethered left thumb web. He was placed on a full-time rehabilitation programme. The left elbow was released 3 months later and the scar on the dorsum of the right hand was excised and grafted. Z-plasty on the thumb–index web, Z-plasty on the left minimus and Z-plasty with scar excision at the left axilla, were all carried out 3 months later. One year after injury the three webs between the fingers of the left hand were divided and closed utilizing local flaps. Throughout this time he alternated between hospital and intensive rehabilitation at the MRU, with oil massage, exercises, games and occupational therapy. On discharge, 13 months after the original burns, he had full movement of all joints.

Case 5.16. This patient sustained severe burns to her face and upper limbs when the aircraft she was piloting caught fire. Extensive skin grafting was required. The problems with regard to the hands were gross stiffness of the metacarpophalangeal and interphalangeal joints and severe deformity (*Figure 5.15a*). Intensive oil massage, slow gentle stretches with padded plasters and active exercises and games gave her reasonable function. Aids to daily living were a vital part of her rehabilitation in restoring independence and therefore morale. Padded cutlery, long-handled combs and toothbrush, button hook (*Figure 5.15b*), Velcro fastenings for clothes, elasticated shoes to avoid tying laces, straws for drinking, and an adapted sponge dishwasher for toilet were all made in the occupational therapy department.

Case 5.17. This patient sustained burns of both hands, legs, face and shoulders in an aircraft crash; the whole of the dorsal surface of the hand and fingers was severely burnt. Stamp grafts were applied 5 days and 12 days after injury, and the patient was admitted to the rehabilitation centre 2 months after the accident. At this stage (*Figure 5.18*) he presented with a rock-like hand and scarring on the whole of the dorsal surface of the left hand. There was no active flexion in any of the fingers, and passive movements amounted to only a few degrees. Palmar flexion was 10 degrees. There were several areas over the back of all the fingers which were slow to heal.

The first objective was to encourage the patient to use the hand and thus improve its circulation to promote healing preparatory to the next operation.

Oil massage four times a day, combined with progressive resistance exercises for the fingers, together with general exercises and games for hand function, were given for 6 weeks. At this stage the circulation was much improved and there was 15 degrees' (180–165 degrees) movement at the metacarpophalangeal joints. Further improvement, however, was prevented by the continual breaking down of the wounds on the dorsal surface of the fingers.

The scars on the back of the hand were then excised and thin skin grafts applied. The patient returned to the rehabilitation centre 5 weeks later, and at this stage movements were as given in *Table 5.1*.

Table 5.1   Finger movements (degrees) of Case 5.17

Finger	*Metacarpo-phalangeal joint*	*Proximal interphalangeal joint*	*Distal interphalangeal joint*
Index	0–30	0–30	0–50
Middle	0–50	0–45	0–90
Ring	0–30	0–50	0–70
Little	0–20	0–10	0–70

There was 30 degrees of flexion at the interphalangeal joint of the thumb, and the thumb could be opposed as far as the ulnar border of the middle finger. Two weeks later stretch splints were started in earnest to encourage flexion, particularly in the little finger. Nineteen weeks after the accident, the webs between the thumb and index finger and the middle and ring fingers were excised and Thiersch grafts were applied. When seen 17 days later, and after 3 weeks' further intensive treatment, full function was restored except for the extremes of opposition of the thumb (*Figure 5.18c*).

This patient thus required 25 weeks' continuous treatment for the severe burns of the hand. He was, however, able to return to full duty in his trade of operations clerk where good free movement of the hand was essential.

The principle of full-time intensive treatment dovetailing with the periodic operations required is calculated to give the best result. Only such a programme can keep pace with and overtake the relentless soft-tissue contractures that are the menace of the burnt hand.

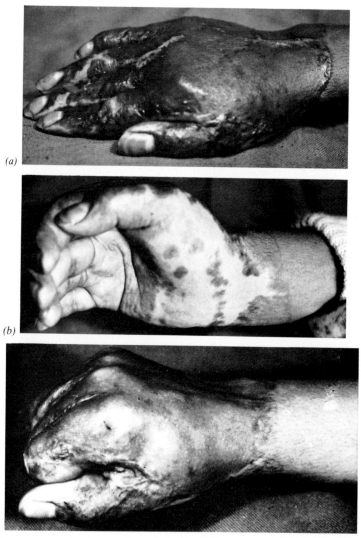

(a)

(b)

(c)

Figure 5.18   Burns of the hand. (a) Dorsal appearance. (b) Maximum finger flexion possible 2 months after accident. (c) Result after 25 weeks' treatment. (Case 5.17)

Case 5.18. This patient sustained third-degree burns of both hands when the lorry he was driving caught fire. The arms were burnt from the elbow to the finger tips on both sides, mainly on the palmar surface. Extensive skin grafting was carried out, and 7 months after the accident he was admitted to the rehabilitation centre. On the left hand there were no movements at any of the interphalangeal joints, and the metacarpophalangeal joints were held in 30 degrees of flexion. The right hand was less seriously affected but there was no palmar flexion and no movement at either of the interphalangeal joints of the ring finger. In both hands there was very adherent and tough scarring, the left hand being considerably worse than the right. After 2 weeks of intensive treatment, involving oil massage six times a day and the usual treatment for burns as described earlier, there was 20 degrees' active movement in the interphalangeal joints of the left hand.

Five months later there was 60 degrees of movement (0–60) at all the proximal interphalangeal joints of the left hand. There was 15 degrees of movement at the terminal interphalangeal joint and 5 degrees at the proximal interphalangeal joint of the ring finger. There was 10 degrees of movement at the interphalangeal joints of the other fingers. In the right hand there was almost perfect function. It was thus 1 year before this patient was able to return to work in a full-time capacity. The important point in this case is that after extensive burns of the palmar surface of both hands, resulting in a great deal of skin loss, the patient was able to return to full work. However expert the surgery, good results cannot be expected unless the operation is followed by intensive, graded and full-time rehabilitation.

SEPTIC FINGERS

General

Formal rehabilitation is necessary when infection occurs in the palmar space, the tendon sheaths, the web space, or when a generalized cellulitis develops. When incisions are made to release pus, and when antibiotic treatment is started early, there is little or no fibrosis and subsequent scarring. Active rehabilitation can therefore start within 4–6 weeks. The average time for the restoration of full function is 2–3 weeks. When, however, early control of infection is not obtained, results as judged by range of movement of the fingers may be poor.

If there has been extensive infection which has been slow to resolve, and several incisions have had to be made, healing may be slow. Considerable pain is caused by active exercise in the early stages of rehabilitation when the necrosed and scarred tissues are present. This inevitably leads to limitation of movement. The problem becomes that of coaxing fibrotic soft tissues into yielding by deep massage and long-continued stretch splinting.

Infections of the palmar space

Unless very extensive and resistant to antibiotic treatment, palmar space infections do well. As the general function of the hand, and particularly the power of grip, suffers considerably after these infections, it is advisable for the patient to have full-time treatment once the infection has resolved and all incisions healed. Although only 2 weeks' treatment is usually required for full function to be obtained, without it the patient may not regain full power of grip because the soft tissues contract extensively in the early days after such infections. It is particularly important for patients to receive rehabilitation when several incisions have been made, when an extensive area of skin has been lost or in long-standing scarring of the palm.

Finger infections

Simple infections do not require rehabilitation, but when the tendon sheath is affected, loss of movement and scarring are sufficiently severe for rehabilitation to be essential. Active exercise should be started as soon as the infection is completely resolved and all incisions healed. This may be as long as 3 weeks after infection.

At this stage the interphalangeal joints may have only 50 per cent of the normal range of movement, and when the tendon sheath has been severely damaged there may be no movement at all. In these cases tendon grafting is advisable unless the soft tissues are so severely damaged that the graft would not take. In such a case arthrodesis of the interphalangeal joint in the functional position, or amputation if the finger gets in the way, is the best course. If the tendon sheath is not too badly damaged and the flexor tendon not affected, 2–3 weeks of rehabilitation will result in full function. For the first week of active treatment, unresisted exercises together with light occupational therapy and light games should be given. By 6 weeks after the infection has resolved, moderately heavy occupational therapy and resistance exercises in the physiotherapy department can be started.

If there is any sign of impaired circulation developing during treatment, resistance should be very carefully graded and no form of heat be used. When there has been much scarring, no more than a few degrees' movement at the terminal interphalangeal joint can be expected. Provided that there is a reasonable range (45 degrees or more at the proximal interphalangeal joint), general function will be good. The lack of movement at the terminal joint need not be a disability. It takes from 6 to 8 weeks for full function to be restored in such cases.

Web-space infections

By 2 weeks after incision of web-space infections, patients are ready for rehabilitation. In all except the mildest cases, 2–3 weeks of intensive rehabilitation are necessary, as there is a tendency for the metacarpophalangeal joints to go into flexion following scarring. Power of grip is also considerably diminished.

General exercises, occupational therapy to encourage grip, and resisted extension exercises to metacarpophalangeal and interphalangeal joints restore full function.

CRUSH INJURIES

Crush injuries produce some of the worst disability seen in the hand and in the last 15 years, we have treated 80 severe crush injuries, caused in industrial accidents by machinery, in road traffic accidents and falls from a height.

In such lesions, bones may be fractured, joints dislocated, blood vessels damaged, nerves severed or crushed, tendons torn and skin broken. But what makes these injuries so much more disabling than each of these lesions on its own is the outpouring of reactive fluid in the soft tissues. This organizes and causes severe fibrosis, leading to a 'frozen hand'. It is impossible to avoid disability due to involvement of tendons, nerves and blood vessels, but a great deal of morbidity can be avoided by insisting on active movements as soon as continuity of the damaged structures has been restored, elevation to prevent oedema, and keeping immobilization to the absolute minimum. Too often X-rays are treated rather than the patient's clinical state – fibrosis is a far more effective internal splint than external plaster, and the dangers of immobilization far exceed those of early mobility. It is impossible to generalize about crush injuries because each case differs, but there is a certain fundamental regimen common to the management of them all.

(1) Oedema must either be prevented by elevation at night on a drip stand or by day in a sling, or reduced by massage in elevation, active exercises and pressure bandaging.

(2) Fibrosis must be attacked by intensive oil massage several times day, and slow stretches followed by appropriate serial plasters.

(3) Active exercises and games for both the hand and the whole upper limb should be introduced as early as possible and should include activities in the occupational therapy department. It is important to devise occupational therapy activities that demand movement of the fingers and not just using the hand as a prop. Carpenters' planes can be given lively spring handles, using Dalzafoam padding, as can the printing press; wrought iron demands hard dynamic work, as does the use of pliers and secateurs.

(4) Special dynamic splints may be needed to produce stronger correction at specific joints, particularly to obtain flexion of the metacarpophalangeal joints from extension or improved power in weakened tendons and muscles.

(5) Great skill must be exercised in judging how far one can press an active approach in the presence of bone infection, non-union and skin loss. Periodic rests for a few days may be necessary between episodes of a more vigorous approach. On the whole, one should err on the side of vigour rather than caution, for the hand is useful only when joints are mobile and tendons active.

(6) In severe and complex lesions, if conservative treatment by itself is insufficient, a long programme of surgical reconstruction is necessary.

In adduction contractures of the thumb web, the interosseus and adductor muscles and the trapezometacarpal joint are all involved; Z-plasty of the skin, division of tendons and reinsertion proximally if muscles are viable, will be necessary if conservative treatment fails.

If a mass of fibrosis is all that is left, complete excision is required. In permanently stiff metacarpophalangeal or proximal interphalangeal joints when intensive rehabilitation has failed, surgery such as ligament resection (Curtis, 1970) will be indicated.

Intensive pre- and postoperative rehabilitation will offer the best conditions for surgery and the best prospect for function. In few other conditions of the locomotor system is a really intensive approach with highly skilled therapy more essential. As these cases present such varied problems, we will discuss them by reference to representative case histories.

Case 5.19. This patient fell from a third floor window, sustaining multiple injuries including dislocations of second, third, fourth and fifth carpometacarpal joints and fracture of the base of the index metacarpal. Skeletal traction was applied but had to be reapplied owing to the position having slipped. Immobilization was necessary for 7 weeks. On starting intensive rehabilitation he had no active or passive movements in the metacarpophalangeal joints or proximal interphalangeal joints. Intensive treatment was given, including passive movements to metacarpophalangeal joints, serial plasters, games in the gymnasium and workshop activities (*Figure 5.19*).

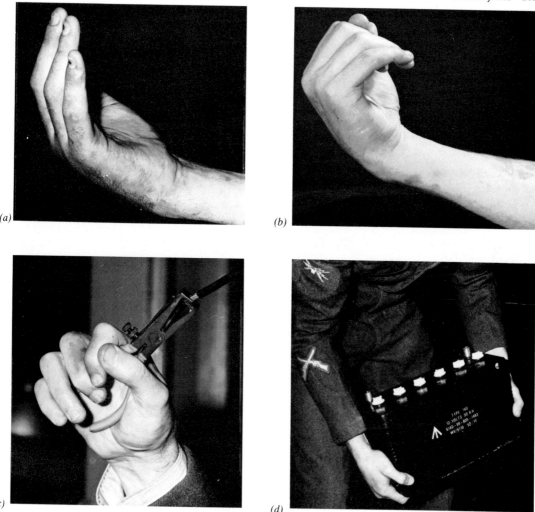

Figure 5.19 Crush injury of hand, dislocation of carpometacarpal joints. (a) Attempted flexion 10 weeks after injury. (b) Flexion 7 months after injury. (c) Use of pliers. (d) Carrying heavy battery. (Case 5.19)

Figure 5.20. This patient caught his right hand in a mechanized press and sustained severe vascular, nervous and bony damage, with fracture subluxation of second, third and fourth metacarpals and destruction of the intrinsic muscles. On admission to the rehabilitation centre, he presented with a frozen hand with no active or passive movements in wrist, metacarpophalangeal or interphalangeal joints. There was gross induration and swelling of the whole hand.

Intensive treatment included the full range of physiotherapy as described – massage in elevation, serial plasters, occupational therapy and games and, in addition, a lively stretch splint to exercise the wrist and increase metacarpophalangeal range when not under formal treatment. The end-result, although not obviously dramatic, allowed the patient to use his hand for most tasks (*Figure 5.20*).

Figure 5.21. This patient was mauled by a lion, sustaining severe infected lacerations of the whole hand and fractures of the carpus, radius and ulna, and middle finger metacarpal. On starting rehabilitation he had a frozen hand with no movement at all. Intensive passive movement with stretches was required, and Plastazote wedges were very useful in increasing passive range of the thumb web and interdigital clefts (*Figure 5.21*).

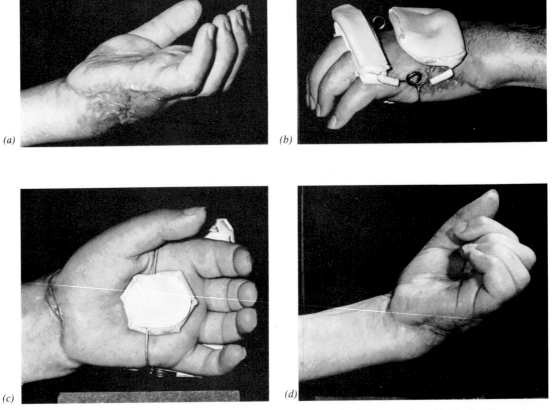

(a)   *(b)*   *(c)*   *(d)*

Figure 5.20 *(a) Ten weeks after severe crush injury. (b, c) Use of lively stretch splint. (d) Flexion 11 months after injury. (Case 5.20)*

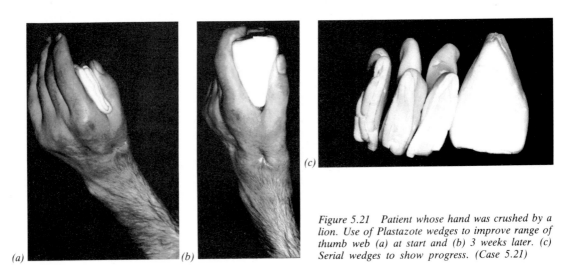

(a)   *(b)*   *(c)*

Figure 5.21 *Patient whose hand was crushed by a lion. Use of Plastazote wedges to improve range of thumb web (a) at start and (b) 3 weeks later. (c) Serial wedges to show progress. (Case 5.21)*

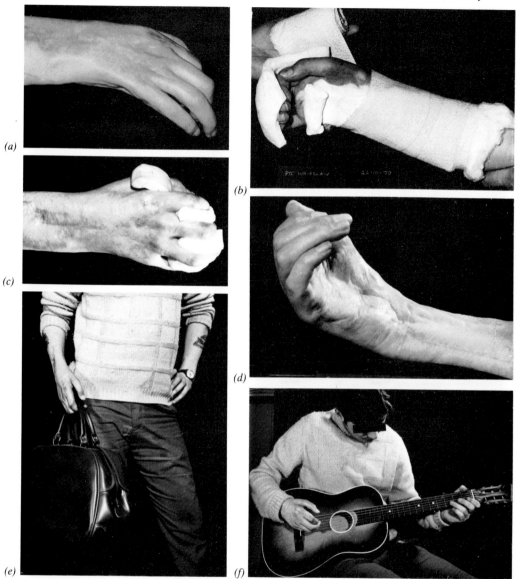

Figure 5.22 Crush injury. (a) Hand at start of treatment. (b) Use of Plastazote stretch splints to increase metacarpophalangeal flexion. (c) Use of Plastazote wedges to increase range of interdigital webs. (d) Active range 3 months after start of treatment. (e) Hook grip. (f) Satisfactory resettlement. (Case 5.23)

Figure 5.22. This patient sustained a severe injury to the right hand, involving the ulnar nerve, flexors carpi ulnaris, radialis, profundus digitorum and palmaris longus; he developed a very stiff hand and shoulder, as he suffered from Parkinson's disease. On starting rehabilitation 6 weeks after secondary nerve suture, he had a range of movement of 0–40 degrees at index metacarpophalangeal joint, 0–50 degrees middle, 0–20 degrees ring, 0–40 degrees little finger, and only 20 degrees at the proximal interphalangeal joints which were flexed to 45 degrees. Intensive oil massage, plasters and stretches were required, and after 7 weeks movements at metacarpophalangeal joints were 0–95 degrees index, 0–75 degrees middle, ring and little fingers. The fingers could be passively flexed down to touch the palm, the ulnar nerve had reinnervated abductor digiti minimi and the patient was discharged back to work.

Case 5.23. A 21-year-old army paratrooper sustained a severe injury to his right elbow and hand when a train door crushed his arm. He had badly lacerated wounds, and the flexor tendons of the fingers and thumbs were divided and crushed; the median nerve was also severed. He had badly displaced fractures of the right radius and ulna and the right elbow.

On admission for rehabilitation the elbow was virtually fixed at 90 degrees. The wrist was held in ulnar deviation with a slight flexion deformity and with about 10 degrees of movement. His metacarpophalangeal joints were virtually fixed in 1–2 degrees of flexion, and the proximal and terminal interphalangeal joints were also fixed in varying degrees of flexion. The basic problem was to mobilize the metacarpophalangeal joints by restoring flexion and opening out the thumb and finger webs. Plastazote wedges, intensive oil massage, exercises and games restored adequate function for him to drive a car, play tennis and perform creditably on the guitar (*Figure 5.22*).

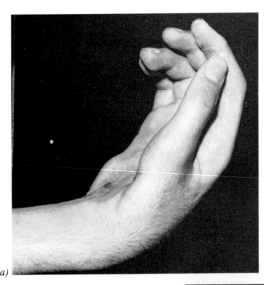

(a)

Figure 5.23   Blast injury to right hand due to firework. (a) Maximum flexion of wrist and fingers at start of rehabilitation. (b) Severe scarring and lack of opposition at the same stage. (Case 5.25)

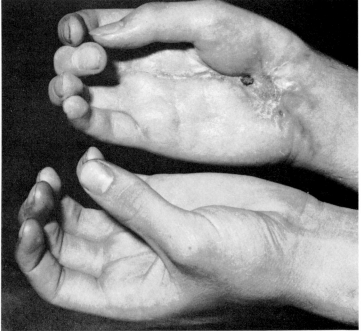

(b)

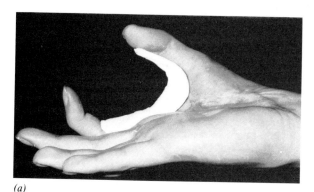
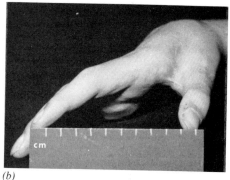

(a)   *(b)*

Figure 5.24   (a) Stretch plaster used to restore thumb web in Case 5.25. (b) Maximum range of thumb web restored by this treatment

Case 5.24.   This patient, a general fitter, caught his left arm in a burn cutter (a type of milling machine), dividing all tendons, arteries and nerves in front of the wrist. Primary tendon suture was effected but owing to skin loss and dirt in the wound the nerve ends were approximated, and abdominal skin flap was required to obtain stable skin cover. He was admitted to the MRU for 3 weeks' intensive preoperative mobilization of the stiff joints and encouragement of maximum power. Three months after injury he was re-explored; the median nerve was sutured, but the ulnar nerve could not be found. Six weeks later he was readmitted to the MRU. After 4 weeks' intensive exercises, occupational therapy and games, the index finger touched the palm, the middle lacked the palm by 0.5 cm, the ring by 4 cm and the little finger by 3 cm. Sensation was beginning to return. At this stage he was tested in the workshops on various tools and found fully fit. Accordingly he returned to duty and in due course made a satisfactory recovery.

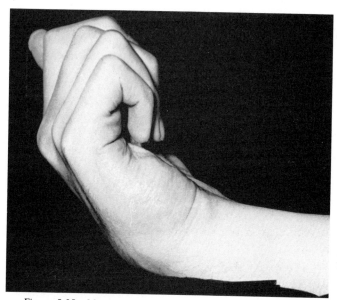

Figure 5.25   Maximum flexion in Case 5.25 on discharge

Case 5.25.   This patient sustained a severe injury to the right hand when a firework that he was making at home exploded in his right hand. He sustained disruption of the palm and thumb web, with partial severing of the thumb at the carpometacarpal joint, destruction of the neurovascular bundle of the thumb and complete destruction of the small muscles of the hand. The digital nerves of the thumb and index fingers were totally divided. The carpus sustained anterior dislocation with fracture-dislocation of the four metacarpals. *Figure 5.23* shows the state of the hand at the start of rehabilitation.

A skin graft was applied and the patient was transferred to the MRU on 10 October 1961, some 3 months after injury, for preoperative mobilization. He had gross scarring of the palm, loss of the web of the thumb, severe limitation of wrist and thumb movements, and sensory loss in the median distribution. There were, of course, no thenar muscles at all. Scar excision was performed on 5 February 1962, and digital nerve suture and further skin grafting to the palm. Full rehabilitation was given for 4 months, when the scar was fully resolved and a good range of passive movement in the thumb web was obtained (*Figures 5.24* and *5.25*). There was reasonable function in the hand but the lack of thumb rotation proved a disability. Six months later, flexor sublimis transfer was carried out and excellent function was obtained.

VASCULAR IMPAIRMENT

General

Impairment of the blood supply to the hand, when caused locally, presents the same problems as discussed under crush injuries, for the disability is due to the scarring and consequent interference with tendon function. Particular care must, of course, be observed to ensure that such patients do not sustain burns, chilblains or the like. Repeated warning should be given about the precautions to be observed in cold weather and in protecting their hands from possible risk of burns.

Sudeck's atrophy

One of the most puzzling and difficult of painful conditions of the upper limb is the so-called reflex sympathetic dystrophy or algodystrophy, often known as Sudeck's atrophy. This condition usually follows mild trauma such as a sprain of the wrist or a simple Colles' fracture, and may result in very severe disability with a painful swollen stiff hand.

Recently, Loh and Nathan (1978) have suggested that both Sudeck's atrophy and causalgia have the same pathophysiological basis and can respond to the same programme of treatment. In causalgia there is disorder of a major nerve, whereas in algodystrophy or Sudeck's atrophy multiple small nerves are involved.

The characteristics of algodystrophy are pain, swelling, stiffness and weakness, trophic skin changes and vasomotor instability (not invariably), osteoporosis (*Figure 5.26*) and occasional thickening of the palmar fascia. In the early stages there is vasodilatation, oedema, raised temperature and sweating. Later, the hand becomes cold and cyanotic, the skin being smooth and shiny with atrophy of the tissues and gross joint stiffness.

Pain is a prominent feature, the patient being loath to move the fingers or use the hand, and hyperpathia is often severe.

Schumacher and Abramson (1949) reviewed 142 male patients with Sudeck's atrophy (111 in the foot, 31 in the hand) and found that 58 followed soft tissue injuries, 19 sprains, 11 crush injuries, 14 compound fractures and 7 simple fractures. Pain was severe in 97, with swelling in 95, cyanosis in 93, cold in 72, excess sweating in 52 and hyperaesthesia in 23. All had weakness and stiffness of the affected part.

It is still a mystery how a trival injury can cause such a devastating disorder which can persist indefinitely if not vigorously treated in the early stages. Clearly there must

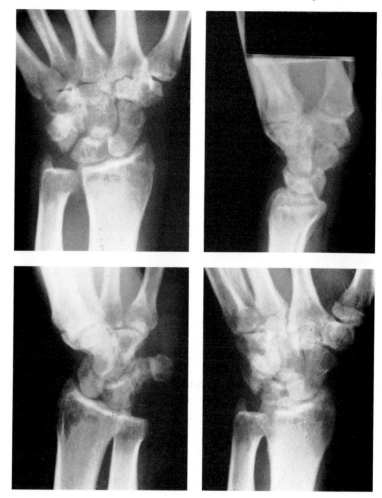

Figure 5.26 Sudeck's atrophy

be an abnormal response to sympathetic output, and we accept Loh and Nathan's view (referred to above) that it is primarily a disorder of peripheral nerve – the common denominator of sympathetic overactivity, hyperpathia and pain to both Sudeck's atrophy and causalgia is very striking. All workers are agreed that if treatment is to be effective it must start as soon as possible, as the keystone of treatment is to urge the patient to use his hand in order to regain joint movement and muscle power and to reduce swelling. The relief of pain is the first priority. Sympathetic block is the most effective means of pain relief.

Sympathectomy has been used for many years in this condition. Drucker and colleagues (1959) reported 26 out of 31 patients (in a series of 61 cases of Sudeck's atrophy) relieved of pain by sympathectomy. Schumacher and Abramson (1949) found 17 of 31 relieved by this procedure. In our view, guanethidine blocks are more effective and, of course, do not involve surgical operations; we therefore favour guanethidine blocks as described for causalgia, and only if they fail do we proceed to stellate blocks or sympathectomy.

Dunningham (1980) compared the results of stellate block and guanethidine in 18 patients with Sudeck's atrophy, and found that guanethidine lasted longer (and was easier to administer). Hannington-Kiff (1974) had very good results in 12 of 17 patients, with guanethidine blocks in Sudeck's atrophy.

Transcutaneous electrical stimulation (TES) helps some patients and is always worth trying. If oedema is present, we insist on elevation 24 hours a day. It is amazing how chronic oedema can resolve in a matter of days by continuous elevation. Sometimes the continuous environmental treatment unit is useful for those patients who cannot tolerate continuous elevation.

It may be necessary to reinforce sympathetic block and electrical stimulation with analgesics; we do not favour oral steroids and are unimpressed by the published reports of their value – the studies, to our mind, being uncontrolled. Passive manipulations of stiff joints are absolutely contraindicated – they always produce more swelling and pain and, therefore, further stiffness. We have seen devastating results of repeated manipulations of the wrist or metacarpophalangeal joints after anaesthesia.

Once pain is reduced and swelling is under control, a vigorous programme of active exercises with progressive resistance is instituted in physiotherapy, occupational therapy and workshops.

We insist that our patients come into hospital to our rehabilitation ward, not the least of the reasons being the frequent necessity of elevation at night. Only by an integrated programme of measures to relieve pain, block sympathetic outflow and encourage use of the upper limb can a good result be expected.

If the patient is seen in the late stage, it may be impossible to achieve a satisfactory result by conservative means, and capsulotomy of stiff metacarpophalangeal and interphalangeal joints will be required. In Schumacher and Abramson's (1949) series, 50 out of 95 patients responded well to such an intensive programme, and the result was directly proportional to the time between injury and the start of rehabilitation. It is important to explain the nature of the condition to the patient so as to enlist his enthusiasm in the rehabilitation programme, and above all to reassure him that he is not mad. There is a belief that a special type of person – sensitive, neurotic, introspective – is liable to succumb to this condition. We no longer subscribe to this view, having been impressed by the dramatic response to effective treatment and the return to normal work and life as soon as pain is relieved.

Shoulder-hand syndrome

The shoulder-hand syndrome is a curious condition in which the patient develops a painful stiff shoulder with a painful swollen hand on the same side. Various terms have been used to describe it, including reflex dystrophy and reflex sympathetic dystrophy. Until the pathophysiology is made clearer, it seems preferable to use the descriptive term 'shoulder-hand syndrome' than a title suggesting a known cause.

Certain precipitating factors are known to precede the onset of the condition, the most important being cardiac infarction and hemiplegia. However, it may follow trivial injuries to the upper limb, and in many cases no exciting cause can be found. The severity of the condition bears no relation to that of the cause and the worst clinical picture may follow a silent infarct. Moreover, the onset may be instantaneous or follow weeks or months after the cause.

The shoulder is painful and very stiff and may in time become completely frozen, with virtually no passive or active range of motion, wasting of the surrounding muscles and severe persistent pain. Radiographs show marked osteoporosis. The hand also is painful and there is marked generalized swelling, particularly obvious on the dorsum of the hand.

The earliest changes are to be seen in the fingers, with thickening round the edges of the nail bed. Later, the skin becomes shiny and trophic changes develop, with ultimate atrophy of the tissues and flexion deformities due to soft-tissue fibrosis and contracture. That this is a vascular disturbance is well shown by the profuse sweating, colour changes and vasodilatation in the skin of the whole hand. Osteoporosis is seen in all the bones of the wrist and fingers.

Diagnosis is usually easy, though it is important not to confuse the stiff shoulder and swollen hand after neglected hemiplegia with the true shoulder-hand syndrome in which obvious vascular changes are to be seen.

MANAGEMENT

The single most important factor in the prevention of this syndrome is the assiduous practice of active exercises to the upper limb in patients, confined to bed, who are suffering from lesions known to provoke the shoulder-hand syndrome; this particularly applies to patients with cardiac infarction and cerebrovascular accidents.

When the condition develops, the patient will require adequate sedation because the pain can be most distressing. Active exercise to shoulder and hand, with elevation and massage to reduce the oedema in the hand, must be instituted immediately. Manipulation of the shoulder is rarely indicated – it may worsen the pain, promote an effusion into the joint and lead to more stiffness.

There is disagreement about the place of stellate ganglion block among experts in this field; most people feel that the results are too disappointing to be worth trial, unlike the results in causalgia.

Prolonged active physiotherapy, encouragement to use the limb and treatment of the underlying condition usually result in a reasonable return of function, though the course may be long and depressing and recovery in a severe case should not be expected in less than 3 months.

Volkmann's contracture

This is a condition of contracture of the forearm muscles and, in severe cases, of the intrinsics also, due to vascular impairment. By far the most common causes are tight plasters constricting the brachial vessels, and fracture-dislocation of the elbow involving the brachial artery.

Three degrees of this condition are recognized: contracture of the forearm muscles with sparing of the intrinsics; contracture of the forearm and intrinsic paralysis – producing the intrinsic minus deformity (claw and ape hand); and, rarely, contracture of the forearm and an intrinsic plus deformity (metacarpophalangeal joints flexed and interphalangeal joints extended) due to contracture of the intrinsics also. Various combinations of forearm contracture and intrinsic paralysis are seen, either the median or the ulnar nerves being predominantly involved. The author has seen two cases in which the radial supplied muscles have also been affected.

In the first type, extension of the fingers is improved by increasing wrist flexion; in the second type the fingers actively extend when the wrist extends, but when an intrinsic plus deformity is also present, proximal interphalangeal flexion increases only when the metacarpophalangeal joints are flexed, as extension of the metacarpophalangeal joints further tightens an already tight extensor mechanism.

In the mild or moderate case it is always worth trying an intensive course of physiotherapy with oil massage to try to loosen scarring and to mobilize the muscles and tendons with slow gentle stretches and serial plasters. If the deformity responds, at a later stage a lively radial splint is worn to encourage the patient to use active dorsiflexion to continue the stretch of the contracted muscles. Recovery of nerve function depends on the degree of intraneural fibrosis produced by the lesion – if spontaneous reinnervation occurs the techniques of re-education described in Chapter 6 will be indicated. If the deformity is corrected but no recovery occurs in the paralysed muscles, tendon transfers and capsulorrhaphy will provide useful function. If the deformity does not respond to conservative measures, or is severe and is clearly beyond physiotherapy, surgical correction is essential. The flexors of the wrist are cut, the flexor pollicis longus extended and all contracted tissues excised. The extensor carpi radialis longus is then transferred to flexor digitorum profundus and brachioradialis to flexor pollicis longus at different levels of the wrist. Zancolli (1979) prefers this procedure to muscle slide operations or bone resection. If, however, the flexor digitorum profundus is spared and strong, then a muscle slide of the wrist flexors can be performed. He uses a splint to stabilize the metacarpophalangeal joints and extend the wrist to stop the patient flexing the interphalangeal joints by tenodesis action when the wrist flexes and the metacarpophalangeal joints hyperextend.

In re-educating the patient, the physiotherapist will support the wrist in extension and the metacarpophalangeal joints in slight flexion to encourage the transfer to work actively. The intrinsic plus deformity is very resistant to conservative treatment, although it is worth a short period of trial even if only to give the surgeon the best condition of the soft tissues on which to operate. In mild cases a triangular resection of the extensor aponeurosis may be adequate, but resection of the interosseus tendons is the only way in which severe deformity can be corrected. This is done at the level of the necks of the metacarpophalangeal joints and tendon transfers are used to provide abduction of the index finger.

The intrinsic plus deformity may involve one or all of the intrinsics (*Figure 5.27*). The small blood vessels are easily compressed in the hand within the flexor sheaths and fascial layers, and the deformity follows crush injuries, tight plasters or even bandages, severe oedema that is allowed to persist, haematoma, direct violence, exposure to X-rays which cause severe fibrosis, scleroderma, and spasticity in lesions of the upper motor neuron.

Case 5.26. This man sustained a fracture of his left elbow at the age of 16 and says that, almost immediately following the injury, he noticed ulnar deviation of the left hand. Eleven years later he complained of pain in the hand due to excess strain in a new job. On examination, he had wasting and weakness of the wrist and finger

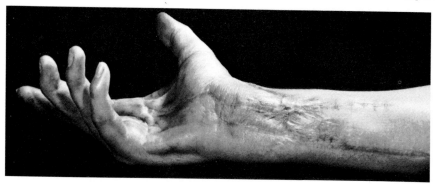

Figure 5.27 Intrinsic plus deformity

extensors, the interossei and the thenar muscles, with scattered sensory loss and hypersensitivity in all three nerves. There was marked ulnar deviation and swan neck deformities of all fingers except the index.

After prolonged effort he could just make a fist. After 2 weeks' intensive exercises his grip was almost normal and function good. In view of this, surgery was postponed to see if he could cope on a lighter job. On review 5 years later sensation had returned to normal and function was excellent with motor grade 4 in all muscles.

Case 5.27. This patient presented a curious story of waking one morning, after a particularly good party, with his right hand painful, swollen and black. There was a possibility that he had fallen asleep with the hand trapped behind a radiator. One month later the hand was still stiff and swollen and he had a marked intrinsic plus deformity. Two months later the contractures of the adductor pollicis and first dorsal interosseus were divided. Six months later he still had a tight thumb web (5 cm less spread than on normal side), a hyperextension of proximal interphalangeal joints and flexion of metacarpophalangeal joints with tight digital webs. Circulation was poor. Wasting of abductor pollicis brevis was present and shown by electromyographic studies to be due to a partial median nerve lesion with a prolonged distal latency at the wrist (9 ms). Intensive oil massage and serial Plastazote wedges restored the web almost to normal and power was adequate for his job as a clerk.

On review, 14 months later, the abductor pollicis brevis was normal. The thumb web measured 12.5 cm, sensation was normal and he could make a full fist, but had some difficulty in holding large objects, as when his metacarpophalangeal joints were extended it was difficult for him to flex the interphalangeal joints. His function was excellent, however, and he was typing at 30 words a minute.

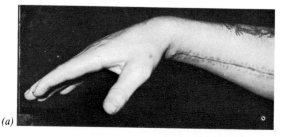

(a)

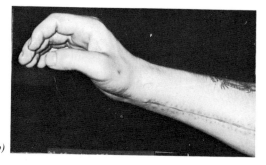

(b)

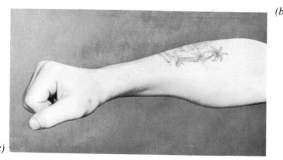

(c)

Figure 5.28 Volkmann's ischaemic contracture of 23 years' duration with contracture of flexors. Surgical release resulted in an excellent tenodesis effect. (a) Full extension with wrist flexed. (b) Beginning of closure of fingers in wrist extension. (c) Full flexion with wrist extended. (Case 5.29)

Case 5.28. A smoke grenade blew up in this man's hand, causing compound fractures of the second and third metacarpals, vascular damage and an intrinsic plus deformity. The avascular muscle was excised and the fractures manipulated. Two months later he started intensive rehabilitation. The range of movement at the metacarpophalangeal joints was 55 index, 60 middle, 65 ring, 45 little, and 60 at the proximal interphalangeal joints. There was a swan neck deformity. Intensive massage, passive and active movements, games and occupational therapy were given and, in view of the recalcitrance of the deformity, a lively stretch splint was provided to assist metacarpophalangeal joint flexion and to prevent hyperextension at the proximal interphalangeal joints. He made an excellent recovery and returned to duty after 9 weeks.

Case 5.29. This patient sustained a Volkmann's ischaemic contracture as a result of an injury as a child. At the age of 30 he began to develop increasing weakness of the arm and hand. At operation atrophied profundus tendons were divided, the profundus tendon to index sutured to sublimis and the remaining profundus tendons sutured to the sublimis. He obtained an excellent result with a good tenodesis effect (*Figure 5.28*).

Case 5.30. This patient, aged 40 years, sustained compound comminuted fractures of the medial epicondyle of the humerus, dislocation of the head of the radius, a fractured shaft of the ulna, gross muscle damage and total skin loss over the right elbow and upper arm when his right arm was trapped beneath an overturned lorry.

Wound toilet was effected and the fractures were reduced and set in plaster.

Two further excisions of devitalized tissues were undertaken 3 days and 11 days later. The median nerve was found to have partially sloughed away, and evidence of ischaemic contracture of the flexors of the wrist and fingers was clearly seen. The whole arm was skin grafted 9 weeks after injury.

Fourteen weeks after injury the patient was transferred to the rehabilitation centre when his condition was as follows.

There was an extremely tough scarred skin all around the elbow and the upper arm. Elbow movements were 80–105 degrees; no rotation was present. The wrist was held in 25 degrees' palmar flexion; 10 degrees of palmar flexion could be obtained passively although not actively. No passive dorsiflexion was possible. All the muscles supplied by the median nerve in the hand were working weakly, but there was no sensation present. The passive movements of the fingers were as given in *Table 5.2*.

Table 5.2   Finger movements (degrees) of Case 5.30

Finger	Metacarpo-phalangeal	Proximal interphalangeal	Distal interphalangeal
Index	25–50	82 fixed	35 fixed
Middle	25–50	63–85	0 fixed
Ring	35–52	20–35	8–12
Little	20–30	20–38	8–18

Thumb: 150–149 in interphalangeal joint

On maximum voluntary wrist and finger flexion, measurements from the finger tips to the wrist crease were: index 19 cm; middle 20 cm; ring 22.5 cm; little 20 cm.

The thumb web measured from the medial border of the thumb nail to the lateral border of the crease proximal to the proximal interphalangeal joint of the index finger was 2.5 cm (*Figure 5.29a, b*).

This was an extremely severe injury, the hand disability being due to a severe contracture of the flexors of the wrist and fingers, with muscle necrosis and a partial median nerve lesion.

Fortunately, the elbow limitation was little handicap as the joint was virtually fixed in the position of function.

Intensive treatment continued for 5 months, comprising oil massage six times a day, serial plaster stretches, active exercises, all varieties of craft work starting with basketry and progressing to heavy carpentry, games in the gymnasium, and efforts to restore morale with outings and recreational activities. The patient was given codeine before each session of stretching.

It was never expected that a spectacular result would be achieved, but the limited objectives aimed for were the hope that the patient would feel that the hand was a part of him again, and that he would regain sufficient active flexion to grip, grasp and lift objects, and be able to manipulate coarse tools, and perhaps write.

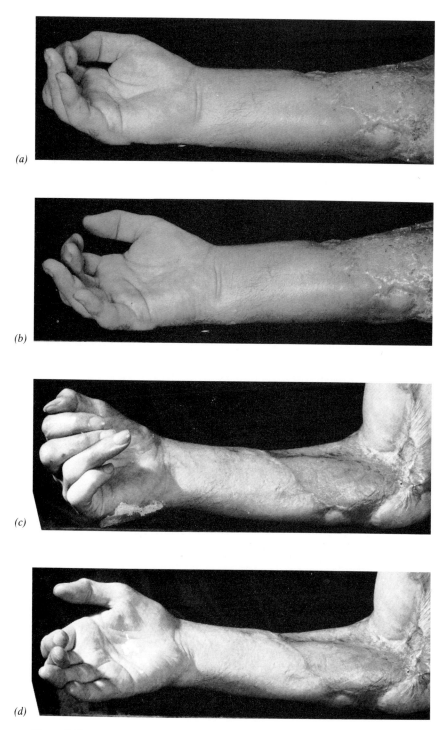

Figure 5.29 Progress of Case 5.30 with ischaemic necrosis of the forearm, the wrist and finger flexors. (a) Maximum flexion and (b) maximum extension after 14 weeks. (c) Maximum flexion and (d) maximum extension after 5 months of intensive rehabilitation

Table 5.3 Finger movements (degrees) before and after intensive treatment of Case 5.30

Finger	Metacarpophalangeal		Proximal interphalangeal		Distal interphalangeal	
	Before	*After*	*Before*	*After*	*Before*	*After*
Index	10–70	+35	82 fixed	+20	35 fixed	No change
Middle	10–70	+35	63–85	+13	0 fixed	No change
Ring	15–60	+28	20–35	+15	8–12	+31
Little	0–35	+25	20–38	+32	8–18	+35

Measurements recorded before and at the end of 5 months' intensive treatment were as shown in *Table 5.3*. There was 30 degrees' palmar flexion and a few degrees' dorsiflexion (*Figure 5.29c, d*). Elbow movements were still 25 degrees and there was no rotation.

This degree of improvement made all the difference to function, for on discharge the patient could grasp most tools, dress easily, grip large objects, carry heavy weights, and he felt the hand once again belonged to him. He was convinced that all the hard work and pain was worth while, and his morale could not have been higher.

FUNCTIONAL DISORDERS OF THE HAND

Psychiatrically determined disorders can affect the hand as they can other parts of the body, imitating organic disease. This may take the form of weakness of grip, sensory loss or paralysis of the hand imitating peripheral nerve disorders. Careful history taking, clinical examinations and electrodiagnosis reveal that the lesion is not organic, and will lead the doctor to the correct diagnosis and treatment. However, it may be possible in patients with *mild* functional disorders and in whom there is no obvious psychiatric illness to obtain full function without recourse to prolonged psychotherapy by exposing them to the atmosphere of the rehabilitation unit. The following case histories illustrate these points.

Case 5.31.   This patient, for reasons best known to herself, deliberately burnt her arm with Lysol. She had an operation to free adhesions following scarring of skin over the wrists. When seen for rehabilitation 3 weeks after surgery she had marked weakness of the hand, grip was only 1.4 kg compared with 5 kg on the normal side. There was stiffness but no true limitation of movement. It was observed both in the physiotherapy and occupational therapy departments, that the patient did not produce the power and function of which she was capable, as she could when taken 'off guard'. She seemed to be a sensible and agreeable person, but was clearly not co-operating. After much encouragement, and after pointing out to her that when not observed she was able to do more than when being observed, she accepted that with time and normal use function would return and she returned to her job. At 3-month follow-up function was normal.

Case 5.32.   This patient presented with weakness, pain, and pins and needles in the left arm for no apparent reason and with no history of trauma. Full examination and investigations, including lumbar puncture, revealed no abnormality. He was admitted to the rehabilitation unit for assessment and treatment. Electrical investigations showed that there was no abnormality in any of the muscles in the upper limb, nor was there any wasting or sensory loss. On examination he held his arm loosely by his side and was unable to lift it or move the hand. Neck radiographs and neck movements were normal. Hysterical paralysis was diagnosed but no convincing reason could be determined for the development of this condition. He was treated by general exercises and games in the gymnasium and was observed discreetly in the occupational therapy department. It was found that when not observed he was able to use the arm normally and when this was put to him he finally accepted that there was no reason why function should not be normal, and returned to duty as a nursing attendant. There has been no further trouble with the arm.

THE SPASTIC UPPER LIMB

Upper motor neuron lesions present the most formidable challenge to rehabilitation and it is distressing to have to record that there is still no answer to the severely spastic hand. By far the most common condition causing spasticity is hemiplegia due to stroke or embolism. An increasing number of patients are being seen now with hemiplegia following head injuries. Other causes include brain tumours and congenital disorders. Cerebral palsy is a specialized problem and will not be considered here. It is estimated that the incidence of hemiplegia is about 2 per 1000 of the population. A district general hospital can expect to see 500 cases a year, of which half will need rehabilitation.

The difficulty in hemiplegia is to determine at an early stage those patients who will benefit from intensive treatment and those who will never recover significant function and should be trained to become one-armed as quickly as possible. We are even more hampered by lack of controlled trials, so it is not clear whether those patients who make functional recovery in the upper limb do so because of physiotherapy or whether partly damaged tissue regains function or healthy tissue substitutes for dead brain tissue.

Enthusiastic and dedicated therapists are convinced that specialized rehabilitation techniques do result in improvement that is not to be explained by spontaneous natural recovery. Their views are to be respected but it still remains true that a long-term prospective controlled trial is urgently needed to establish the exact role of the newer techniques and the type of patient who should be encouraged to attend for many weeks or months for intensive treatment. Experience with head injuries has shown us that recovery of physical and intellectual functions can occur several years after injury and that a multidisciplinary approach to such patients, using physiotherapy, occupational therapy, speech therapy and memory retraining on an intensive basis, is eminently worth while. It is likely that damage in head injuries is diffuse and incomplete and unlike the localized lesion in cerebrovascular accidents, and that other areas of the brain can take over lost function. It is therefore worth persevering with rehabilitation for many months, even in patients with an apparently hopeless prognosis. One of the most important factors in recovery is constant and diverse stimulation of the patient by all members of the team in their different spheres. Controlled trials are not needed to prove that some rehabilitation is better than none at all – those patients who return to a protected environment after head injury and who are never encouraged to aim for independence, remain vegetables. But here, too, much work is required to determine those patients who are likely to acquire skills adequate for employment and who will never be independent, so that the efforts of the therapeutic staff can be concentrated on those who will benefit most. Where hemiplegia is due to cerebrovascular accidents the picture is a little clearer. Hurwitz and Adams (1972) have specified good and bad prognostic factors. Of 100 patients with hemiplegia, 10 per cent fail to survive 2 months, 30 per cent will be permanently chairbound and 60 per cent will make some degree of recovery, of which one-third will achieve independence. It is usually accepted that the likely prognosis will not become clear for at least 12 weeks.

Although severe dysphasia and dementia are likely to be a serious bar to rehabilitation, it is important to reasses at 3 months because some patients may have improved by then and be ready for rehabilitation. Surprisingly, age is no bar to successful rehabilitation and, although the sooner rehabilitation is started the better, it is still worth attempting even if there has been a long delay.

Careful assessment of the patient's prestroke condition is essential, for if there has been intellectual deterioration, sensory deficit or impaired postural control before the illness the outlook is poor. This means finding out from the relatives what the patient's personality, outlook, motivation and physical function were before the stroke. Old patients have muscular weakness anyway, and if there has been a history of angina, coronary thrombosis, arthritis or pulmonary disease, these will all limit the objectives at which rehabilitation is aimed. The occupational therapist, nursing staff and, if necessary, clinical psychologist, will need to assess the mental and speech functions. Loss of body image, difficulty in concentration, lack of insight or poor orientation in time and space will hinder rehabilitation. Receptive aphasia is more serious than expressive aphasia and loss of recent memory may be the most serious bar of all to employment or even personal independence. Continued incontinence is a bad sign.

In the early flaccid stage, the aims of treatment are to prevent contractures and to keep the paralysed joints mobile. The hand must be elevated to prevent oedema, using a folded pillow. All joints must be put through a full range of movement several times a day, which the patient is encouraged to do himself. A sling is worn as soon as the patient is allowed out of bed, usually after 48 hours.

In the small number of patients who develop the shoulder-hand syndrome, vigorous mobilization is essential. The condition can be recognized by the pink, swollen, glossy hand and the stiff and markedly painful shoulder, more painful than the stiff shoulder to be expected with hemiplegia.

Not only is there a danger of permanent stiffness if mobilization is not carried out early, but calcification in the ligaments overlying the elbow may occur. If the shoulder becomes stiff due to neglect, previous rotator cuff degeneration or actual damage in a fall when smitten by the cerebrovascular accident, intra-articular steroid injection is well worth trying, followed by active and passive exercise. Two or 3 weeks after the stroke the patient will develop spasticity, with the typical adducted internally rotated shoulder, flexed elbow, pronated forearm, flexed wrist and fingers, and adducted thumb. Prognosis for return of function in the hand is bad if spasticity is severe, if sensory deficit is pronounced, motivation poor, intellect imparied, dysphasia receptive and severe, hemianopia present, difficulty with balance and grossly stiff shoulder.

Sensory loss is of the central type – the patient can feel a pin-prick, touch, and can differentiate hot and cold but he cannot synthesize sensations into meaningful terms; thus he cannot recognize objects, textures or shapes. The simplest test of central sensory loss is to draw numbers and letters on the patient's hand when blindfolded and ask him to identify them. Loss of two-point discrimination is a bad sign but less functional than recognition of letters, numbers, objects and textures. There is no evidence as yet to suggest that retraining can affect serious central sensory loss, and recovery of fine hand function will not occur.

The minimum aim of treatment is for the patient to be able to walk, to be socially reliable and to achieve personal independence. In the upper limb, there should be mobility and stability of the shoulder, use of the upper limb for support and possibly retraining of the hand for grasp. A few patients will regain fine function of the hand, but only if sensation is normal, mobility good and spasticity mild.

It is imperative for attainable objectives to be set and for the patient to understand what can be expected and what cannot. Often, intelligent patients find it hard to accept their physical restrictions, and great tact and persuasion is necessary to help them adjust so as to avoid depression, frustration and refusal of treatment. Hurwitz and Adams (1972), in their excellent paper, stress that the important factors in management are constant effort to communicate with the patient, reassurance, stimulation of sensory input and intensive retraining of balance. Support from relatives, satisfactory reintegration into the community, appropriate housing and adaptions in the house, and encouragement to be independent and to undertake some useful activity, are all obviously essential for the best results.

Physiotherapy

RANGE OF MOVEMENT

It is generally agreed that proximal stability is an essential prerequisite for any possibility of distal function. Full passive range in the shoulder should have been maintained during the flaccid stage and passive movements should continue in the spastic stage. Stiffness is treated in the usual way with active assisted exercises, pulley exercises, slings and multiple slow stretches, avoiding anything like a manipulation. Similarly, range should be maintained or regained in the elbow, wrist and fingers, although gross spasticity makes this very difficult.

RE-EDUCATION OF MOVEMENT

As Bobath (1978) points out, normal postural reflex mechanisms are the basis for all normal voluntary movement. The hemiplegic has lost his postural reactions on the affected side and one must therefore start by treating the trunk, shoulder and hip. Because spasticity inhibits the action of anti-gravity muscles, one must restore the normal reflex mechanism first. Thus she recommends elevating the arm until the spasticity disappears or is reduced, and then asks the patient to hold the arm at various levels. From her long experience, Bobath finds that the degree of spasticity varies from day to day and from one joint position to another. Assessment and treatment therefore must progress *pari passu* – the conventional MRC grading of power is useless; much more relevant is the assessment of the degree of spasticity in different movement patterns. Muscles function in a great number of patterns and therefore they must be tested in different activities; for example, the patient is asked to attempt opening the hand with the wrist flexed, extended, pronated and supinated, and with adduction and abduction of the fingers.

As patterns are abnormal in hemiplegia, the aim is first to suppress these abnormal patterns and then to introduce normal patterns. Resistance exercises and propriocep-tive neuromuscular facilitation techniques, using the principle of irradiation, increase the spasticity and are therefore contraindicated. As muscles are involved in movement, the patient is trained during movement and not on held positions. Reflex inhibitory patterns are used to release spasticity – extension of the neck and spine produce external rotation of the arm and elbow. When this has been achieved, extension of the wrist and abduction of the thumb are added. The discovery of the correct patterns in which spasticity is reduced and function obtained is the key to treatments and these vary from patient to patient. Each time the patient is made to feel the normal functional movement, and then each component is separated and trained individually.

In the flaccid stage, primitive movements are encouraged – such as rolling, taking care to avoid spastic patterns. All voluntary movements other than those of the spastic pattern (i.e. flexion, internal rotation and adduction) are encouraged. The arm is positioned in the patterns opposite to those of spasticity and the patient is encouraged to hold them. For example, with the shoulder externally rotated in the supine position the patient holds the arm in abduction at various levels, always opposing retraction of the scapula. The patient then supports himself on his sound arm and tries to move his weight to the affected side whilst the head is flexed to the sound side to elicit the positive extensor supporting reaction in the other arm. When spasticity has supervened, the patient is treated lying on his side, the arm is elevated, flexed at the elbow and the palm put on the top of the head. Flexion and extension are then trained with the arm held in elevation. The arm is held at various heights with the elbow in varying degrees of flexion and extension, thus mimicking the movements of dressing and feeding. The scapula is pulled away from the spine as much as possible throughout this manoeuvre.

In prone lying, the patient supports himself on his forearm with the wrist flexed and the thumb extended and abducted, and then practises transferring his weight from one arm to the other.

When finger release is difficult it is worth trying the effect of putting the arm behind the body in internal or external rotation. Much depends on the particular patterns that are found by experience to be effective and, above all, by rapport between therapist and patient. Sensory stimuli are always used and the patient is worked from proximal to distal. Cold can be useful in the form of crushed ice in towels applied to the flexor surface of the arm. No exaggerated claims are made that these techniques will, for example, restore intrinsic action in the hand in severe spasticity, but there seems no doubt that they are logical, make sense to the patient and do allow muscle function during treatment which is not possible with conventional techniques.

Phenol blocks

The technique of injecting the motor point of the spastic muscle with 2–3 per cent phenol has proved useful in selected cases. Originally it was believed that there was a selective destructive effect on the gamma-efferent fibres, releasing the alpha fibres to normal function. It is now known that this is not so and the effect is to destroy all types of fibre. The technique has been described in detail by Copp and Keenan (1972). Briefly, a needle is inserted into the motor point, a stimulus being passed down the needle from a square wave stimulator. When there is a maximal contraction of the muscle with minimal current, the injection is given slowly, stopping every few minutes to observe the effect. It is wise to infiltrate with local anaesthetic first to establish if the deformity is due to contracture (when phenol block will be useless) or spasticity. Tightly flexed fingers can be released, making the appearance of the hand more acceptable and preventing pressure sores. Injection of the musculocutaneous nerve can release severe elbow flexor spasticity. The most useful results are cosmetic, easing of nursing and limited increase in muscle action – dramatic improvement in function is not to be expected.

Surgery

Surgery in spasticity is useful in certain well defined situations. Some voluntary control is essential – there must be extension of the fingers even with the wrist flexed. Lamb (1971) gives as contraindications: athetosis, sensory loss, age, poor emotional control and apraxia. He finds that the best results are obtained in cervical cord lesions where there is no intellectual impairment and sensation is intact.

Zancolli (1979) has classified the spastic hand into three types.

(1) The patient can extend his fingers with the wrist in the neutral position.
(2) The fingers can be actively extended only with flexion of the wrist.
(3) There is no active extension of the fingers even with maximal wrist flexion.

In these patients, flexing the wrist often helps to release the hand and provide some function, and it is important not to arthrodese the wrist. If the patient cannot flex the wrist and the fingers remain flexed, surgery is useless.

In the first group, where the patient can extend his fingers with the wrist in the neutral position, the usual procedure is a tenotomy of the flexor carpi ulnaris; generally, nothing more is needed.

In group (2) when the fingers can be actively extended but only with flexion of the wrist, the flexors are released in the forearm, a tenotomy is carried out on the flexor carpi ulnaris and the thumb deformity is corrected by excision of the adductor mass.

In this second group there are some patients who cannot actively extend with flexion of the wrist. In these, the flexor carpi ulnaris is transferred to the extensor carpi radialis brevis to give some active extension. To correct the thumb deformity, the adductor insertion is divided and the first metacarpal stabilized by an abductor tenodesis. The proximal end of the abductor pollicis longus is divided and put into the radius rather than the brachioradialis tendon. If there is marked hyperextensibility of the metacarpophalangeal joint of the thumb then a metacarpophalangeal capsuloplasty is done. The adductor is released and the brachioradialis is transferred to the extensor pollicis longus.

In group (3), reduction of deformity may help the patient but elongation of the flexors is all that can be undertaken. This may improve the cosmetic appearance and the patient may find the hand less clumsy, but little in the way of functional improvement can be expected.

The problem of the thumb held against the palm can be tackled by releasing the long flexor, dividing the first dorsal interosseus, partially releasing the adductors and sometimes a Z-plasty of the skin. It is usually necessary to put brachioradialis to extensor pollicis longus and to reroute extensor pollicis longus through the extensor carpi radialis tunnel. The proximal end of abductor pollicis longus is fixed to the radial side of the radius and so a tenodesis action is produced during ulnar deviation of the wrist.

Preoperative block of the median nerve establishes if there is any element of contracture which will militate against successful surgery.

All the skills of a modern occupational therapy department may need to be deployed to provide aids to daily living, and to retrain the patient in activities of everyday life (see Chapter 6).

Painful shoulder in spastic upper limb

Sometimes there is persistent pain from the shoulder, due to spasticity of the adductors and internal rotators. If there is no response to intensive physiotherapy and steroid injections, it is sometimes worth resecting the tendons of pectoralis major and subscapularis, but leaving the capsule intact. Exercises in passive abduction and external rotation are started at 5 days.

A variety of procedures have been described for the tight elbow: biceps lengthening; resection of the fascia of brachialis and brachioradialis; partial transection of brachialis; release of the flexor pronator origin; capsulectomy and removal of ectopic bone. The results are variable and complications, if they arise, can be disastrous.

CEREBRAL PALSY

The management of this sad disorder is complex and demands a highly specialized team. The techniques developed by Bobath (1978) are often of considerable help in breaking up abnormal patterns and allowing more natural movements. Much depends on the exact nature of the deficit – athetosis, for example, has a notoriously bad prognosis, while 'pure' spasticity responds better to both physiotherapeutic and surgical techniques. The position and function of the hand are dependent on the total body patterns – both trunk and shoulder patterns determining those of the elbow, wrist and hand.

Repeated evaluation by the therapeutic team is necessary to watch the natural history of the disorder unfold and to assess the patient's intellectual status and motivation as well as that of the family, who play such an important part in rehabilitation. The child is observed at play and in the various daily activities. Function of the upper limb must be assessed in a variety of postural sets – for example, neck extension and flexion, trunk position, and in lying, sitting and standing.

Smith (1977) has summarized well the status of surgery in cerebral palsy. He stresses the importance of operating stage by stage, for release of one group may allow the antagonist to recover some function. He finds, as do most authorities in this field, that splinting excites more spasticity or stops the child using the limb.

(1)   When the wrist is flexed and ulnar deviated, a well tried procedure is to transfer flexor carpi ulnaris to extensor carpi radialis longus. It will be effective only if

the child can extend the fingers when the wrist is put into dorsiflexion. The transfer corrects the deformity and encourages dorsiflexion of the wrist. Plaster is worn for 2 months and then active exercises are encouraged. A night splint is worn for 6 months.

(2) When the fingers and wrist are held in severe flexion, the flexors and pronators are slid down the forearm. The tendon can be lengthened or combined with tendon transfers. Smith splints in full extension for 3 months and uses a night splint for a further 3 months.

(3) When the thumb is held adducted into the palm with the metacarpal acutely flexed, an adductor release is performed and often combined with transfer of brachioradialis to the abductor pollicis longus. Plaster is worn for 6 weeks and a splint for 6 months to keep the thumb web open.

(4) Hyperextension of the proximal interphalangeal joint with flexion of the metacarpophalangeal joint occurs due to distal displacement of the hood. As the metacarpophalangeal joints flex, the deformity worsens. Smith cuts the extensor communis tendon at the level of the middle of the proximal phalnx, splits it into two and puts through drill holes laterally and looped, to be sutured to the extensor tendon just distal to the metacarpophalangeal joint. Thus he makes the extensor tendon work only on the metacarpophalangeal joint and the hyperextension deformity is corrected.

PARTIAL AMPUTATIONS

Amputations involving the whole hand are considered in Chapter 7; here we are concerned with partial loss of fingers or thumb.

The most valuable contributions the rehabilitation centre can offer to a patient with an amputation of one or more fingers or thumb, is the opportunity to find out to what extent he is truly disabled by giving him a variety of tasks to undertake so that he can discover what he can or cannot do. Our experience comprises 74 patients with loss of one or more digits. It is surprising how little disability the loss of one or two fingers may produce.

The patient illustrated in *Figure 5.30* merely required 3 weeks' intensive work to build up full power and to regain his confidence, and he was able to return to work fully fit. If the amputation stump is tender, tapping several times a day for 5 minutes, first by the therapist and later by the patient himself, is sometimes successful. When severe pain is a feature, all the methods described on pages 130 *et seq.* for painful peripheral nerve disorders are appropriate. On the other hand, a patient may lose so many digits that some form of prosthesis is required. Under these circumstances the prosthesis must be made to cater for the particular activity that the patient requires, and if he has a variety of activities in his job and hobbies it may be necessary to make a range of prostheses for each situation. The prosthesis must be light, simple, easily put on and taken off, should be durable, waterproof and therefore washable, and be easily fitted under a glove. A variety of materials are available for the manufacture of hand prostheses; at our MRU we find fibreglass most valuable – it is extremely strong and will stand screws and appliances drilled into the material without weakening it. It is easily kept clean, cheap and easily made. Each patient must be judged on his own

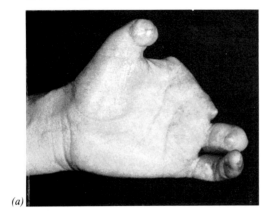

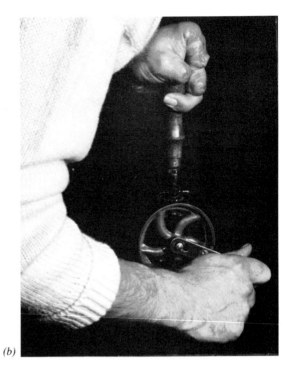

Figure 5.30   Result of traumatic amputation   *(b)*

merits; it is no use trying to replace the normal hand with an elaborate prosthesis. Either a prosthesis will be cosmetically acceptable but functionally useless, or it is likely to be functionally valuable but cosmetically not attractive. Therefore one should make the patient a dress hand which he wears under a glove and provide him with a range of prostheses to fit the particular functions he requires.

For example, the patient illustrated in *Figure 5.31a* had lost all four fingers, and required a dress hand (*Figure 5.31b*) and some device which would allow him to hold

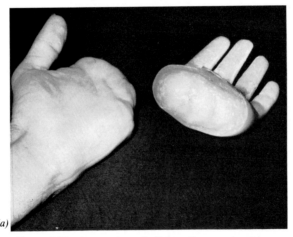

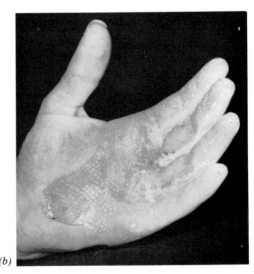

Figure 5.31   Amputation of all four fingers, showing fibreglass dress hand   *(b)*

heavy objects (*Figure 5.32*). Similarly, the patient illustrated in *Figure 5.33* wanted to hold a tennis racket, as that game was his hobby. The prosthesis allowed him to hold his racket and he was able to play an excellent game of tennis.

Case 5.33. This patient sustained traumatic amputations of index, middle and ring fingers through the proximal interphalangeal joints. Neuromata were excised 3 months later from the tips of the ring and middle fingers. He was referred to the MRU, and after 10 days' intensive occupational therapy and games he was assessed in his job as a mechanic by asking him to strip and reassemble an engine. This he was able to do with no trouble and he returned to full duties 4 months after injury.

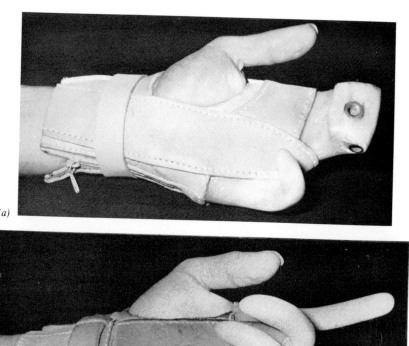

(a)

(b)

Figure 5.32　*Working prostheses*

Case 5.34. This patient crushed the middle finger of the left hand in a car door, and it had to be amputated through the metacarpophalangeal joint. One year later he was complaining of severe tenderness over the stump which interfered with his job as a driver. Two weeks' intensive exercises and games, and several sessions daily of tapping the stump by the physiotherapist, completely relieved symptoms.

Case 5.35. A detonator exploded in this patient's hand and he sustained disarticulation at the proximal interphalangeal joint of the thumb, amputation of the index finger at the proximal interphalangeal joint and disarticulation of the middle finger at the metacarpophalangeal joint. He required excision of the scarred thumb web, and after a short spell of work at the MRU to build up power he was fit for work as a capstan operator. No prostheses were required (*Figure 5.34*).

Case 5.36. This patient sustained a traumatic amputation of the left index finger through the proximal interphalangeal joint. Because he was a teleprinter operator, a fibreglass prosthesis was made to give him the correct finger length and he returned to full duty, having been assessed on his job and found fully fit (*Figure 5.35*).

Case 5.37. This patient sustained traumatic amputation of index, middle and ring fingers just distal to the metacarpophalangeal joints and at the proximal interphalangeal joint of the little finger. After 3 weeks' intensive rehabilitation he had excellent function, being able to grip between the thumb and stump of the little finger. He was retrained as a radio engineer, and was provided with a dress hand at his own request.

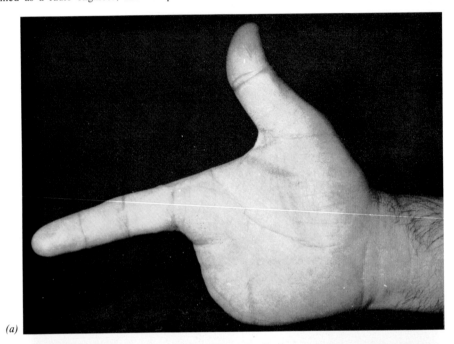

(a)

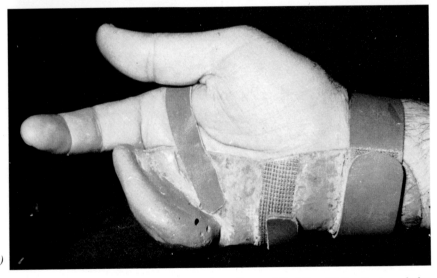

(b)

Figure 5.33   Traumatic amputations of the hand. (a) Extent of disability. (b) Prosthesis made for tennis

(continued)

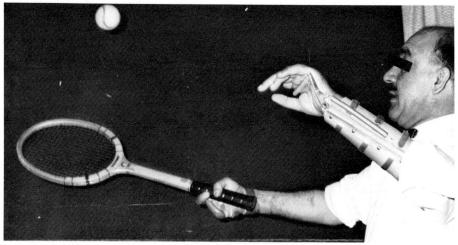

Figure 5.33 (cont.)   (c) Prosthesis in action. (We would now use a much lighter splint for the dropped wrist)

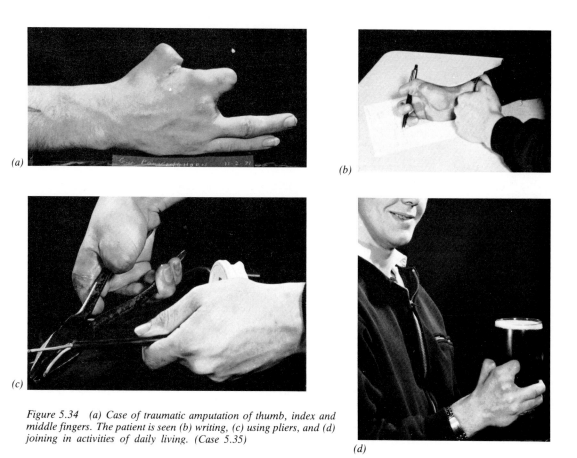

(a)

(b)

(c)

(d)

Figure 5.34   (a) Case of traumatic amputation of thumb, index and middle fingers. The patient is seen (b) writing, (c) using pliers, and (d) joining in activities of daily living. (Case 5.35)

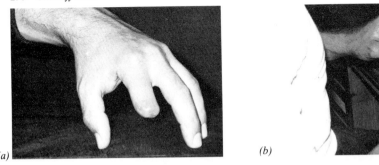

(a)   (b)

Figure 5.35   (a) Amputation of tip of index finger. (b) Fibreglass prosthesis for teleprinter operator. (Case 5.36)

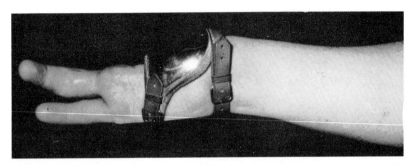

Figure 5.36   Prosthesis which helped this seaman with his wire splicing. (Case 5.38)

Case 5.38. An ammunition hoist fell onto this patient's right hand, amputating the right thumb and index and middle fingers. After 3 weeks at the MRU, this man proved that he could carry out all the duties of his trade of gunner at sea. The occupational therapist went to the ship with him and satisfied herself and the gunnery officer that he was completely fit for full duty. A prosthesis (*Figure 5.36*) helped him with wire splicing.

Case 5.39. This patient sustained a traumatic amputation of the right little finger. A light and a heavy prosthesis allowed him to cook without symptoms from the tender stump (*Figure 5.37*).

APPENDIX A

Passive mobilization techniques

These should be carried out: (1) through the range normally under the patient's active control; or (2) through the accessory range of movement, or joint play – this includes rotation, and anteroposterior and lateral gliding.

In the crushed hand, movements are both stiff and painful due to the oedema which splints the subcutaneous tissues. It is important to maintain the joint structures in a supple condition, whilst using all methods available to reduce the oedema. Maintaining the accessory range helps to accomplish this. It is essential to recover the joint play when attempting to mobilize a very stiff hand.

Small oscillatory movements at a slowish speed should be carried out as far as the painful range, and just into the stiff range of movement.

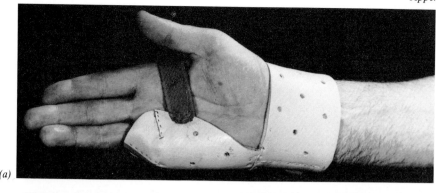

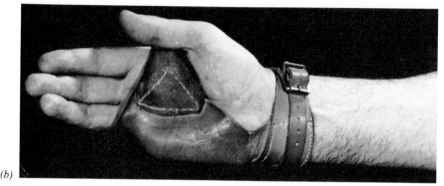

Figure 5.37   Amputation of little finger in a cook. Tenderness of stump militated against firm grip. (a) Prosthesis for cooking and (b) heavier prosthesis for butchery. (Case 5.39)

Extension of the wrist mostly occurs at the mid-carpal joint and is harder to regain than wrist flexion, which occurs mainly at the radiocarpal joint. Therefore, special attention should be paid to the gliding and traction movements of the intercarpal joints in the posteroanterior plane.

The intermetacarpal joints are involved in cupping of the palm and this is increased by the parallel gliding of one metacarpal on its neighbour.

The metacarpophalangeal and interphalangeal joints should have traction and counter-traction applied, and rotation and anteroposterior and lateral gliding movements should be carried out.

The treatment of the thumb metacarpophalangeal and interphalangeal joints is similar to that in the fingers. At the carpometacarpal joint, however, abduction, adduction and rotary oscillations should be performed. The physiotherapist stabilizes the carpus with one hand whilst moving the metacarpal with the other.

APPENDIX B

Stretch plasters for metacarpophalangeal joints fixed in extension

There are two stages in the correction of the rigidly extended metacarpophalangeal joints – the first to achieve approximately 50 degrees of flexion, and the second to increase the flexion from 50 to 60 degrees.

Stage 1

The method used is similar to the procedures already described to stretch a flexion deformity into extension but with the plaster applied to the dorsal instead of the palmar surface. If the interphalangeal joints are also rigid, then these are also stretched into maximum flexion and the plaster is allowed to set in this position. The plaster is again applied with a cotton wool lining and over the dorsum of the fingers, and the splint held in place with a crêpe bandage. A new plaster is made as soon as an increase of flexion is gained.

Stage 2

An increasing pull is applied over the proximal phalanges, or if necessary over the proximal interphalangeal joints, to increase the flexion of the fingers towards the palm, as illustrated in *Figure 5.22*, the splint having two parts. A cock-up plaster splint is made for the wrist joint, cutting away a semicircular piece for the thumb and ensuring that, in the palm, the splint ends well proximal to the metacarpal heads to allow the joints to flex. After the first six layers of plaster have been applied, a 10 cm strip of duralumin is bent to a right angle 3.8 cm from its end, and the longer length placed on the plaster at the level of the wrist joint. The final six layers of plaster are placed over the metal.

Reinforced moulded Plastazote is used for the other part of the splint. Two identical pieces of 3 mm Plastazote are cut, the length being 3.8 cm longer than the middle finger from tip to metacarpophalangeal joint when the finger is flexed. The width is the same as that of the metacarpophalangeal joints. One end of each piece is then trimmed to the shape of the finger tips. A piece of 3 mm Perspex, or other suitable material, is cut 1.3 cm smaller all round than the Plastazote. The Perspex, evenly spaced, is then laid between the two layers of Plastazote, which in turn are placed for 5 minutes in the oven, preheated to a temperature of 60°C (140°F). When the Plastazote is soft and malleable, these three layers should be gently compressed, removed from the oven and placed directly on the dorsum of the fingers, the metacarpophalangeal joints, and over the distal 3.8 cm of the metacarpals. A stretch is maintained for a few minutes to obtain maximum flexion, until the Plastazote has cooled and set in position. When applied to the patient, the plaster cock-up splint should be lined with cotton wool as described earlier, and this section bandaged to the patient's forearm. The Plastazote piece is then applied direct to the dorsum of the hand, without a lining. A bandage is placed over the Plastazote and then round the metal hook in the cock-up. A stretch should be put on the bandage to obtain the maximum flexion of the patient's fingers, especially at the metacarpophalangeal joints.

Plastazote web stretches

Thumb and finger webs following burns or lengthy immobilization need to be stretched passively, and for this to be most effective the degree of stretch obtained should be maintained overnight by Plastazote wedges. In the exceptionally contracted state, sometimes only 3 mm Plastazote, or the same thickness folded double, can be inserted between the fingers. This should he heated at 60°C (140°F) until malleable, placed between the fingers and allowed to shape itself while the fingers are held in maximum stretch by the physiotherapist.

For the thumb, there is usually sufficient space to introduce a wedge cut from 2.5 cm Plastazote. It is again heated in the oven and inserted between thumb and index finger, the physiotherapist maintaining the stretch until the Plastazote has cooled. Care should be taken to apply the stretch between the heads of the metacarpals of thumb and index finger. If the proximal phalanges are forced apart, the metacarpophalangeal joints are hyperextended and the web itself will not be stretched. This could lead to these particular joints becoming painful and flail.

APPENDIX C

Prostheses

In certain conditions where a dress hand, or a simple working prosthesis, is required, fibreglass, by virtue of its durability, can be very successful. It is not intended that the prosthesis should be movable or mechanical in any way since this would then become the work of a highly skilled prosthetic technician, but there are occasions when the prosthesis is a small, simple extension for part or all of the hand, and therefore the work entailed in its construction could well be undertaken by the occupational therapist.

A DRESS HAND MADE IN FIBREGLASS

A fibreglass prosthesis of the fingers was made for a patient (see *Figure 5.31*) who had a traumatic amputation of all digits at the level of the metacarpophalangeal joints, with his thumb left uninjured and fully active. He was a carpenter by trade, and intended to become an instructor. His requirements were a dress hand and three working hands for his job, enabling him to hold tools freely. These were: one to support tool handles in a 'grip'; one into which the handles of his small tools could be screwed; and one with an extended index finger and flexed digits, to serve a dual purpose of pointing on the blackboard while lecturing, and to use the flexed fingers for holding objects with looped handles.

Procedure

Several plaster casts were made of his hand and forearm to allow work to continue simultaneously on the various prostheses in order to save time. Since each fibreglass 'hand' had to be stitched manually onto a firmly fitted leather glove, it can be appreciated how useful it was to have a number of casts.

Since it was impossible to take a cast of the amputated fingers, a patient was found who had an identical size of hand and a complete cast of it was made. Only the digits of the cast were intended to be used, the idea being that these could then be superimposed on one of the patient's own casts, and the work could be done on them.

Since the addition of fibreglass digits would not give him a firm 'hand', the fibreglass had to be continued up the palm, on dorsal and palmar surfaces (to avoid anterior and posterior movement) by making a hollow shell into which he could place most of the remainder of his hand, and leave his thumb free. Once the fibreglass of the hand minus the fingers was completed, the problem was then to place the fingers on the end of this 'shell' and so make a whole hand. A fibreglass mixture was made up and poured into the cast of the fingers. This was then superimposed on the fibreglass 'shell' and contact made with more mixture. The result was a complete hand with fingers and a container for the palmar and dorsal surfaces of the patient's metacarpals.

The next stage was to attach this to a neat-fitting glove. In order to do this the edge of the 'shell' part of the prosthesis had to be drilled for stitching, using a 1.7 mm ($^1/_{16}$ inch) drill bit. It was found that the fibreglass was easy to drill and presented no difficulties. The plaster cast of the hand now came in useful for shaping the glove. A pattern was first made in cotton, one for each of the dorsal and palmar surfaces. The pattern was tacked into position on the cast and, while there, the finished 'palm' and fingers were placed over the top, and a line marked on the cotton where the stitching had to take place on to the leather. The pattern was then cut out in the leather and completed in saddle stitch using a strong linen thread. Constant fittings were made on the patient's hand to ensure that it was firm and neat-fitting. An opening was made along the ulnar side of the little finger, and a zip fastener inserted. The stitching of the leather on to the 'palm' part of the prosthesis had to be done with curved surgical needles, since there was not room inside the shell for a straight needle. The inside of the entire prosthesis was then lined with chamois.

APPENDIX D

Fibreglass spint for stabilization of the carpometacarpal joint or of the metacarpophalangeal joint of the thumb

This is a light, comfortable splint which rests these joints but will still enable the patient to use his hand by means of the fingers flexing to the thumb instead of the thumb flexing to the fingers. It is easily applied and easy to keep clean. There are no buckles to fasten since the leather is attached to the fibreglass in such a way as to double back on itself and finally close with the Velcro fastener. A soft pliable leather should be used for this reason, preferably with a shiny surface, since that type of surface does not become dirty as quickly as a suede finish. Should the leather part become really soiled, a saturated solution of salts of sorrel will make it like new if brushed over the leather surface on a pad of cotton wool.

A plaster cast must first be made of the patient's thumb, hand and wrist. The wrist should be held in a comfortable position of function for the patient (about 15–20 degrees of extension). The position of the thumb should be that which gives the patient most relief from pain, bearing in mind that there must be no passive strain on small ligaments round the joints. The fingers should be able to flex downwards on to the thumb.

The area to be made in fibreglass extends, on the palmar surface, from midline, level with the proximal palmar crease, over the web, to the dorsal surface in line with the lateral border of the second metacarpal, and stretching proximally to 2.5 cm beyond the distal wrist crease. For stabilization of the carpometacarpal joint, the fibreglass must extend just beyond the metacarpophalangeal joint, but for stabilization of the metacarpophalangeal joint, it must extend up to the distal end of the proximal phalanx of the thumb so as just to allow slight flexion of the terminal joint for function. In other words, the thenar eminence is completely covered on the palmar surface, and the metacarpal area on the dorsal surface (*Figure 5.38*).

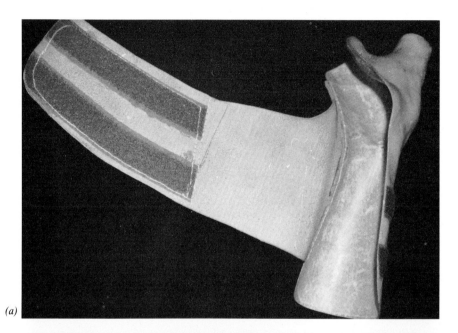

(a)

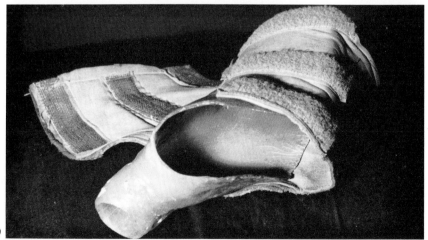

(b)

Figure 5.38   Two views of the fibreglass splint for stabilization of the carpometacarpal or metacarpophalangeal joint of the thumb

REFERENCES AND BIBLIOGRAPHY

Bassot, M. J. (1965). Traitement de la maladie de Dupuytren par exercise pharmacodynamique. Isole's ou completee par un temps plastique uniquement cutané. *Lille Chirurgical* **20**, 38–39

Baxter, H., Schiller, C., Johnson, L. H., Whiteside, J. M. and Randall, R. E. (1952). 'Cortisone therapy in Dupuytren's contracture. *Plastic and Reconstructive Surgery* **9**, 261–273

Bobath, B. (1978). *Adult Hemiplegia: evaluation and treatment*, 2nd edn. London: Heinemann Medical

Carroll, R. E. and Taber, T. H. (1954). Digital arthroplasty of proximal interphalangeal joint. *Journal of Bone and Joint Surgery* **36A**, 912–920

Clarkson, P. W. and Pelly, A. (1962). *The General and Plastic Surgery of the Hand*. Oxford: Blackwell

Copp, E. P. and Keenan, J. (1972). Phenol nerve and motor point block in spasticity. *Rheumatology and Physical Medicine* **11**, 287–292

Curtis, R. M. (1970). Surgery for the stiff finger. Communication to Members of the American Society for Surgery of the Hand

Drucker, W. R., Hubay, C. A., Holden, W. D. and Bukovnic, J. A. (1959). Pathogenesis of post traumatic dystrophy. *American Journal of Surgery* **97**, 454–465

Dunningham, T. H. (1980). The treatment of Sudeck's atrophy in the upper limb by sympathetic blockade. *Injury,* **12,** 139–144

Fisk, G. (1971). Carpal instability and scaphoid fractures. *Traumatismes Osteoarticulaires de la Main*. Paris: Expansion Scientifique Francaise

Hannington-Kiff, J. (1974). Intravenous regional block with guanethidine. *Lancet* **1**, 1019

Hannington-Kiff, J. (1977). Relief of Sudeck's atrophy by regional intravenous guanethidine. *Lancet* **1**, 1132–1133

Hueston, J. T. (1971). Enzymic fasciotomy. *The Hand* **3**, 38–40

Hueston, J. T. and Tubiana, R. (Eds) (1974). *Dupuytren's Disease*, 2nd edn. Edinburgh and London: Livingstone

Hurwitz, L. J. and Adams, G. P. (1972). Rehabilitation of hemiplegia. Indices of assessment and prognosis. *British Medical Journal* **1**, 94–98

Kolar, J. and Vrabec, R. (1959). Periarticular soft-tissue changes as a late consquence of burns. *Journal of Bone and Joint Surgery* **41A**, 103–111

Lamb, D. W. (1971). The hand in quadriplegia. *The Hand* **3**, 31–37

Loh, L. and Nathan, P. W. (1978). Painful peripheral states and sympathetic blocks. *Journal of Neurology, Neurosurgery and Psychiatry* **41**, 664–671

Plewes, L. W. (1953). Physiotherapy in industry, with special reference to Sudeck's atrophy. *Physiotherapy* **39**, 325

Robins, R. H. C. (1961). *Injuries and Infections of the Hand*. London: Edward Arnold

Schumacher, H. B. and Abramson, D. I. (1949). Post traumatic vasomotor disorders. *Surgery, Gynecology and Obstetrics* **88**, 417–434

Skoog, T. (1948). Dupuytren's contraction, with special reference to aetiology and improved surgical treatment, its occurrence in epileptics, note on knuckle pads. *Acta Chirurgica Scandinavica* **96**, Suppl. 139

Smith, R. J. (1977). Surgery of the hand in cerebral palsy. In *Operative Surgery*: vol. *The Hand*, pp. 215–230. Ed. by R. G. Pulvertaft. London: Butterworths

Stack, G. H. (1969). Mallet finger. *The Hand* **1**, 83

Tauras, A. P. and Frackleton, W. H. (1967). Silicone capping of nerve stumps in the problem of partial neuromas. *Surgical Forum* **18**, 504–505

Zancolli, E. A. (1979). *Structural and Dynamic Bases of Hand Surgery*, 2nd edn. Philadelphia, Pa: Lippincott

Principles of Rehabilitation　　6

INTRODUCTION

If patients with severe injuries to the hand are to regain maximum function as quickly as possible, intensive treatment for several hours a day is required from a highly skilled therapeutic staff, under the direction of a doctor with specialized knowledge of all aspects of the problem. There are various ways of providing such facilities – in a special rehabilitation centre for locomotor disorders, in hostel accommodation within the hospital grounds, or daily attendance at the rehabilitation department of the district general hospital. Ideally, the same surgical team should have direct supervision of the patient throughout the whole course of treatment; however, in many instances surgeons are so busy that they simply cannot afford the time to give the detailed attention to the minutiae of rehabilitation that is required, and they may delegate the supervision of rehabilitation to a colleague in rehabilitation medicine. In Great Britain the training of such a doctor has been agreed by the Royal Colleges. He should have a sound background in general medicine and in the medical disorders of the locomotor system, for within the sphere of his practice he will be dealing with patients with a wide variety of disorders, including the rheumatic diseases, neurological disability such as hemiplegia and paraplegia, multiple sclerosis, head injuries, and general medical disorders such as metabolic bone disease and endocrine malfunction that produce locomotor disability. He should have a sound understanding of the general principles of orthopaedics as they relate to trauma and the surgery of locomotor disease such as inflammatory and degenerative arthritis, and finally a thorough knowledge of the practice of the professions supplementary to medicine – physiotherapy, occupational therapy, remedial gymnastics – and the services (both statutory and voluntary) for resettlement.

The overall final responsibility, however, rests with the surgeon. There is no question that when a surgeon, who believes in the value of expert rehabilitation, works together with a physician in rehabilitation medicine, who fully understands the surgical problems involved, a happy and efficient service results, with mutual respect between all members of the team.

In Britain the district general hospitals usually have on their staff a rheumatologist with experience in rehabilitation who can assume managerial responsibility for the rehabilitation department and advise his colleagues on difficult problems. There is always likely to be a place for a few specialized centres for the rehabilitation of locomotor disorders on a regional basis, where difficult problems can receive long-term intensive treatment and where all the various problems presented by disability can be solved on a multidisciplinary basis. Such units as Mary Marlborough Lodge, Oxford, provide invaluable facilities for studying the problems of severe disability in depth (Nichols, 1971). Ideally these centres should be within the hospital grounds, in hostel accommodation, so that continuity of treatment can be maintained. At the Royal National Orthopaedic Hospital there is a mini-care ward accommodating patients from Monday to Friday. Patients spend the day in the various treatment departments and they may stay up until 9 p.m.; they go home at week-ends. The ward is much cheaper to run than an acute ward, and promotes an atmosphere for progressive return to normal life. At a later stage patients can return home and attend as outpatients on a full-time or part-time basis. However, local conditions or the considerable demands of multiple disabilities on the rehabilitation services may prove too much for the district general hospital and special residential centres, such as those pioneered by the Royal Air Force during World War II and subsequently developed in the National Health Service in such places as Odstock Hospital, Salisbury, Garston Manor, Passmore Edwards Rehabilitation Centre, Clacton, and Farnham Park, may be the answer. In a large city, a day centre serving several hospitals in the area may provide the solution – such as the Camden Road Day Centre in London, which provides facilities for rehabilitation on a full-time basis.

The value of such residential centres is that they offer the whole range of facilities for physiotherapy, occupational therapy, games and workshop activities, for both recovery of function and assessment for work; in addition, they provide an atmosphere of optimism, and confidence can be engendered in a way that is difficult in an acute hospital. A certain amount of friendly rivalry between patients who compete with each other to get better more quickly and the realization that there are others worse off than themselves are all conducive to good morale. Moreover, the regular assessment of progress and the setting of objectives gives the patients the feeling that recovery is being steadily achieved. Above all, the staff try to create the feeling that although rehabilitation means hard work, it should also be fun. Dances, film shows, discussions and outings are all as much a part of rehabilitation for long-term disability as remedial treatment. All this is much easier to accomplish in an environment totally given over to detailed after-care, than in the hospital.

Originally the Services rehabilitation units were designed for orthopaedic disorders, but their work has expanded to take in patients with rheumatological, neurological and general medical problems – in short, any patient with a locomotor disorder who would benefit from intensive full-time expert rehabilitation. Those with simple locomotor problems such as meniscectomy and uncomplicated fractures are treated as outpatients by the hospital rehabilitation services where physiotherapists, remedial gymnasts and occupational therapists work under the direction of the surgeon. As the RAF is required to provide hospital services on a regional basis near operational stations, it is uneconomic to set up full-scale medical rehabilitation units in connection with each hospital and therefore rehabilitation of long-term complex cases is centralized in the two Medical Rehabilitation Units (MRUs). These are within a few miles of each other, close to London, and are visited regularly by orthopaedic and neurological consultants. The staff of the MRUs in turn visit the hospitals regularly and so a close rapport exists between all members of the team, despite their geographial separation. Facilities include large gymnasia where exercises and games are supervised by remedial gymnasts, active intensive physiotherapy and realistic occupational therapy, swimming and hydrotherapy.

Because most servicemen are highly skilled tradesmen, facilities are now provided for trade rehabilitation so that patients may use tools of their trade to regain power and range of movement, and have detailed assessments at the end of their stay. An education officer provides continued education for long-stay patients preparing for higher examinations and trade tests. A welfare officer is on the staff to solve domestic, social and financial problems, there is a speech therapist, and a disablement resettlement officer visits the weekly resettlement clinics to prepare severely disabled patients, who are unable to continue in the Service, for civilian life.

At the Royal National Orthopaedic Hospital, the rehabilitation department is housed in the same building as the outpatient block, well away from the wards. It contains a large open physiotherapy department, a warm pool and gymnasium, an occupational therapy department (comprising kitchen, bathroom, bedroom, interview room, large open work area and workshop with carpentry and metal work and a games area), offices for the two rehabilitation (resettlement) officers and speech therapist and an office for the director.

Very close by is the social work department and adjoining is the limb fitting centre. There is thus an integrated comprehensive rehabilitation organization serving the whole hospital. Educational assessments and continued educational and vocational counselling are provided by the large school – whose main purpose is the education of long-stay children with scoliosis, tuberculosis, etc., but whose staff give an invaluable service to young men and women whose disability is severe enough to have to seek other employment. The Graham Hill Assessment Unit is separated from the rehabilitation unit by some 180 metres (200 yards). It consists of a model flat equipped for the disabled and a house built to a standard local council design, with all of the features of housing that make life difficult for the handicapped.

At a certain stage of rehabilitation, it is important to determine what problems the disabled patient will face on return to the community. In this unit the patient has the opportunity to live for a few days, either on his or her own or with spouse or relatives, as relevant. The patient shops from the hospital shop, cooks, cleans and is generally fully independent. Each day the rehabilitation staff assess the problems as they arise and can then offer solutions in the patient's own home. These assessments are, of course, related to home visits if the patient lives in the area or, if from far away, a comprehensive report can be sent to the domiciliary occupational therapist. By this means patients can bridge the often unnerving gap between hospital and home.

We believe that this type of unit offers a more realistic setting than the occupational therapy department alone – though it is still invaluable for training purposes. The unit is also valuable as a means of assessing the actual problems the patient encounters at home, and can be used to provide the surgeon with the information he needs in planning a reconstructive surgical programme.

Severe hand injuries, like other severe locomotor problems (e.g. head injuries, multiple fractures and burns), need a wide spectrum of facilities for successful rehabilitation: skilled physiotherapy (many times a day), hydrotherapy, realistic graded occupational therapy to regain muscle power, joint range and co-ordination, the immediate provision of splints (corrective and dynamic), appliances, gadgets, prostheses, assessment by skilled technicians at various stages to pin-point specific disability in relation to the job, games and class exercises to regain general arm function and full physical fitness, social and industrial resettlement and, above all, detailed overall assessment of remaining physical abilities and the temperament and outlook of the patient.

Such requirements demand a full-time programme and must be taken seriously. When it is realized that it costs nearly a million pounds sterling to train the pilot of a modern high-performance aircraft, the economic value of spending time and money to return him to full duty after injury becomes obvious. The more highly skilled the individual, the more capital investment he represents and a greater loss to the community, as well as to his family, will result if adequate rehabilitation is not given. Most hand surgeons have realized this, and rightly demand the development of an adequate rehabilitation programme for their patients; they insist that trainee surgeons must be indoctrinated into the principles of after-care. It is hoped that before long all concerned with the problems of the injured hand will see to it that every patient who needs it is given every opportunity to receive such care. Resources both in staff and space are limited, but much can be done by the rationalization of existing resources to ensure that only those patients who really need physiotherapy and occupational therapy for restoration of function are referred for treatment and that the departments are not used as social clubs for geriatric patients or dumping grounds for undiagnosed 'rheumatic' disorders. Moreover, therapists should be used as therapists, not as telephone operators, transport officers, clerical workers or welfare officers. There is considerable scope for the use of aides who can dress and undress patients, prepare them for treatment, help in walking re-education, put on calipers, arrange appointments and generally ensure that the therapists are free to practise their specific skills. Occupational therapy, too, should be dynamic, realistic and related to patients' skills, jobs and hobbies. It is essential that the physiotherapy and occupational therapy departments adjoin each other and that their staff work closely together. Class work and group therapy are an efficient means of treatment, enjoyed by all patients, and saves the therapists' time. Regular consultations with the senior medical staff will ensure that no unnecessary treatment is given and that treatment stops as soon as it has become effective or proved to be non-effective. The participation of the therapeutic staff in ward rounds and attendance at operations, and the encouragement by the doctors to the staff to offer suggestions and ideas, all make for an efficient and harmonious team.

Modern physiotherapists and occupational therapists are highly skilled personnel whose full potential can only be realized if encouraged and challenged. In recent years physiotherapists have taken part in some excellent research projects and have been commendably critical of some of the traditional outdated treatments that have become the legacy of a more leisurely past, when physiotherapy was a palliative for pain rather than a dynamic force for quick recovery. Occupational therapists are becoming more and more concerned with problems of disability in the home and industry, and the image of diversionary feminine craftwork is fast receding.

Previous editions of this book have been critized for including too much material on physiotherapy which is common knowledge and to be found in textbooks for therapists. The following section will therefore deal only with recent advances and techniques, specific to problems of the hand and upper limb, and of methods of treatment with which doctors concerned with the hand ought to be aware and would not normally find in medical textbooks.

PHYSIOTHERAPY

Exercises

Exercise techniques aim at increasing strength, endurance and co-ordination of weak muscles. Strength can be defined as the maximum tension which a muscle is capable of generating in a single contraction. It can be measured by a spring balance, strain gauge dynamometer or a grip dynamometer (see *Figure 1.9*). Endurance is the ability of a muscle to continue to work against a load, and can be measured by estimating the time taken before the performance falls off – usually judged as a proportion of its maximum strength. Co-ordination is the ability to perform a movement or series of movements rapidly and correctly and can be measured by devising tasks of varying complexity, such as correct assembly of mechanical parts or negotiation of a complicated shape (*Figure 6.1*). Each parameter should be measured regularly throughout treatment, both as a guide to the staff of progress and as encouragement to the patient. One cannot assess function properly in the clinic. It is not sufficient to measure grip strength; muscles are required for endurance and this, together with dexterity, work tolerance, application and motivation, can only be assessed under close supervision in the appropriate department. Reports must be presented at the

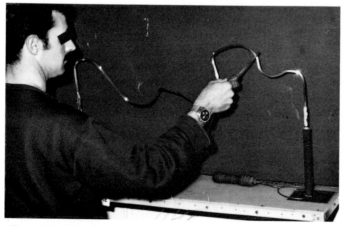

Figure 6.1   Test of co-ordination — note different sized loops. The frame can be wired to a buzzer so that a sound or a flash of light is emitted whenever the loop touches the frame

review clinic so that a full picture of the patient's situation can be obtained – including progressive ranges of movement recorded accurately by goniometry or by studying serial plasters, grip strength, endurance curves, workshop assessments and educational standards.

Muscles which are too weak to work against gravity (below 3 on the MRC scale) must be re-educated with support – this can be provided by the therapist herself, by slings, boards or in water. Proprioceptive neuromuscular facilitation techniques are particularly suitable for weak or inhibited muscles.

Proprioceptive neuromuscular facilitation techniques

These have been considered in Chapter 3, but for ease of reference they are considered again here. They represent a comparatively recent development in physiotherapy and are a logical and functional way of exercising a muscle. They are well established and widely accepted as an essential part of routine physiotherapy. Consequently, all physiotherapists now have a mastery of these methods but, since many doctors are still unfamiliar with them, a brief explanation of their rationale will be presented here.

Maximum activity in a muscle depends on maximum discharge of the anterior horn cells which supply that muscle. In order to obtain maximum discharge of the anterior horn cells, all available influences must be brought to bear on them. When a muscle has been immobilized for any length of time, such as after a tendon graft or whilst in plaster after a fracture, the central inhibitory state is heightened in the anterior horn cells which supply that muscle, and it is therefore more difficult to excite; for example, after knee injuries the quadriceps may be markedly inhibited. It is therefore important to try to make available all possible influences on the anterior horn cell to lower its heightened inhibitory state. Increasing sensory flow and irradiation of activity from neighbouring anterior horn cells are the two most valuable methods.

Increased sensory inflow

This can be produced by any of the following.

(1) Stretch – increasing stretch activates the muscle spindle system, resulting in an inflow of afferent impulses into the cord, and sets the bias of the spindle system to a more sensitive level, reducing the central inhibitory state.
(2) Pressure on the proprioceptive end-organs in tendon and joint, as well as traction on the joint.
(3) Visual effects – the patient is asked to watch the movements and 'feel' the pattern that is being encouraged; this is reinforced by the physiotherapists's commands, given in a forceful, positive manner.
(4) Ice cubes rubbed on the muscle – this can be useful, provided sensation is normal.
(5) Stroking the muscle with a soft brush for 1–2 minutes is highly effective as a sensory stimulus.

Irradiation

If the anterior horn cells lying adjacent to those supplying the muscle to be treated are stimulated to discharge, there will be an overflow of electrical activity which will lower the central inhibitory state. This is known as irradiation. A well known example of this is in the re-education of a weak quadriceps muscle, when the patient is asked to dorsiflex the ankle as he tries to contract the quadriceps. The cell columns supplying the anterior tibialis lie close to those supplying the quadriceps and their electrical activity irradiates to those cells supplying the quadriceps and increases their discharge.

When the finger extensors are weak, a stronger contraction can be elicited by irradiation from cells supplying the extensors of elbow, wrist and thumb than by a simple prime mover action (*Figure 6.2*).

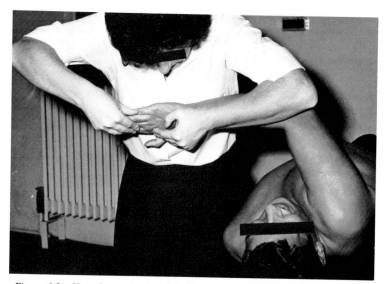

Figure 6.2   Use of proprioceptive facilitation techniques to re-educate extensor tendon suture

Successive induction

When there has been maximum voluntary contraction of an antagonist, there is facilitation of the agonist. Thus, after a strong maximum contraction of the wrist and finger flexors, it is easier for the extensors to contract, as there has been an alteration of central inhibitory and excitatory states in the spinal cord.

Pattern re-education

Muscles normally work in spiral and diagonal patterns. Thus, bringing the hand to the mouth involves a diagonal movement from the side across the body, and almost all functional activities such as dressing, using tools and swishing rackets or clubs involve rotational movements and diagonal patterns. The 'Swedish drill' types of exercise that were popular in the earlier part of this century were unphysiological as well as boring – the new proprioceptive techniques are physiological and capture the patient's interest as he can see clearly how they relate to daily life. Moreover, it is possible to exhaust a patient in a few minutes and thus these manoeuvres are highly efficient for both physiotherapists' and patients' time.

TECHNIQUES

Irradiation is always from strong muscles to weak and so in re-educating weak hand muscles the shoulder and elbow are worked first and then the wrist, fingers and thumb. Furthermore, the moving part is felt by the patient most and thus the shoulder is pivoted and fixed. Maximum movement is encouraged distally, as the manoeuvre increases in force, so that only the weak part is allowed to move. Thus, in re-educating weak finger flexors, as after suture or graft, the diagonal flexion adduction internal rotation pattern is used and at the start the whole upper limb is brought across the body and then out away from the body in extension abduction external rotation. Next, the shoulder is fixed and the power concentrated on the elbow, then the wrist and finally the fingers.

Repeated contractions are used to reinforce the activity of the weak muscles. 'Hold/relax techniques' allow relaxation between each isometric maximum contraction, thus reinforcing each contraction. Each patient has his own best line of activity or 'groove' and, since the diagonal patterns vary slightly from patient to patient, the physiotherapist has to find the groove for each patient which varies with his body structure. For opposition of the thumb the best position to work in is extension, adduction and internal rotation; for adduction of the thumb flexion, adduction and external rotation; and for palmar abduction of the thumb in extension, abduction and internal rotation.

For re-education of the fingers, the index and middle fingers are worked as a unit, as are the ring and little fingers. As all the fingers rotate towards the thumb in flexion and derotate in extension, they must be worked in a diagonal pattern.

At a later stage, when power 4 or 5 is needed, progressive resistance is provided. This can be against the therapist's resistance (proprioceptive neuromuscular facilitation can be adapted well for this), against springs, against resistance in water, with games, and finally, if really strong power is required, by circuit training. This is most appropriate following generalized weakness of the upper limb.

Heat

Heat can be useful to accelerate healing in local infections, but its main value is in relaxation of muscle spasm and it is a pleasant preparation for making an exercise or passive manoeuvre, such as stretching, less painful and therefore more effective.

Wax, infrared irradiation and hot soaks all have their advocates. If there is weakness or stiffness of the limb as a whole, a short spell in the warm pool is the most effective of all.

Ultrasound

This modality is especially useful in the treatment of acute strains and sprains and in ligamentous inflammations – such as tenosynovitis and de Quervain's syndrome.

It is widely used in chronic scarring – such as after burns, crush injuries and fibrosis following chronic oedema. No control studies have been reported to substantiate its claims in this sphere, nor is it easy to see how they could be conducted since measurement of scarring presents formidable difficulties. We have routinely used ultrasound in the rehabilitation of the stiffly scarred hand as well as oil massage and exercises and so it is not possible to say which is the effective agent. Extrapolating from its undoubted effect in active inflammation, it seems reasonable to use it if there is any inflammatory element. The modality is easy to use, safe, the apparatus not expensive and the treatment taking only a few minutes to give. It is very doubtful if it has any effect on chronic tough scars such as in Dupuytren's contracture.

Ultraviolet

There is undoubtedly a place for ultraviolet irradiation to attack local infections which systemic antibiotic treatment does not affect. Using applicators with the Kromayer technique, sinuses can be effectively treated.

Massage

There is no place for massage to reduce muscle spasm, relieve pain or improve circulation.

Ice, heat and exercises are the best means of reducing spasm; pain is more efficiently and far more cheaply relieved by transcutaneous electrical stimulation (TES) or by analgesics which, on rare occasions, can be prescribed an hour or so before a potentially painful treatment; active exercises are infinitely more efficient at increasing circulation than massage.

Massage finds its most effective role in 'breaking down' adhesions, mobilizing scars and helping to reduce oedema. Massage is invaluable, therefore, in tendon adherence, burns, crush injuries and in any condition where oedema of the hand and forearm is limiting function or militating against the use of active physiotherapy.

Ice

Ice treatment is useful in reducing oedema, spasticity and pain before other therapeutic techniques, such as stretches and exercises.

The easiest way of applying cold to the hand is by ice dips. A mixture of a large proportion of ice and a smaller quantity of water, producing a stiff consistency at 10°C (50°F) or less is found most effective. The patient dips his hand into this mixture, taking it out when the cold is uncomfortable, drying it and reinserting his hand for a total of 3 minutes. The procedure may then be repeated during treatment sessions if necessary. This treatment is contraindicated in anaesthetic hands, owing to the danger of ice burns and damage to an already poor circulation.

Bad Ragaz techniques

These techniques, which were originated in Switzerland at Bad Ragaz, are found most useful for mobilizing and exercising the larger joints in water – in this case the shoulder. Techniques very similar to those of proprioceptive neuromuscular facilitation may be used. The patient floats on his back in the water, supported by air rings round his waist, under his knees and round his neck. This means that he may move completely through the water, for the physiotherapist gives him a fulcrum from which to move.

With the patient lying supine, the physiotherapist places her hands on the dorsum of the hand and the lateral border of the arm. The patient is instructed to push his arm against the therapist's hands; the therapist keeps her hand still, and the patient's body has to move away through the water. Abduction occurs at the shoulder joint. The therapist then moves close to the patient again and the movement is repeated. To increase the resistance in this movement, while the patient is pushing his arm away, the therapist keeps moving towards the patient and a greater water resistance is built up. The speed of the movement may also be increased.

Bilateral arm movements may be carried out. The patient lies supine, with both arms in full elevation, and grasping the hands of the physiotherapist, who stands behind his head. The patient pulls on the hands of the therapist, then thrusts away, so that the patient's body moves backwards and forwards through the water while the therapist remains still.

Various proprioceptive neuromuscular facilitation patterns may be carried out in the water, either supine or prone. If the physiotherapist does not allow her hands to move, the patient's body will move away when he lifts his arm. A variety of movements may be adapted for this form of treatment and the principles of the mobilizing techniques utilized.

Serial plaster stretches

These plasters are used to maintain the correction resulting from passive stretches as described on page 37. They are particularly useful in overcoming flexion deformities due to flexor tendon adherence at the wrist, extra-articular contractures of the metacarpophalangeal and interphalangeal joints, and to obtain flexion of the metacarpophalangeal joints when they are held in stiff extension.

The materials required are: 10-cm plaster of Paris bandage; 30-cm bowl with hot water – this is used to gain the fastest possible set; 7.5-cm crêpe bandage; petroleum jelly; large scissors; a Formica-topped table with adjustable height; a chair for the patient and one for the therapist, placed on either side of the table. The patient sits with the forearm resting on the table, with the palm upwards and the elbow flexed. A plaster bandage is cut so as to extend 10–15 cm above the wrist to just beyond the tip of the middle finger. The length will vary slightly according to the patient's skin condition and degree of scarring, and the severity of the contracture. Twelve layers of plaster are usually needed to produce the required thickness of the splint.

TECHNIQUES OF TREATMENT

A semicircular-shaped piece of plaster is removed from the thumb side so that opposition will not be limited. Petroleum jelly is then applied to the patient's skin, if hairy, to prevent the plaster adhering to it. Stockinette is not used, as this tends to wrinkle when the plaster is applied. The patient is then given one more stretch to make sure the greatest possible mobility has been obtained.

It is most important that the physiotherpist treating the patient makes the plaster, as the therapist will know the range of movement that has been gained during treatment. The layers of plaster are then soaked in the warm water in the bowl, squeezed out well and smoothed so that there are no wrinkles, and the plaster applied to the patient's arm (*Figure 6.3a*). Parallel grooves are made for each finger by gently squeezing up the plaster between the finger webs. The plaster may then be held in position with the crêpe bandage, leaving both hands of the therapist free for gaining the correct position. When the required degree of wrist extension has been obtained, the tendency to ulnar deviation must be corrected. The metacarpophalangeal joints are held in a slight degree of flexion and the proximal and terminal interphalangeal joints in the required degree of extension. When the pull of adherent tendons is very

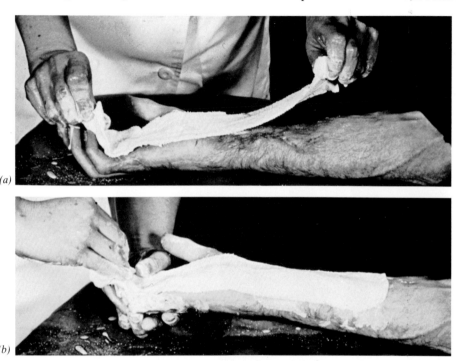

Figure 6.3 Use of stretch plasters in a patient with a severe crush injury resulting in stiff metacarpophalangeal and interphalangeal joints. (a) Plaster being applied. (b) Slow stretch being applied as the plaster sets — note support of hand

strong, the hand must be maintained in pronation while the plaster is setting (*Figure 6.3b*). If a supinated position were to be held while making the splint, the patient would be able to relax the tension when the plaster was later applied, by pronating the hand. This is due to the diagonal direction in which the muscles lie across the forearm between origin and insertion. The position is held by the therapist until the plaster is dry; the crêpe bandage is then removed, and the inside is well smoothed with plaster so that there are no projections. This is most important when a splint has to be applied over an anaesthetic area of skin. The splint is then dried in a warm place, but preferably not under direct heat as this tends to reduce the strength of the plaster and to make it crack.

APPLICATION OF THE PLASTER

The plaster is lined with a thin layer of cotton wool, and cotton wool is also placed over the extensor aspect of the hand and between the fingers. The plaster is applied with a 7.5-cm crêpe bandage. The patient places the forearm and wrist in the plaster, which is held in position by two or three turns of bandage; then the fingers are actively extended on to the splint where possible. The bandage is then fixed over the fingers but the terminal phalanges are not covered, so that the patient can check the colour of the fingers and the temperature if the limb is anaesthetic. The first splint should be applied at a time when the patient can return to the department for its removal. It is best to apply it before lunch and have the patient return for treatment immediately after lunch. A new splint is never given to a patient who cannot have the plaster checked soon after wearing it. A new stretch plaster may be made at daily intervals if the patient is able to lift the fingers from the splints, with the wrist maintained in extension. The patient should sleep in the previous day's splint, which is not therefore at maximum correction; a splint for full correction would be too painful to wear all night. The usual timetable followed is to wear the splint from 12.30 to 1.15 p.m. and then from 4 to 5.30 p.m.; this may be extended if the patient experiences no undue discomfort.

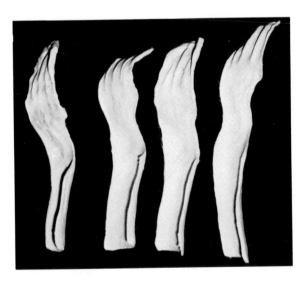

Figure 6.4 Serial plasters for correction of tendon adherence in patient illustrated in Figure 3.17. Note grooves for individual fingers

Should there be a great deal of difference in contracture between one finger and the next, it is difficult to apply a plaster which stretches each finger to the required degree. It is then useful to cut down the length of each finger of the first eight layers of plaster and apply these initially so that a different degree of correction may be given to each finger (*Figure 6.4*). The remaining uncut plaster should then be applied on top of the previous layers to maintain the position achieved.

General

Following a session of intensive treatment in the physiotherapy department, the patient should then carry on restoration of power and range of movement in the gymnasium or occupational therapy department, and treatments should be co-ordinated to provide maximum efficiency of each department's contribution. Physiotherapists and occupational therapists should be constantly in and out of each other's department, discussing progress, graduating treatment and producing combined functional assessments. There is no place for divisive trade unionism in the rehabilitation of the severely handicapped; either therapist should be capable of retraining in activities of daily living and in assessing function.

OCCUPATIONAL THERAPY

The role of occupational therapy is still under-rated in many parts of the world. An efficient rehabilitation organization cannot operate without an occupational therapy department with facilities for light and heavy work.

There are four main contributions that a department of occupational therapy can make.

(1) The provision of work in order to improve the range of movement of joints, increase muscle power and restore co-ordination. This work must be as realistic as possible and related to the patient's hobbies or work.
(2) The provision of facilities for assessing fitness for work and to decide if there is any adjustment required to tools or to the work situation.
(3) The ability to provide vocational guidance if a patient's disability precludes him from returning to his original work.
(4) The provision of aids to daily living in order to make patients as independent as possible. This will include such devices as Velcro fastening to replace buttons for people with intrinsic muscle weakness, or padded handles for spoons, forks and knives for patients with limitation of grip due to crush injury of the hand or tendon weakness. There are a wide range of gadgets and appliances which are now available for all types of disability (see page 330).

The type of work that can be offered in a department depends very much on the local situation. If the hospital or rehabilitation unit is sited in or near a large industrial town, it is usually possible to make arrangements with local industry whereby some form of productive work can be produced by the patients which can be remunerative and the proceeds can be ploughed back into the department. If, however, the hospital or unit is in the country then some form of craft may be necessary, as there may be no industrial potential available.

In the past patients spent their time in occupational therapy departments in such pursuits as weaving, leather work, basket work and making felt animals, all of which had limited value for restoration of function and little appeal to men. In recent years a number of techniques have been developed which are particularly applicable for injuries of the hand and which can contribute to productive work for the hospital or for outside industry. The following activities have been found most valuable for hand disabilities: printing, which includes guillotining and typesetting; stool-seating, which is popular because the goods can be useful in the patient's home – this provides both narrow and wide grips, a good deal of rotation movement, and can be performed in elevation if the patient is suffering from oedema of the hand; brush making and wire twisting; packing, labelling and sorting – in our rehabilitation unit, for example, we pack, label and sort high quality pepper for a local firm; polyethylene bag sealing which is useful for covering books and documents, involving cutting out and stapling and demanding considerable co-ordination; rug hooking; carpentry; model making; mosaic work and marquetry; radio assembly; wrought iron work; cross-cut sawing; cement mixing; indoor gardening and, later, outdoor gardening; all forms of bench work, involving metal filing; lathe work; foot-operated wood turning; and watch repairing (*Figure 6.5*).

For retraining of rapid co-ordinated intrinsic muscle activity, piano playing, typing or playing musical instruments are all of great value.

The Morse code training set provides a variety of skilled movements demanding precision, power and co-ordination. The fingers of the left hand have to stabilize the springs while the thumb pushes the wire through from under the board. The right

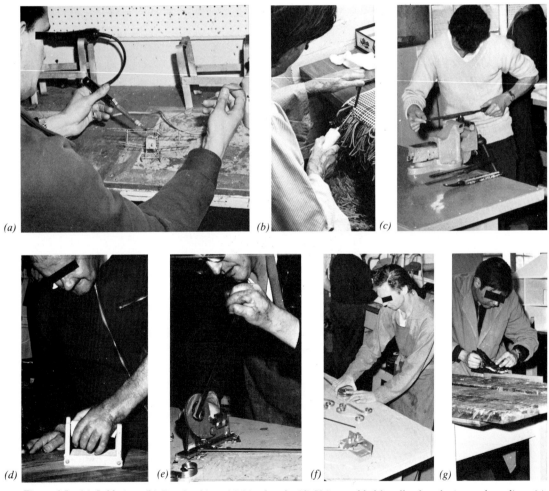

Figure 6.5   (a) Soldering. (b) Rug hooking. (c) Metalwork. (d) Using padded handles for planing and sanding. (e) Wrought iron work for metacarpophalangeal range (f) Wrought iron work for power of fingers. (g) Carpentry

hand threads wire above and below the board; adjusting and stabilizing is required by each finger. Wire must be uncoiled and cut, knobs screwed on and wire fixed to terminals with firm rotatory movements. Every type of hand movement is required, not only range and stability but power – the radio assembly set provides the same movements but on a smaller scale, thus demanding more precision, as well as soldering.

Assessment

One of the most important contributions the deparment can make is an accurate assessment of the patient's ability for work. This will involve testing in a variety of activities, using different ranges of tools, preparing reports on the patient's ability to carry out the movements required, his work tolerance, the standard of work produced, the time taken and his motivation. These assessments can be made at various stages of treatment and provide a valuable index of progress and encouragement to the patient. They will also indicate specific problems that need attention – a particular range of movement may be limited or a muscle group lacking in power and this will direct the attention of the physiotherapist to specific treatments required.

Before leaving the rehabilitation centre a full report is prepared by a thorough assessment that may take 2 or more days. This will ensure that the patient is confident that he can do his job when he returns to work, or will indicate what modifications may be required to tools or with the work situation. It will also indicate to his employer that, despite an apparent deformity, function has been proved to be satisfactory on the patient's particular job. The work report used at Joint Services Medical Rehabilitation Unit, Chessington, is illustrated in *Figure 6.6*.

There are almost as many assessment forms as there are occupational therapy departments. Attempts to provide a uniform assessment form for all hospitals has never succeeded because types of disability and patient vary so much.

Figure 6.7 shows the standard assessment used at the Joint Services Medical Rehabilitation Unit, Chessington. Barthel's index (Mahoney and Barthel, 1965) has the attraction of simplicity. It assesses disability from 0 to 100 – the cumulative score of a patient in nine activities: feeding, transfer, hygiene, bathing, mobility, stair climbing, dressing, bowel control, bladder control. It does not, however, measure the ability to run a home or the patient's social attitudes.

Sheikh and colleagues (1979) use a scheme for measuring disability with 17 items of activities of daily living: transfer from floor to chair; transfer from chair to bed; walking indoors; walking outdoors; ascending a flight of stairs; descending a flight of stairs; dressing; washing; bathing; using the lavatory; continence; grooming; brushing teeth; preparing for making tea; making tea; using taps; feeding. They find there is no significant inter-observer variability and suggest that the scheme is sufficiently repeatable and valid for the assessment of patients with chronic disease.

It is standard practice for the occupational therapist to provide a range of alterations to household and kitchen utensils for disabled housewives, and for her to visit the patient in the home to study the situation and advise on alteration of heights of kitchen apparatus or suggest techniques and gadgets to cope with particular

OCCUPATIONAL THERAPY DEPARTMENT
JOINT SERVICES MEDICAL REHABILITATION UNIT

ROYAL AIR FORCE
CHESSINGTON
SURREY

WORKSHOP ASSESSMENT REPORT   DATE:

NAME OF PATIENT .... MEDICAL OFFICER ....

INJURY ....

PRESENT FUNCTIONAL DISABILITY ....

....

DOMINANT HAND ....

SERVICE TRADE ....

DETAILS OF TRADE ....

....

ASSESSMENT FOR: ....

WORKSHOP TEST (APTITUDE) ....

....

TOOLS USED IN THE TEST   HAMMER ....   OTHER SPECIFIC TOOLS

FILES ....   OR EQUIPMENT

SAWS ....   REQUIRED ....

SOLDERING IRON ....

DRILLS ELECTRIC ....

DRILLS HAND ....

SCREW DRIVER ....

PUNCHES ....

TIN SHEARS ....

PLIERS ....

SPANNERS ....

MATHEMATICS ABILITY TEST ....

POWER ....

WORK TOLERANCE (FATIGUE) ....

ATTITUDE TO TEST/WORK ....

STANDARD OF COMPLETED WORK ....

SUITABLE/UNSUITABLE FOR R.T.U./TRAINING ....

OPINION:

SIGNED:.................

Figure 6.6

JOINT SERVICES MEDICAL REHABILITATION UNIT
RAF CHESSINGTON

AIDS TO DAILY LIVING (ADL)
ASSESSMENT CHART

KEY   0: impossible   3: can manage with minimal
    1: with much assistance   difficulty
    2: with little assistance   4: normal

DATE					COMMENTS
WASHING AND TOILET					
Turn taps					
Wash and dry hands, face and neck					
Wash and dry extremities					
Wash and dry back					
Clean teeth					
File/cut finger- and toe-nails					
Shave					
Brush/comb hair					
Wash hair					
Cope with bathing					
Get on/off lavatory					
Manage on lavatory					
EATING AND DRINKING					
Drink from cup/glass					
Eat with spoon and/or fork					
Butter bread					
Eat with knife and fork					
Pour tea					
Stir tea					
Manage boiled egg					
Serve self					
Cut meat					

Figure 6.7

DATE					COMMENTS
DRESSING AND UNDRESSING					Time taken:
Manage track suit on/off					
Vest					
Pants					
Shirt					
Trousers					
Tie					
Jacket					
Socks					
Shoes					
Tie shoe laces					
Boots					
Hat					
Overcoat					
Gloves					
Caliper/artificial limb					
Manage all fastenings					
MOBILITY					
Getting in and out of bed					
Manage in and out of chairs (low, high, with/without arms)					
Stand safely					
Walk (distance)					
Manage stairs					
Manage wheelchair					
Manage public/private transport					

Figure 6.7 (cont.)

DATE					COMMENTS
COMMUNICATION					
Talking					
Writing					
Reading					
Using telephone					
Typing					
GENERAL ACTIVITIES					
Pick up objects from floor					
Carry objects					
Open/close doors					
Manage keys					
Open/close windows					
Make bed					
Manage light switches					
Manage electric plugs					
Open letter					
Handle money					
Strike matches					
Wind watch					
Open/close drawers					
Clean shoes					

Figure 6.7 (cont.)

HOBBIES:

HOME CONDITIONS:

OTHER A.D.L. PROBLEMS:

AIDS PROVIDED:

Signature

Figure 6.7 (cont.)

disabilities. Indeed, occupational therapists should be encouraged to visit patients at their work to study the actual working conditions, and advise on alteration of the work situation or provision of necessary gadgets, appliances or alteration of tools. Indeed, there is only a limited place for assessment of the patient in the clinic; far more can be learnt about the patient's potentialities and capabilities by seeing him under treatment in the various departments and at work.

This means a close relationship between the rehabilitation team and local industry, either directly or through a rehabilitation officer.

Surprisingly, severe disabilities are compatible with excellent function, and mild disabilities can be associated with surprisingly poor function – this may be a problem of motivation or unhappy work or social background which needs time and careful assessment to unravel. The closest possible liaison between occupational therapists, physiotherapists, gymnasts, social workers and welfare officers is essential if the patient is to benefit to the full. A physiotherapist will be able to indicate to the occupational therapist which particular requirement needs to be satisfied in a particular stage of rehabilitation.

The physiotherapist will, for example in a patient with a crush hand, provide intensive oil massage to loosen up the scarring, passive movements to try to increase range, and then send the patient to the occupational therapist who will reinforce this activity by giving the patient work involving active flexion of the fingers against resistance.

Following this, the patient can then have a period in the gymnasium playing games using a racket with a padded handle, continuing to build up power of the hand and general function of the upper limb.

Aids for daily living

There are a whole host of aids and gadgets available for patients in the home, with weakness of the upper limbs. In the kitchen these include non-slip place mats using rubber or plastic foam, two-handled cups, the Crayleigh cooker safeguard with built-up sides to prevent pots and pans slipping, platforms over the sink, strainer lids on pans for one-handed people, a wire pastry blender, egg separator and whisk, needing light touch only, one-handed peelers, graters clipped to the wall, bread boards with spikes to hold the bread, non-spill measuring spoons and jugs, one-handed tin openers and suction cups on the bottom of bowls. Special types of irons and ironing boards are available for one-handed people, flexible mops, extending brushes, pick-up sticks, grips to cover small keys. T-shaped key handles, large handles on taps or lever tap handles, door-knob turners, swing-top wastebins and magnetic catches for shutting doors. For clothing, Velcro fastenings, zips, dressing sticks, long tongs, ties knotted on hat elastic, zips under arm seams, clip-on aprons, boot removers, elasticated shoes, knitting aids, one-handed darners and card holders.

In the garden, the Wolfe handle grip makes tools easier to manoeuvre, using metal guttering with a grip on the tool. One-handed weeders, hoes, spray bottles and cutters are all available and special pruners for patients with weak hands.

For patients with severe shoulder weakness, slings can be used to support the forearm either from a steel, free-standing support or with an overhead frame from the chair; mobile gantries with slings for bilateral weakness are available. A most useful device for severe upper limb weakness is a tilting forearm support with a rolling swivelling action for eating. Ballbearing arm supports take the weight of the upper limb on freely moving levers mounted on ball races. The residual power utilizes a slight displacement of the upper limb which tilts the balanced hand up or down without the need of elbow function. A bracket on the wheel chair carries the support. A heavy model is available in which all joints are friction-controlled for spasticity.

The flexor hinge hand splint (*Figure 6.8*)

Dr P. J. R. Nichols kindly provided the following description of this most useful splint.*

The purpose of the splint is to increase the function of a weak or flaccid hand by providing a three-point prehension grasp between the thumb and the index and

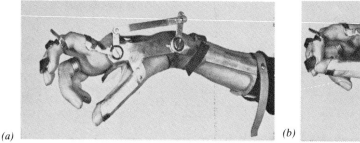 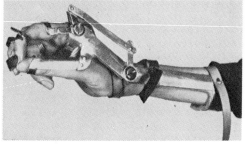

(a)   *(b)*

Figure 6.8   Flexor hinge splint. (a) In position with wrist flexed and grip open. (b) Wrist extended and grip closed

middle fingers. It provides stability of the wrist, thumb and interphalangeal joints of the index and middle fingers in a functional position, and allows a 'hinge' movement at the metacarpophalangeal joints of these two fingers. It supports the palmar arch.

The thumb is stabilized in a position of palmar abduction. The index and middle fingers are held together in a finger cage which allows movements at the metacarpophalangeal joints, but no movement at the interphalangeal joints. The two fingers move in flexion to meet the fixed thumb.

The splint may be worked by residual muscle power of the wrist or fingers, not less than grade 4 strength, or it may be driven by external power.

Thus the types of flexor hinge splint are:

(1) Finger flexor driven – fixed wrist, spring return at metacarpophalangeal joints to open.
(2) Finger extensor driven – fixed wrist, spring return at metacarpophalangeal joints to close.

---

* Kits supplied by: Orthopedic Supplies Inc., Firestone Boulevard, Downey, Los Angeles, California, USA; and Jaeco Orthopedic Specialities, PO Box 75, Hot Springs, Arkansas, USA.

(3) Wrist flexor driven – hinged wrist with spring return.
(4) Wrist extensor driven – hinged wrist, no spring.
(5) Power driven – fixed wrist, spring return at metacarpophalangeal joints to open.

The most generally useful is the wrist extensor driven splint, particularly in cases of cervical cord lesion.

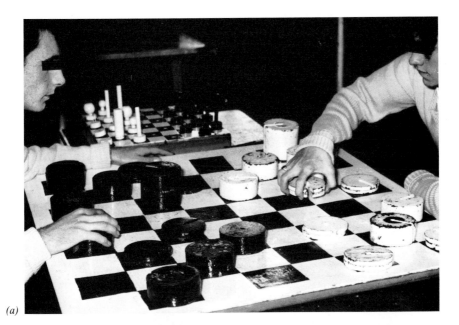

(a)

(b)

Figure 6.9   Draughts. (a) Heavy. (b) Magnetic

In all cases it is essential to have a good free range of movement at the metacarpophalangeal joints of the index and middle fingers and a wide supple thumb web. Active pronation also needs to be as full as possible and it is necessary that either elbow flexion is present or that substitute equipment to produce elbow flexion is fitted.

These splints are not suitable for patients with severe spasticity. If the patient is unable to relax consistently, he may also be unable to tolerate and use a flexor hinge splint.

The actual assembly and fitting of the splint is a highly skilled job and individual to each patient. When loss of sensation is involved, a continual watch should be kept for pressure areas developing. Training in use of the splint should be intensive.

Games used in occupational therapy

Games are, of course, popular with patients and can be modified to encourage function, as well as being entertaining.

DRAUGHTS

Draughts is still one of the more popular games among patients. Boards should be of at least three different sizes: normal, 60 cm square and 90 cm square. The size of the pucks should range from normal up to 12.5 cm in diameter; the weight should vary from light up to as heavy as possible; the shape – flat round discs.

The board can be elevated on a stand which is adjustable in height. Hooks are fixed to each square and weights are used as pucks to improve shoulder elevation and elbow extension. The board can be made magnetic and placed vertically for shoulder elevation (*Figure 6.9*).

COMPETITIVE BLOW FOOTBALL

The patients squeeze the rubber bulb of a syringe, thus blowing out air which propels a ping-pong ball along a table. A penalty is awarded against a player who touches the ball with the end of the syringe. The game can be played standing (*Figure 6.10*) or sitting, when a circular pitch is used (*Figure 6.11*).

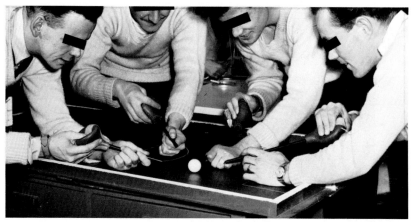

Figure 6.10   Blow football

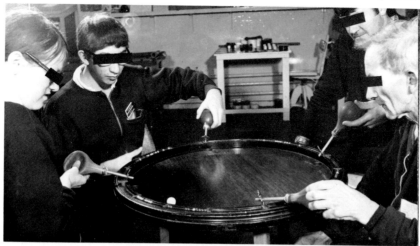

Figure 6.11 Sitting table blow football

Construction of the pitch

The table should be constructed, with a rim all round, approximately 150 × 90 cm. This can be larger or smaller according to the space available. Corners should be rounded, otherwise the ping-pong ball is inclined to get stuck in a corner. Markings and goals can be on a smaller scale than those on a football field, and rules as judged suitable by the therapist to the needs of the patients. The bulbs are those used for drawing up distilled water, and can be bought at a garage tool shop. For much lighter work for the hands, bulbs used by florists for spraying flowers are recommended.

Timing

Fatigue develops quickly and, as a guide, the first efforts should not exceed 1 minute – 30 seconds using the affected hand, then 15 seconds with the normal hand and finally the last 15 seconds with the affected hand again.

Positions of holding the bulb

(1) In the palm of the hand for all types of grip and general muscle work. (2) For encouraging action in the long and short flexors to the thumb and adduction and abduction of the fingers, the neck of the bulb is held between the index and middle fingers with the thumb on the crown of the bulb (see *Figure 6.10*).

FLIP FOOTBALL

This game is useful for extension of the metacarpophalangeal joints and wrist, and is similar to blow football in all but the apparatus used. In place of the bulb, a square leather bag is made to fit over the patient's hand to cover the fingers and grip above the metacarpophalangeal joints. The bag should be at least 5 cm longer than the fingers, and should not be too stiff – plenty of extension is needed to carry the momentum of the leather 'flip' action.

Finger extension is used for play, and only the edge of the leather is allowed to touch the board, otherwise the fingers will be used to push the puck (a flat puck is used in place of the ping-pong ball) instead of using the 'flip' action.

BAR FOOTBALL

Bar football can be adapted to offer various types of grip (*Figure 6.12*).

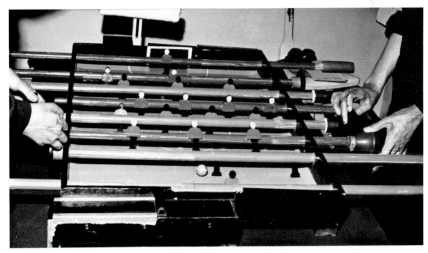

Figure 6.12   Bar football

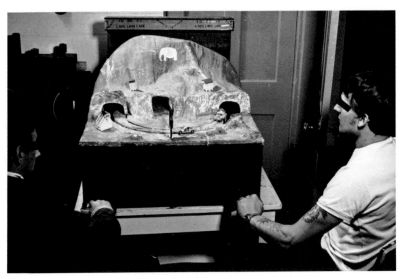

Figure 6.13   Car race game

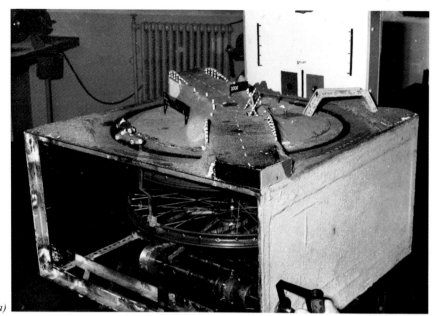

(a)

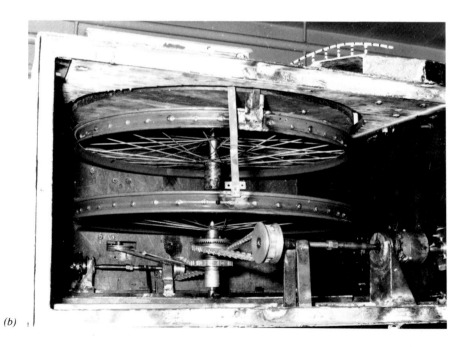

(b)

Figure 6.14   (a) The car race game interior. (b) The wheel drive

CAR RACE GAME FOR PRONATION AND SUPINATION

This game is constructed from a large box approximately 1 metre square by 35 cm high. The upper surface is designed as a circular car racing track, with a groove cut out in which two small model cars can move around the track. The internal mechanism is basically a simple bicycle wheel drive with adaptations. The cars are attached to a metal rod which is fixed to a handle with an inner bar grip. The handles are on opposite sides of the track, and two patients compete. The cars are rotated round the track by pronating or supinating the handles. Each lap is recorded on an indicator at the back of the track, the winner of the race being the 'driver' whose indicator finally shows a chequered disc. It is important to see that the starting position of the patient's arm is correct, or the movement will not be pure pronation and supination. The patients should adjust the chair they are sitting on until the wrist and elbow are in a lime with the handle, and the upper arm at right angles to the forearm. The elbows should be held close to the sides. The mechanism of the handle is such that unless a firm grip is held on the inner bar against the main handle, the cars cannot be rotated round the track during pronation or supination (*Figures 6.13* and *6.14*).

BEAT THE CLOCK HAND GAME

This consists of a strong wooden box measuring 1.2 m long × 30 cm high × 30 cm broad. A 3.8-cm groove is cut in the centre of the top of the box, extending from one end to the other. A metal lever stick is fixed to one end of the groove, and can be moved to the opposite end. At intervals along this groove metal gates are placed which impede the forward movement of the lever, but, by manipulating the handles of these gates, the lever can pass onwards. Releasing the lever at the start automatically sets the electric clock in action. The object of the game is to move the lever through all the gates from one end to the other in the shortest possible time. The gates are attached to handles requiring a variety of grips, and varying in power and range. Thus, wrist flexion and extension, rotation, flexion of the interphalangeal joint of the thumb and mass flexor action of the fingers can be provided (*Figure 6.15*). Any number of 'gates' can be added to the box. Any number of players can compete, all attempting to beat the time taken by the previous player. Apart from its use as a competitive game, it is most useful in the assessment of hand function.

In most cases of injury to the hand, some degree of weakness of muscle or stiffness of joints develops in the upper limb as a whole, particularly where there has been prolonged immobilization. Moreover, the patient's general fitness may well suffer and it is important to restore him or her to at least the premorbid state of physical fitness and in many cases to a higher standard – many of our patients admit to being fitter than ever before on discharge.

Appendix A of this chapter lists the exercise tables used in the classes in the gymnasium under the close supervision of remedial gymnasts.

Games are interspersed between exercises and may include relay races, cricket, tennis, squash, badminton (with padded rackets when appropriate), croquet, golf, putting, table-tennis and bar skittles. For fine hand control, darts, pick-a-stick, draughts and chess are useful.

In the final stages of rehabilitation, when the aim is a high degree of fitness, circuit training is ideal, since it provides training of cardiorespiratory reserve as well as development of specific muscle power (Appendix B in this chapter).

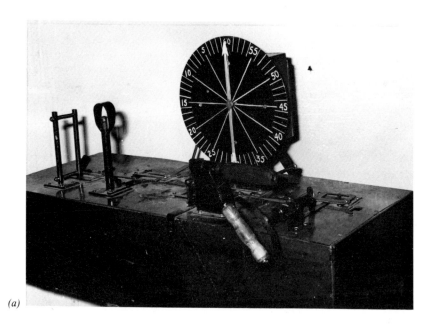

(a)

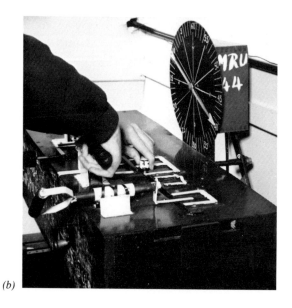

(b)

Figure 6.15 Beat the clock hand game

APPENDIX A: EXERCISE TABLES

Shoulder free exercise routine – about 20 minutes

EARLY STAGE – LAX STOOP STAND OR LAX STOOP SIT

(1) Arm swinging forwards and backwards.
(2) Arm swinging side to side.
(3) Arm swinging circling.
(4) Arm swinging:
    (*a*) forwards to hold in position statically;
    (*b*) sideways to hold in position statically;
    (*c*) backwards to hold in position statically.
(5) Standing/sitting; static contraction against other hand resistance:
    (*a*) sideways (abduction);
    (*b*) forwards (flexion);
    (*c*) backwards (extension).
(6) Lying: arms bent, hands together; arms raising upwards.
(7) Lying: arms straight upwards, hands together:
    (*a*) arms bending to touch top of head;
    (*b*) as in (*a*) with hands reaching backwards along floor.
(8) Lying: arms sliding sideways to given position.
(9) Fist bend prone lying:
    (*a*) move hands upwards along ground;
    (*b*) move hands sideways along ground.
(10) Prone lying:
    (*a*) slide hands down to sides;
    (*b*) slide hands up above head.
(11) Lying: arms straight, hands clenched; arms raising to given position.
(12) Lying: arms bent by sides; alternate arm reaching to touch shoulder.
(13) Side lying: arm reaching forwards and backwards.
(14) Side lying:
    (*a*) arm bent raising upwards.
    (*b*) arm raising upwards.
(15) Lying: alternate arms raising upwards.

INTERMEDIATE AND LATE STAGES (STANDING)

(1) Stride standing	Hands clasped in front of chest	Arms reach forwards	
(2) Stride standing	Hands clasped in front of chest	Arms reach upwards	
(3) Stride standing	Hands clasped in front of chest	(*a*) Swing side to side, followed by	
		(*b*) a large circle (right and left)	
(4) Stride standing	Hands turning outwards and inwards.		

(5) Stride standing	Arms swinging sideways, one arm pressing in front the other behind the body.
(6) Stride standing	Arms swinging forwards, bending to touch shoulders.
(7) Stride standing	Alternate arm reaching to opposite shoulder, one in front the other behind.
(8) Fist bend stride standing	(*a*) Arms reach forwards to horizontal. (*b*) Arms reach sideways to horizontal. (*c*) Combination. (*d*) With skip jumps.
(9) Bend standing	Elbows raising sideways.
(10) Reach standing	Hands opening and closing (static shoulder act).
(11) Stride standing	Arms raising sideways to given position.
(12) Stride standing	Arms swinging forwards to given height.
(13) Across bend standing	Elbows circling: (*a*) Backwards. (*b*) Forwards. (*c*) Co-ordination of both.
(14) Stride standing	Arms bending behind neck.
(15) Stride standing	Alternate arms swing forwards and upwards with rhythmical presses in inner range.
(16) Stride standing	(*a*) Arms reaching sideways and upwards. (*b*) Combined with astride jumping. (*c*) Combined (15) + (16).

Elbow free exercise routine

STRIDE STANDING

(1) Hands held together, arms straight in front of body; arms bending to touch chest with hands.

(2) Hands together, arms above head; arms bending backwards to touch back of neck with hands.

(3) Arms bent to sides, palms facing upwards; turning palms downwards then upwards.

(4) Arms to sides, palms facing backwards; arms bending with hands turning forwards to touch shoulders.

(5) Stride standing; arms swinging downwards to cross body, alternating one in front one behind.

(6) Arms bent, hands clenched at waist, static tension (5 seconds) for elbow flexors and extensors.

(7) Stride standing; arms bending to reach behind head.

(8) Fist bend stride standing; static tension with slow movement within range pushing action.

(9) Fist bend stride standing; followed by grip and pulling action.

(10) Stride standing; arms swinging backwards with elbows raising upwards.
(11) Wing stride standing; moving hands up body as far as possible in easy stages.
(12) Wing stride standing; followed by downward movement as far as possible. NB: hands to stay in contact with body.
(13) Walk forward standing; static tension with slow movement within range drawing back bow and arrow and release.
(14) Cross arm bend stride standing; palms together:
    (*a*) arms stretching forwards;
    (*b*) arms stretching upwards;
    (*c*) arms stretching downwards.

Hand free exercise routine – about 30 minutes

ALL EXERCISES SEATED AROUND TABLE/PLINTH

(1) Arms bent, hands supinated; wrist bending forwards.
(2) Arms bent, hands pronated; wrist bending backwards.
(3) Arms bent; hands circling to right then left.
(4) Arms bent, hands pronated; bending and stretching fingers and thumb to make fist.
(5) Arms bent; as in (4), with supination on close and pronation on opening of fingers/thumb.
(6) Arms bent (forearms rested), opposition of thumb to each finger tip in turn:
    (*a*) slowly;
    (*b*) with eyes shut;
    (*c*) fast in game form.
(7) Arms bent, hands supinated; interphalangeal joints bending and stretching:
    (*a*) individually;
    (*b*) combined movement.
(8) Arms bent, palms on table; hand shortening (bend metacarpophalangeal joints).
(9) Arms bent, hands pronated; finger parting and closing:
    (*a*) combined movement;
    (*b*) individual side to side;
    (*c*) individual and pair control.
(10) Arms bent, palms on table; finger raising:
    (*a*) individually;
    (*b*) combination and co-ordinated movement.

Use of small light objects in exercise and games

BALL

(1) Hand supinated holding light airflow ball; throwing up to catch.
(2) Hand pronated holding light airflow ball; dropping to catch.
(3) Alternate catch and bouncing ball from hand to hand.
(4) Collective game; each with ball rolling round table to next patient in circle. *Loser* = first to drop a ball or to collect more than one ball.

SMALL STICKS/PENCILS

(1) Finger tips together with stick balanced on index fingers, bend index fingers to drop object to fingers below. Once on little fingers, manipulate back to index fingers.
(2) Rolling object between fingers over the back and up the front for complete turn. NB: this can also be done with pennies, dominoes, etc.
(3) Using rubber hoops for flexor strength:
  (*a*) pick up hoop with finger tips;
  (*b*) pick up hoop with middle phalanges and squeeze;
  (*c*) place hoop in hand for full grip with proximal phalanges.
(4) Use of rope to tie knots, various.
(5) Use of various tools:
  (*a*) screwdriver;
  (*b*) scissors;
  (*c*) pliers.
  NB: all strength exercises which give resistance – i.e. (3) and (5) – are subject to the stage of the patient's treatment, especially nerve/tendon sutures or any graft.

APPENDIX B: CIRCUIT TRAINING

The circuit comprises eight activities which follow straight on, one after the other. The 'white' circuit demands that each activity is performed three times, the blue five times, the green seven times and the red nine times.

The target is 5 minutes for the white course, 6½ minutes for the blue, 8½ minutes for the green, 10 minutes for the red.

When each target is achieved, the subject moves up to the next colour.

Before assigning the patient to the circuit, the instructor will assess the patient's general fitness by asking him to perform a few of the circuit tasks to see how he responds and gain a good idea of his exercise tolerance.

These circuits are very popular as the patient can watch his progress against himself.

(1) Shuttle run 18 m performed six times = 108 m.
(2) Three dips on the parallel bars.
(3) Three sit-ups.
(4) Three bench squats, the bench being lifted to a height of 2.4 m from knees bent position.
(5) Three 'beat' heaves, heaving the chest up to the beam from the hanging position.
(6) Astride jumps on and off bench: 10 for white, 12 for blue, 14 for green, 18 for red.
(7) Three 'burpees'. From standing to press-up position and return as fast as possible.
(8) Step-ups on bench: 10 for white, 12 for blue, 14 for green, 18 for red.

The circuit can be started at any one of these activities and proceed round, so that eight patients can be taking part at one time.

REFERENCES AND BIBLIOGRAPHY

Brewerton, D. A. and Daniel, J. W. (1969). Return to work after injury. *The Hand* **1,** 125–128

British Medical Association (1968). *Aids for the Disabled*. London: BMA

Mahoney, F. I. and Barthel, D. W. (1965). Function evaluation. The Barthel index. *Maryland Medical Journal* **14,** 61

Mattingly, S. (Ed.) (1977). *Rehabilitation Today*. London: Update

Nichols, P. J. R. (1971). *Rehabilitation of the Severely Disabled*. London: Butterworths

Rusk, H. (Ed.) (1977). *Rehabilitation Medicine*, 4th edn. London: Kimpton

Sheik, K., Smith, D. S., Meade, T. W., Goldenberg, E., Brennan, P. J. and Kinsella, G. (1979). Activities of daily living index in studies of chronic disability. *International Journal of Rehabilitation Medicine* **1,** 51–57

Aids for the disabled are on display at:

Disabled Living Foundation, 380 Harrow Road, London W9 2HU

Royal Association for Disability and Rehabilitation (RADAR), 25 Mortimer Street, London W1

Amputations of the Upper Limb 7

Ian Fletcher

INTRODUCTION

Causes

In Great Britain the most common cause of an upper limb amputation is trauma and about 80 per cent of these injuries occur in industry.

A small percentage are due to road traffic accidents while electric burns are responsible for a fair proportion of very high arm amputations in young children and linesmen, some of whom may lose both arms.

The premature detonation of home-made explosives accounts for quite a few one-handed youths while some even less fortunate youngsters suffer bilateral loss, frequently associated with eye injuries.

Despite skilful surgery and modern antibiotics, many severely crushed or mutilated arms and hands will fail to recover sufficiently to allow an industrial worker to resume his former occupation or any other bimanual activity. However, an amputation and the subsequent fitting of a prosthesis may well permit an early and active return to industry.

It is not unknown for drug addicts to lose a limb as a sequel to accidental injection into an artery.

A small percentage of upper limb amputations have to be performed to remove malignant tumours and these include the forequarter and shoulder disarticulation.

Complete and permanent paralysis of the upper limb is often an indication for ablation. This is accepted more often by the patient who has suffered an irreparable traction lesion of the brachial plexus than by the victim of poliomyelitis who regards the affected limb as a living member, due to the retained sensibility. The former individual, however, often considers his flail and anaesthetic limb to be a dead and useless burden.

The patients

It is clear, therefore, that the majority of upper limb amputees are young active males. Most of them wish to return to their former level of activity whether as an industrial worker, motor-cyclist or adventurous schoolboy. Each one hopes to take his place in equal competition alongside an able-bodied counterpart. It is therefore of paramount importance that they all receive correct and continual rehabilitation from the day of injury (or diagnosis of disease) to that of return to normal life, which usually means their former occupation.

As in rehabilitation for other conditions, it is essential to consider the amputee not only as a 'bread-winner', who must return either to his original employment or to some other suitable occupation, but also as a human being. His social life and pastimes may be seriously affected; psychological problems are likely to arise and must be foreseen in order to deal with them promptly. An amputation is permanent, irrevocable and mutilating but, because of its finality, it usually presents a challenge to its victim who, amazingly enough, accepts the new situation very philosophically. He cheerfully sets about proving to himself and to others that not only is he equal to them but that he is better!

Although encouragement is essential from the beginning, it is very unwise to overemphasize the value of an artificial limb. There must be no doubt that it is considerably inferior to the human structure it attempts to replace. No mechanical hand, however ingenious its design, can compete with nature's creation until tactile sensibility of a very high order is incorporated.

The Limb Fitting Service

Those eligible to benefit under the National Health Service in the UK may, at the discretion of the medical officer concerned, be supplied with two prostheses for each missing limb whether due to an amputation or of congenital origin. There is no cost to the wearer for the supply or repair of the prostheses or of any terminal appliance which may also be issued to an upper limb amputee. In special circumstances a patient may be supplied with a non-standard appliance, made for his or her particular needs.

In England the Limb Fitting Service is administered by the Department of Health and Social Security* which has 29 centres† situated in various cities and large towns.

Training of amputees

Instruction in the use of an artificial limb is arranged for amputees by each centre dealing with prostheses. The actual arm training, however, is underaken at only a few centres because of the comparatively small number of upper limb amputations performed. Nearly all the establishments with training facilities are situated adjacent

---

*The Scottish Home and Health Department is responsible for the Limb Fitting Service in Scotland, and the Welsh Office for the Service in Wales.

†Most of the establishments outside London are designated 'Artificial Limb and Appliance Centres'. At these the Department's medical officers (who are professional civil servants) not only deal with prostheses but also assess patients who are referred for the consideration and supply of wheelchairs and motorized vehicles. At the Appliance Centres war pensioners may also be fitted with any surgical appliance which is prescribed for their attributable disabilities.

Because of the enormity of the population in and around Greater London there are three Appliance Centres within the metropolis and one Limb Fitting Centre (Roehamptom, in south-west London).

to a hospital where patients may be accommodated, free of charge, during the period of tuition should they live too far away to attend daily. It is usual for arm training units to accept patients from about four or five peripheral centres which are basically responsible for the supply and maintenance of the prostheses and periodic review of the amputees.

Although an arm training unit at each centre would seem to be ideal, expertise would be lacking with so few patients and it would be soul destroying to be the only person undergoing training even if the occupational therapist were the most charming person in the world! Competition with other amputees is essential if training and rehabilitation are to be successful.

SITES OF AMPUTATION AND PROSTHESES

The forequarter amputation

The most mutilating of all upper limb amputations is the forequarter (*Figure 7.1*). It is usually a planned operation for the eradication of malignant disease and so skin flaps may be carefully fashioned in order to provide adequate cover to the rib cage. Sometimes, however, these amputations are the result of electric burns or other forms of severe trauma which necessitate skin grafting of the chest wall. In such cases considerable difficulty may be experienced by the artificial limb fitter in obtaining a satisfactory shoulder 'cap' which will not cause chafing of the insensitive skin graft due to body movement. Although the lining of the prosthesis is normally of soft chamois, it is necessary, in these traumatic cases, to have a layer of polyethylene sponge 3 mm

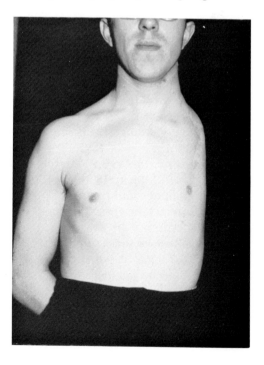

Figure 7.1 Forequarter amputation

thick underneath the whole of the lining. Not until the prosthesis has been worn for an hour or more may it become evident that there is a 'high spot' in the 'cap' which is causing friction. If this occurs then an immediate adjustment is indicated. Because of these hazards it is important to ensure that the amputees have very limited activity during their early training with the prosthesis, and frequent inspection is essential.

The forequarter prosthesis

For such a high and unsightly amputation the main purpose of the prosthesis is to restore the shoulder contour and protect the amputation site. It is unlikely that the patient will obtain much functional ability with the new limb and many are content to have nothing more than a shoulder restoration which permits the clothing to hang correctly. This partial prosthesis is made of soft polyethylene foam contained within a nylon jacket which fits the body like the upper half of a waistcoat. The foam contour is easily removed when the jacket needs washing.

Those patients requiring the full limb replacement – either as an additional prosthesis to the above or as their main limb for everyday use – have a blocked leather shoulder cap which has been moulded on a plaster cast of the amputation area. Over most of this is fitted an additional leather or plastic cap which has been made to match the contour of the sound shoulder. It is extended downwards in one piece to form the arm. An elbow mechanism is attached and contains a device which permits the wearer to rotate the flexed forearm internally and externally.

Concealed side steels connect the forearm to the elbow spindle, which also incorporates a manually operated elbow locking device operated from a lever set in the middle of the forearm. This allows the wearer to flex the forearm with the sound hand and at the same time select the desired locking position (*Figure 7.2*).

The artificial hand may either be detachable at the mid-forearm (or wrist), or be made continuous with the forearm, thus lessening the weight of the prosthesis distally – an important factor in high-level amputations.

If desired, a two-way hinge may be fitted into the shoulder to allow flexion and abduction of the arm. This is useful only for dressing and can be a nuisance to the wearer when walking because he may lose control of the limb, which tends to swing into abduction.

The hands may be rigid with either articulated or fixed fingers to be worn with an outdoor glove. Alternatively, they may be made of a firm foam with a malleable wire core in each finger and thumb and covered with a flesh-like plastic glove in which the normal skin markings are represented. The digits may be positioned according to the wearer's preference.

The prosthesis is secured to the patient by means of webbing straps. One, which is riveted to the back of the cap, passes horizontally around the body, close under the sound axilla, to be fastened to a buckle having a double V-like attachment to the cap anteriorly. Prior to securing the prosthesis the wearer threads the end of the under-arm strap through a loop on a second strap which passes vertically upwards and over the sound shoulder from its posterior attachment to the first strap. On the front of this second strap is another buckle and strap-end, purely for adjustment purposes.

Very muscular patients may be able to achieve active elbow flexion by means of a leather cord attached posteriorly and passing over a pulley set behind the artificial shoulder. This 'flexion cord' then passes down the medial side of the arm and through an eyelet fitted to the inner side of the forearm, about 2.5 cm below the elbow joint. A leather extension thong may be added to operate with the mechanical thumb lever or other terminal devices.

Velcro fastening may be used instead of a buckle should the patient so wish. Sometimes it is necessary to extend the shoulder cap posteriorly across the neck and over the opposite shoulder to form a yoke. The end of it is finished as a strap which

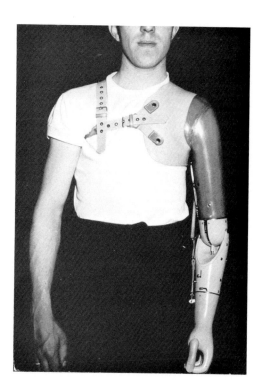

Figure 7.2 Same patient as shown in Figure 7.1, wearing prosthesis. Note: a flexion cord and extension thong, which are rarely used on these prostheses, have been supplied for this patient

takes the place of the second strap previously mentioned. The yoke provides more support than the double strap fixation but in the course of time the leather tends to become distorted in the neck region and results in an unacceptable appearance, the only remedy being renewal of the leather section.

There is a limited number of terminal appliances which may be used successfully by these amputees who are ever-conscious of the presence of the prosthesis and any additional weight, especially in the region of the hand. Women, particularly, value an appliance for holding meat or vegetables when preparing food in the kitchen, and also an appliance for holding needlework. These are simple and light.

A simple dress arm, known as the endoskeletal prosthesis, may be supplied as an alternative for adult amputees (see page 339).

The shoulder amputation and prosthesis

Removal of the arm from the shoulder joint is far less disfiguring than the forequarter amputation. Following this procedure, however, the acromion process becomes extremely prominent (*Figure 7.3*). Great care is needed when fitting the prosthesis in order to prevent chafing of the overlying skin by the shoulder cap when worn for long periods.

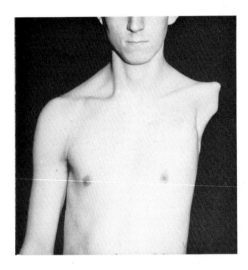

Figure 7.3   Disarticulation of the shoulder. Note the very prominent acromion process

When this operation is performed for malignant disease, the condition dictates the level of amputation. If, however, a patient suffers a traumatic amputation through the neck of the humerus the surgeon should endeavour to retain the head, as this will help to provide a rounded shoulder which makes for greater comfort in a prosthesis.

The artificial limb is very similar in design to that just described for the forequarter amputation, except for the extent of the shoulder cap and the material from which it is made. Plastic or leather may be chosen. When a disarticulation has been performed and the acromion process is particularly prominent, it is advisable to prescribe a leather cap and provision for the bony prominence is then made by removing a complete section from the overlying part. This 'window' is hidden within by the chamois lining and without by a thin layer of Persian calf, which is normally used as a finishing cover on all leather shoulder caps (*Figure 7.4*).

Plastic shoulder caps are not recommended for this amputation but may be used when the humeral head has been preserved.

The remainder of the prosthesis, apart from its suspension, may be similar in design to the foregoing. Alternatively, a more functional type can be supplied. This has an elbow unit with an internal locking mechanism for eight positions and is manually operated from a strap on the locking lever which is set just above the elbow joint. The upper end of this strap is fastened to the shoulder cap by the rivet holding the front suspension section of the harness. The latter is made of webbing and has a V-shaped attachment to the back of the cap to which it is anchored by two rivets.

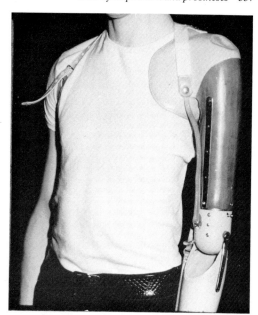

Figure 7.4 Same patient as shown in Figure 7.3, wearing prosthesis. Note the section of cap which has been cut away over the acromion process

A flexion control cord is usually supplied and in place of the standard eyelet, on the 'flexion lever' fixed to the forearm, a double roller lever is fitted through which the cord is fed prior to its being attached to the extension thong. This is used to open appliances such as tweezers, split hook, pliers, etc.

When the amputee 'rounds' his shoulders, tension is applied to the flexion cord which pulls the forearm into flexion, provided the elbow joint is free. When it is locked, the tension on the cord is transmitted to the extension thong which pulls on the lever arm of whatever appliance is fitted. The roller lever at the elbow reduces the inevitable friction on the cord and is particularly useful when the forearm is flexed to 90 degrees or more.

Some patients with a disarticulation at the shoulder have insufficient power to operate the flexion cord and its extension. They may prefer to use the prosthesis simply as a sleeve-filler and wear a cosmetic hand. Others, however, may have lost the contralateral limb or have sustained severe injury to it which necessitates active use of the shoulder prosthesis. In these cases a shaped leather waist belt may be supplied to provide a suitable anchor point for the flexion cord which is then operated by elevating the shoulder. This is usually more effective than the shoulder 'rounding' and often results in greater excursion of the cord. A 5 cm travel is the minimum for operating many terminal devices.

The above-elbow amputation and prosthesis

In order to obtain useful function from a prosthesis with an amputation performed through any part of the humerus there must be a minimum bone length of 8.8 cm (measured from the tip of the acromion process). About 18–20 cm is considered to be the ideal length for the sectioned bone in an adult of average height. Although it may reasonably be assumed that a long stump affords greater leverage, experience has proved that a 20-cm stump, with normal shoulder movement and musculature, is more than adequate. A very long stump deprives the amputee of the fitment of a prosthesis having a self-contained automatic elbow and rotational mechanism. This unit is 11.4 cm long and there must therefore be a minimum clearance of 12 cm from the position of the natural olecranon, otherwise the artificial elbow will be set too low.

When possible, the skin flaps should be fashioned to provide for either a terminal or a posterior scar since it is the lower and anterior aspect of the stump which exerts pressure against the socket to activate the prosthesis. It is also advisable to provide a stump end with normal skin whenever possible. Surgeons have been known to apply split-thickness skin grafts over the entire circumference of an excessively long stump in order to preserve maximum length. Such treatment may be condoned when the bone is only 8.8–10 cm long and there is insufficient skin cover, but it is not to be recommended when it is possible to provide natural skin flaps on a longer stump.

The prosthesis may be made with either a plastic or a leather socket. The latter is to be preferred when there are bony prominences because leather will 'give' during alterations of posture. Women, with their usual subcutaneous layer of fat around the shoulder, favour plastic sockets, which are both lighter and neater in appearance. An inner 'cup' socket is added to the main socket when the stump is either short or very tapered. In the former case it is necessary to extend the cup socket well over the shoulder so that the rim lies on the supraspinatus and trapezius muscles (*Figures 7.5* and *7.6*). Longer stumps need only have a socket fitted up to the tip of the acromion.

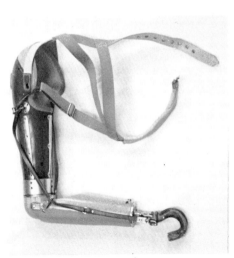

Figure 7.5   Prosthesis for left above-elbow amputa- tion. This shows a leather inner 'cup' socket extend- ing beyond the outer leather socket. The former is of a lighter colour. The flexion cord is clearly shown with the extension thong reaching to the split hook

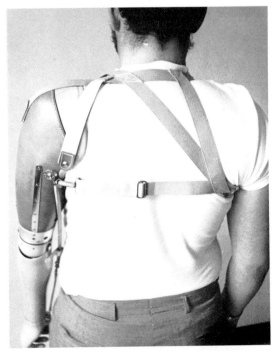

Figure 7.6   An above-elbow amputee wearing the same type of prosthesis as shown in Figure 7.5 and displaying the harness suspension

The prosthesis is provided with an elbow unit permitting passive internal and external rotation and a digitally operated locking system for the various positions available. In addition, there are eight positions in which the elbow may be locked from full extension to full flexion. A thin leather strap extends up from the lock lever, sited on the front of the elbow mechanism, to be attached to a webbing section of the main harness. There is a three-point fixation of the harness to the socket: anterior, superior and posterior. The superior webbing strap is the main one and this lies between the other two. From its attachment on the socket it passes horizontally across the back of the neck and curves over the opposite shoulder to terminate in a tab end with eyelet holes. The posterior attachment is made of stout elastic and it meets the anterior strap on top of the shoulder, where they are both stitched to the long superior one. The webbing section of the lock strap runs over the shoulder, medial to the attachment of the other three straps, to pass obliquely downwards to the back of the opposite axilla, under which it passes, to end in a buckle anteriorly. When putting on the prosthesis the amputee fastens the two ends so that the buckle lies snugly in the infraclavicular fossa. To prevent the superior strap from riding up the neck, it is held down by a check strap which is attached to the 'axillary' strap at the position where it curves forwards under the arm. Attached to the same point is another horizontal strap and this extends from the axilla of the sound arm posteriorly to within about 5 cm of the back of the socket. Here a stout leather 'flexion cord' is fixed prior to passing over a pulley set on the posteromedial aspect of the socket and in line with the axilla. This cord, with the necessary extension thong for terminal device operation, is then secured as described for the foregoing prostheses (*Figure 7.5*).

The endoskeletal prosthesis

A lightweight and purely cosmetic prosthesis has been designed by the sole manufacturer of upper limb prostheses.* This is suitable for adults who have lost an arm at least 10 cm above the elbow (including shoulder disarticulation and forequarter amputation).

The socket (or shoulder cap) is made of the same material as that used for the conventional prosthesis but the distal construction is essentially modular. The forearm and upper arm each contain a metal tube connected at the elbow to form a freely moving joint. This has a locking mechanism, manually operated by means of a press button situated in the middle of the forearm tube. Above the elbow is a passively manipulated rotating device. (This has to be omitted when fitting long stumps in which the bone end is between 5 and 10 cm from the joint.)

The proximal end of the upper tube is fixed to the socket or shoulder cap of the appropriate prosthesis. The whole limb is then encased within a shaped section of tubular polyethylene foam extending from wrist to the mid-upper arm and covered by flesh-coloured stockinette. A hand of firmer foam with wired fingers and thumb and cosmetic glove is then attached. Suitable appendage straps are riveted to the finished limb. It is possible for many women to have very lightweight straps but this depends

*Hugh Steeper Ltd, Roehampton.

upon their physique! Occasionally, the prosthesis can be secured to a brassiere and the patient may then wear dresses with a lower neck line than is possible with the conventional suspension.

The elbow disarticulation and prosthesis

Disarticulation of the elbow is an operation which should be avoided! Because of the expanded epicondyles the prosthesis is, of necessity, very bulky in the elbow region. Not only does it have to contain the wide stump end with slight clearance, but jointed side steels have to be fitted externally since there is no space for any internal elbow mechanism as previously described. One of the jointed steels, usually the medial, has an elbow lock fitted which also adds to the width of the elbow (*Figure 7.7*).

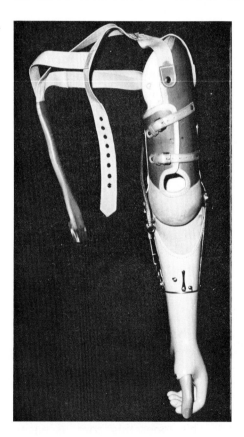

Figure 7.7   Prosthesis for an elbow disarticulation. Note the locking rod on the medial side of the forearm. Also the mid-forearm bisection and the hand with lower forearm made in one piece

These amputees, fortunately, are able to utilize their natural humeral rotation because no such device can be conveniently incorporated. This is about the only advantage the elbow disarticulation amputee has over the patient with an arm off at the recommended level above the elbow. Whereas the latter is fitted with an essentially cylindrical socket, the former usually has to be provided with a leather socket, which is open down the front to permit access of the wide distal end of the humerus and then secured by two cross-straps and buckles.

The harness and the rest of the prosthesis, distal to the elbow, are the same as those used for above-elbow amputees.

The prosthesis for long above-elbow stumps

If the stump is longer than recommended, the prosthesis cannot be fitted with the standard elbow mechanism, incorporating elbow locks and rotational device. A modified limb has to be made with a socket similar to that used on the conventional above-elbow amputee but finished with a dome-end to accommodate the tip of the stump. Jointed side steels with an external lock are fitted, as on the elbow disarticulation type. Again, the harness is of the same pattern.

The below-elbow amputation and prosthesis

For the below-elbow amputee to make practical use of the stump it should not be longer than 20 cm or shorter than 8.8 cm (measured from the olecranon to the cut end of the longer forearm bone). The criteria concerning scars and skin cover are the same as those outlined for above-elbow amputations. Ideally, the stump length for an adult should be 18 cm. This provides for adequate leverage, comfortable fitting and neat wrist mechanism. There should be good biceps and triceps power, the latter muscle being the activator of terminal devices.

Sockets may be of leather or plastic and the same form of harness suspension is used on each. This consists of webbing or one of the man-made fibres. One main suspension strap is situated along the front of the arm. About 7.5–8.8 cm above the elbow crease it is connected to an inverted V-shaped strap which straddles the front of the elbow, to be attached to a posterior arrangement of narrow webbing shaped to cradle the elbow just proximal to the epicondyles and then anchored to two D-rings set either side of the top of the socket and in line with the elbow joint. A posterior suspension strap is fixed to the centre of the 'cradle' and this exends obliquely up the back of the arm to meet the front strap after this has passed over the shoulder. The two then cross in the midline, in the region of the second or third thoracic vertebra. They continue to follow an oblique course until they encircle the opposite axilla where they are joined by means of a 'strap end' and buckle, respectively, as described for the above-elbow prosthesis. Near the cross-over at the back another, adjustable, strap is attached and this lies below and almost parallel to the posterior suspension strap. At the end of this is fastened a stout leather cord which passes through a guide ring situated below the medial socket-suspension ring. This 'operating cord' is easily connected to any of the activated terminal appliances worn by the amputee.

When the patient has a very short stump it is necessary for the main socket to be fitted with an inner 'cup' socket which not only provides for a snug fit but is also extended over the back of the olecranon for greater security and leverage. The top front edge of the prosthesis needs to be high to prevent the stump from slipping out when the elbow is fully extended. The high front will, inevitably, limit flexion due to the position of the biceps tendon; the fitting of such sockets is therefore very critical and calls for considerable skill on the part of the prosthetist. It is also usual for stumps, less than 12.7 cm long, to be fitted with short sockets in order to lessen the effect of leverage. The correct length of the finished limb is achieved by providing the artificial hand with a lower forearm section continuous with the wrist. As for the majority of prostheses for amputations at different levels, the artificial hand – or hand and section – is made detachable from the forearm so that it may be exchanged for one of the many terminal appliances referred to later in this chapter.

The below-elbow amputee activates the appropriate terminal device by contracting the triceps of the affected limb and, at the same time, stabilizes his shoulder or flexes it slightly. This produces a powerful pull upon the 'operating cord' and an extremely delicate degree of control is achieved very quickly by the amputee.

The wrist disarticulation and prosthesis

When an amputation has been performed through the wrist joint, leaving intact the very important articular disc, pronation and supination should be unaffected. When such a stump is contained within a socket reaching to the elbow, as just described, all rotation movement is lost. A split socket is therefore used, having a transverse gap of about 3.8–5 cm between the proximal and distal halves (*Figure 7.8*). The length of the distal socket is critical. It must be long enough to have a secure grip upon the end of the stump when appliances are being used but must not extend proximally beyond the mid-forearm, otherwise pronation–supination movements will be impeded and

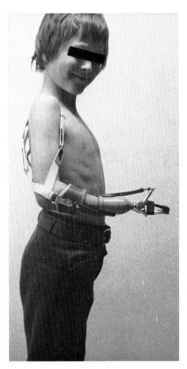

Figure 7.8 Split-socket prosthesis for a wrist disarticulation

uncomfortable to attempt. The two halves of the prosthesis are connected by strong side suspension straps which are easily detached to allow a 'dress' hand to be worn in place of the distal socket. (A hand fitted to the prosthesis in the conventional way would be unsightly due to the length of the stump.)

The harness and operating cord attachment are of the same pattern as those used on the forearm amputee.

The transcarpal and carpometacarpal amputations

A similar type of prosthesis to that just described may be fitted to either of these amputations but they are usually less comfortable and the 'dress' hands for these longer stumps are bulky and less cosmetically acceptable. It will therefore be apparent that neither of these amputations is to be recommended.*

The wrist or mid-forearm rotary mechanism

From the above descriptions it will be noted that the majority of these artificial limbs have a detachable hand. The mechanism fitted to the forearm of these prostheses is known as 'the rotary'. At the time of writing there are two types with essentially the same action: one, with a single knob control, is of modern design and is superseding the two-knob version which has been in use since World War I.

The old type has a knob on a lever arm which is connected to a sliding blade – the snap-catch blade. This is responsible for holding the hand or other terminal device securely in place onto the forearm. The method of fixing the device into the prosthesis is by means of a tapered metal stem which has a deep circular groove cut into it near its point. As the taper enters the central hole of the rotary, it pushes the snap-catch blade to one side until it is opposite the grooved portion; then it snaps into place to provide a firm hold.

Around the periphery of the rotary face (which is at right angles to the long axis of the forearm) are three small spring-loaded balls which engage into three of 12 holes drilled in the opposing face of the hand-plate (or adaptor, as it is called when fitted to an appliance).

The central stem with its groove permits easy rotation of the hand or other terminal devices and the three balls enable 12 different positions of rotation to be selected. On the old rotary there is a second, ball-headed, lever arm which operates a lock against rotation. This is simply a small blunt-ended metal rod which engages in whichever hole happens to be opposite it at the time the lever is turned. The modern rotary has one lever, for locking and releasing the hand or appliance. It operates by means of a sideways push (by the wearer's thumb) after the knob has been slightly depressed into the forearm. Then pressure to the left releases the snap-catch blade and the spring-loaded balls eject the device from the rotary. Pressure to the right engages the locking 'pin'.

---

*These comments apply *only* when patients are able to be fitted with a prosthesis. In countries where, for economic or other reasons, no prosthesis can be supplied, then the additional length of stump could prove beneficial.

To upper limb amputees who are likely to perform heavy manual work – whether it be in their respective occupations or pastimes, such as digging the garden – leverage upon the prosthesis is all-important. Above-elbow amputees benefit from a very short upper forearm section to which a digging appliance may be fitted. The same applies to forearm amputees with a short stump. In both cases the prostheses are fitted with what is termed a 'mid-forearm bisection'. This is where the rotary mechanism is incorporated. Should an appliance need to reach to the normal hand level then an extension bar may be added. The sedentary worker is usually supplied with a wrist bisection and this facilitates speedy changes of appliances since the rotary controls are under the cuff.

Terminal appliances

There is an extensive range of appliances which may be fitted on to the various types of upper limb prostheses. Some are fairly standard tools adapted for an amputee; for example, pliers, hammer, tweezers and eating utensils such as knife, fork and spoon. Then there are items which have been made to hold standard articles, such as saw, plane, chisel, brace and welding tools, to name but a few. Many years ago bilateral arm amputees were supplied with a box containing a fantastic array of appliances for day-to-day use, such as a toothbrush holder, and others for shaving brush, hairbrush, comb, razor, fork, spoon and drinking glass. Apart from the greater difficulty these people had compared with unilateral amputees in changing appliances, it must have made them feel really handicapped. These days bilateral amputees are trained with a pair of split hooks, the most versatile of all appliances. With these they can be completely independent for the majority of, if not all, day-to-day activities. Ordinary cutlery can be used and no longer do they take dirty knives and forks away from restaurants after a meal!

The split hook has two curved jaws, one of which is movable and attached to a lever arm which is pulled open by tension on the appropriate cord of the prosthesis. The jaws are closed by either strong elastic bands or springs, according to the type of split hook in use. There is a variety of shapes but the two jaws may be likened to the index and middle fingers held in a semi-flexed position and are 'opened' and 'closed' by interosseous action.

Only a few of the appliances are activated; for example, pliers of various sorts, tweezers, a sailing device, the split hooks and toilet appliances. The thumb on a standard hand may have a lever arm fitted so that a pull on the cord will result in slight opening. Unfortunately, the opening is insufficient to be of much practical use.

Partial hand amputations

The loss of one or more fingers presents a greater problem to the surgeon than the removal of the whole hand. How much to remove and how much to leave is not necessarily answered by the old adage 'save all possible'. Not only the *function* of the hand but its *appearance* is of great importance to both men and women. A severely mutilated hand which is capable of reasonable function, following surgery, may well be kept hidden in a pocket or covered by a glove and not used because it is considered unsightly by the patient.

Many patients attend limb fitting centres, requesting a plastic skin-like glove to cover a hand damaged by comparatively minor trauma.

It is the surgeon's duty to consider this aspect of the problem when faced with a grossly injured hand and to discuss the matter with the patient.

When either the index or the little finger has been traumatically amputated and the head of the respective metacarpal can be saved, the hand will retain more strength of grip than when the distal half of the metacarpal has been removed. The cosmetic effect of the latter operation is considerably better than the former and the patient's wishes should be sought before embarking upon either procedure.

When all the fingers and thumb on one or both hands have to be amputated, the surgeon should seriously consider amputation through the wrist because this is far more likely to give a good functional and cosmetic result. There are many bilateral forearm and hand amputees in heavy industry who also enjoy a full and active home life.

The hand and finger prostheses

Although finger and hand prostheses can be fitted, it is an ironic fact that the less there is to be replaced the more difficult it is to achieve a satisfactory result.

A cosmetic prosthesis for the complete or partial loss of a single digit is usually an embarrassment to function and since the hand is constantly changing colour a perfect match is rarely obtained and the join is not easily masked.

When part of the hand and two or more fingers have been amputated, requests are often made for a complete glove covering. Although this may be supplied, it must be

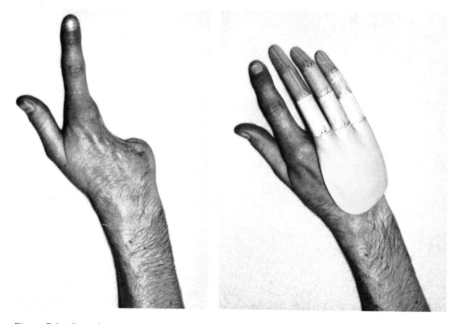

Figure 7.9   Partial amputation of the hand and 'dress' replacement, designed to be worn with an ordinary glove. It has three wooden fingers, articulated at all joints

appreciated that the surviving digits are unlikely to be comfortable if contained within a plastic glove for any length of time. Function of the intact portion of the hand must inevitably suffer while it is encased. Sweating is also a troublesome feature while a plastic glove is being worn over any part of the natural hand and it is advisable for the patient to be supplied with at least two chamois glove linings which may be worn alternately.

It is unlikely that a standard cosmetic glove could be supplied if the shape of the hand or finger remnants were distorted, either by trauma or surgery; for example, malunion of metacarpal and phalangeal fractures, deepening of web spaces and transposition of digits.

The gloves are made from a variety of stock moulds and the cost of a specially made 'one-off' article would be prohibitive.

There are other types of 'dress hand' prostheses which may be worn inside an *ordinary* glove and these are very acceptable. They consist of the requisite hand replacement with either rigid, curved fingers or jointed fingers (*Figure 7.9*). There must be sufficient space between the cut end of bone and normal joint position for an articulation to be incorporated in the prosthesis. These movable fingers are made in wood or plastic; the latter are more durable but the former are neater and more suited to people wearing thin gloves.

In addition to the dress replacements, patients may require a 'working' prosthesis when a major portion of the hand has been lost. This type usually consists of a blocked leather palm case suitably padded and lined; then a partial covering of metal provides substantial protection for use in industry.

When the fingers have been amputated and a mobile thumb survives, a metal opposition plate is also added.

A screw nipple fitting may also be incorporated should the patient wish to fit certain tools into the prosthesis.

When the thumb and at least one finger survive it is rarely necessary to provide any terminal appliance but the protective covering may still be advantageous to an industrial worker.

The complete loss of the thumb is best treated surgically or left entirely alone. These amputees are rarely improved functionally by artificial aids.

If required, a dress thumb made of plastic can be supplied to the patient for use when wearing an ordinary glove. Such a prosthesis is referred to as a 'thimble' fitting thumb. Similarly, thimble fitting plastic fingers are made, straight or curved, according to individual requirements, to be worn within a glove.

Children's prostheses

Prostheses designed for children are, essentially, scaled-down models of the adult versions.

The commonest congenital limb deficiency is absence of the hand and most of the forearm, the left side being affected twice as often as the right.

The first prosthesis, which is cosmetic and in one piece, should be supplied at about 6–8 months of age. This is followed by a working type, similar to that described on page 341, which is fitted at about 18–20 months. The mother and child then receive instruction in its use. The hand is detachable from the wrist and a little pair of 'grippers' may be substituted and operated by means of a thin Perlon cord. The suspension straps are made of Cushlon with Velcro fastenings and are of similar design to the adult version. It is, however, necessary to fit a strap across the front of the chest during the very early years to prevent the harness slipping over the shoulder.

Myoelectric prostheses

Since the mid-1950s Britain has been engaged in the development of electrically controlled forearm prostheses.

Because the activating impulse originates in the remains of the appropriate forearm muscles, the term 'myoelectric' was coined by those working in this field of research. The amount of electrical energy generated by the contraction of a group of muscle fibres is infinitesimal, so the current produced has to be very considerably amplified by means of batteries.

The prosthesis is operated by suitable electrodes on the skin overlying flexor and extensor muscle remnants. A compact storage battery, worn by the amputee is connected to the prosthesis and when he wishes to open the artificial hand he 'thinks' of opening the phantom hand and so contracts the extensor muscles. Likewise, contraction of the long flexor group results in closure of the hand.

Although a variety of myoelectric prostheses have been made both in Britain and abroad, and worn for trial periods by a small selected group of forearm amputees, they have not been well accepted. The mechanism contained within the hand and wrist is heavy. The weight of the various hands ranges between 950 g and 2 kg (the human hand weighs approximately 450 g).

Apart from the appearance, which is reasonable provided care is taken of the cosmetic glove covering, the hands are less efficient than a split hook. For general use, such as picking up and handling pens, eating utensils and money, there is no comparison with the efficacy of the latter appliance. The hands, however, do achieve a better grip on round objects.

In the autumn of 1978 a few Swedish myoelectric hands were imported into Britain. These were suitable for quite young children with below-elbow stumps. A trial of these little prostheses was therefore undertaken in children between the ages of 3½ and 4½ years. Stump lengths varied from 5 to 12 cm. It must, however, be stressed that these prostheses are not suitable for stumps extending to wrist level.

The prosthesis consists of a plastic socket with a German (Münster) type fitting without an intervening sock and no suspension straps. There is a passively manipulated wrist unit which is an integral part of the hand. There are only two fingers – index and middle – and these are joined at the base to pivot as a single unit at the metacarpophalangeal joint position. The thumb is in opposition with the tips of the fingers and jointed at the base. The fingers and thumb movement have a ratio of 1:1 and a gripping power of 1.5 kg.

The hand mechanism is encased in a plastic shell which in turn is covered by a cosmetic plastic glove with the full complement of fingers, the ulnar two having light filling and therefore flail. At the upper end of the socket and sited directly over the extensor and flexor muscle mass just below the elbow are the respective electrodes.

These are gold plated and in contact with the skin. They both have an easily regulated sensitizer so that the hand action may be made to respond quicker or slower to the muscle current. It has no effect on speed of movement or grip. The electrodes are connected to the hand and to a 6-V rechargeable battery, carried somewhere on the child's body. An average daily consumption is in the order of 6 hours.

Surprising to relate, the children learned to control the hand within a few minutes although those with short stumps were conscious of the weight for some days. The complete prosthesis weighs approximately 370 g; the hand alone is 200 g. A conventional prosthesis for a child of the same age weighs 283 g, including a cosmetic hand, but only 227 g with a split hook. Unfortunately, the hand is not designed to hold a table knife, the fingers being set too close to permit the blade to slide between them.

Inevitable problems include frequent breakages of the wire, either at the battery connection or at the electrode. The glove is easily damaged, particularly the two flail fingers. Malfunction of the hand mechanism was also a common occurrence during the early days of its introduction.

SEVERE LESIONS OF THE BRACHIAL PLEXUS

There may come a time when amputation is considered for a patient with an irrecoverable lesion of the brachial plexus. For many this has proved to be an extremely worthwhile and acceptable form of treatment. When performed, it is essential to combine the operation with an arthrodesis of the shoulder if it is paralysed and not already ankylosed. Occasionally, some power exists in the pectoral muscles on the affected side and this may tempt the surgeon to leave the shoulder alone. Unless the antagonists are working, the humerus will adduct and internally rotate, particularly if the biceps is acting. If teres major and latissimus dorsi have reasonable power (4 or 5), a Zachary transplant may be worth contemplating. If it is undertaken then an external rotation osteotomy of the humerus is also advisable. The latter operation is often of greater benefit than the transplant and may prove to be sufficient as an isolated procedure, should active flexion of the humerus be possible.

Before discussing removal of the limb with the patient it is of paramount importance to ensure that he clearly understands that no further *useful* recovery is possible. If he remains in any doubt it is extremely unwise to recommend amputation. The next step is for the clinician to ascertain the type of occupation the patient wishes to pursue so that he may be advised accordingly about the value or otherwise of a prosthesis.

It must be stressed, however, that prostheses have their limitations; therefore it would be worth the patient's while to visit a limb fitting centre where he may discuss every aspect with a doctor fully conversant with prosthetics. Many aspects of the patient's life must be taken into account before a correct decision can be made: factors such as the length of time since the original injury; previous or present employment, if any; the patient's aspirations and whether these can be attained with or without an amputation; how much the existing one-handed condition affects him and how much the appearance of the withered limb.

Not only the occupation but also the patient's pastimes must be considered. It may be of interest to know that, with a simple attachment for a cricket bat, a teenager became captain of cricket despite the loss of an arm and leg and, on leaving school, he played for his university. Swimming is easier with an amputated limb than with a flail one.

The hand is prone to injury, particularly burns which are extremely slow to heal. In many instances the fingers become swollen and unsightly and difficult to cover with a glove. Pain is a fairly common feature and it usually affects the hand which patients describe as 'being held in a vice'. When severe it may prove to be a contraindication to amputation, and in any event the patient *must* be made to understand that amputation will *not* rid him of the pain, the cause being avulsion of one or more roots from within the spinal cord.

The people most likely to benefit from amputation are those contemplating return to industry, because a prosthesis can be very helpful in a variety of manual occupations. An example may be quoted of a man with an above-elbow amputation combined with an arthrodesis of the shoulder who is a full-time motor mechanic. He frequently carries gear boxes with his prosthesis, which is also used for a variety of other tasks. Another similarly affected man frequently needs to lift objects weighing 25–30 kg, which he does with the prosthesis and a split hook.

Sites of amputation

Only two sites of amputation need be considered: above the elbow and below the elbow.

In the non-paralytic below-elbow amputee the terminal devices which may be fitted into a prosthesis are activated by triceps action combined with either slight flexion of the same shoulder or its active stabilization.

A below-elbow amputation without reasonable triceps power is of doubtful value, and obviously a forearm amputation with weak elbow flexion and no active extension has nothing to offer. Even a Clark's transfer (of pectoralis major to biceps) to reinforce flexion power has been of insufficient help to many a prospective industrial worker, alternative occupations having to be found. In these cases the standard type of prosthesis can be of no more use than a sleeve filler. To provide some practical advantage it is necessary to fit it with jointed side steels which are connected, above the elbow, to a leather 'corset' which encircles the arm for a distance of about 10–12.5 cm and is fastened by two or three straps and buckles. A hand-operated spoke-lock is fitted, usually to the inner steels, and to prevent a torque from occurring in the various locking positions (8, 51, 94 and 128 degrees) a broad steel band is used to connect the two side steels where they are riveted to the corset. A padded shoulder saddle with running strap and webbing appendage is added. When the triceps is weak or completely paralysed, a Bowden cable system is utilized to obtain terminal device operation, the two fixed points for the cable being on the metal arm-band posteriorly and the middle of the forearm socket, respectively. The cable is routed to the lateral side of the elbow. Flexion of the humerus then provides the power to activate the thumb and any of the gripping tools used as terminal devices, hence the need for an arthrodesis of the shoulder should natural active flexion be weak or absent.

Since many of the forearm amputation stumps are partly or totally anaesthetic in patients with brachial plexus lesions, it is usually necessary to supply a leather cup socket extended posteriorly over the olecranon so that a snug fit is obtained.

The below-elbow amputation stump should have a bone length of approximately 15–18 cm (measured from the tip of the olecranon). The position of the scar is not of great importance. A posterior or terminal transverse scar is to be preferred if normal sensation is present. Obviously normal skin is better than either hyperaesthesia or anaesthesia. Stump length, however, should not be sacrificed in order to provide a fully sensitive end, since short stumps in patients with brachial plexus lesions are prone to develop flexion contractures when, so often, the biceps is stronger than the triceps.

An above-elbow amputation is to be recommended when there is doubt about the strength of the biceps and triceps being adequate for the occupation and, possibly, the pastimes of the patient concerned. In these amputations bone length should be approximately 20 cm (measured from the acromion process). Leaving longer stumps in either the above- or below-elbow amputations is a dis-service to the patient because the respective elbow and wrist mechanisms cannot be conveniently incorporated, as mentioned on page 341. The remarks above, concerning skin sensibility, apply also to the above-elbow stumps. When these higher amputations are indicated it is nearly always necessary to perform an arthrodesis of the shoulder, and the position of the humerus relative to the scapula varies slightly according to the build of the patient. It is, however, necessary to allow a considerable amount of abduction to permit the socket of the prosthesis to fit comfortably between the arm and the chest wall. This means approximately 20–25 degrees of abduction in the average individual. About 15–20 degrees of humeral flexion is also essential for successful prosthetic wearing (*Figure 7.10*). (A stump set *vertically* after an arthrodesis of the shoulder has insufficient range of movement to flex the prosthetic forearm to its fullest extent.)

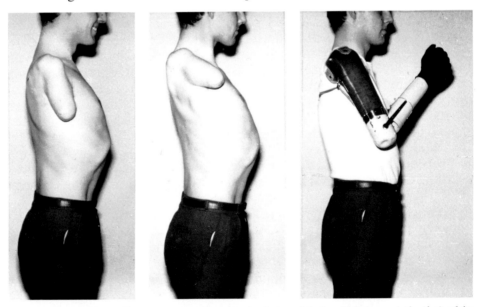

Figure 7.10   (a) Above-elbow amputation after complete lesion of the brachial plexus. Arthrodesis of the shoulder with stump set in 15 degrees of flexion. (b) Maximum elevation of the stump following shoulder arthrodesis. (This is more than adequate for activating a prosthesis.) (c) Active flexion of the prosthetic elbow is achieved by the forward movement of the arthrodesed stump. (Reproduced by courtesy of the Editor of The Hand)

The built-in external and internal rotation device, above the elbow mechanism, is of particular advantage when the shoulder has been fused.

Since a leather socket is normally prescribed for these particular above-elbow amputees, it is usual to have an additional inner cup socket. This is made from a cast of the shoulder and stump and, as there is gross wasting and narrowing of the shoulder following the arthrodesis, the outer socket can be built to conform to the sound shoulder and the inner one is then fully contained, with the exception of an extension over the shoulder. The patients are very conscious of the appearance of the shoulder when dressed and they are usually well satisfied with the restoration which is provided by the above-elbow prosthesis.

It must be clearly recognized that the majority of patients with an amputation, above or below the elbow, combined with an arthrodesis of the shoulder, have considerably less active control of a prosthesis than do amputees with normal stump control. Nevertheless, a prosthesis has proved to be of great value to a large number of young men who suffered irreparable plexus lesions. Without the amputation they would not have been able to have returned to industry.

Some victims with a permanent palsy, affecting their non-dominant hand, were engaged in a sedentary occupation prior to injury and when it became clear, after lengthy discussions, that an amputation was not likely to prove beneficial they were advised against ablation. Many continued their former mode of existence quite happily but only after being in full possession of the facts concerning the prognosis and possibilities available to them.

Pain following brachial plexus lesions

One of the most distressing features of this terrible injury is severe pain. It is very different from the well recognized phantom limb pain which occasionally occurs after amputation. Many of the victims of brachial plexus lesions have both hyperaesthesia and anaesthesia affecting different parts of the limb. They may or may not have the additional excruciating pain, most severe in the hand, which is caused by cord damage due to avulsion of one or more nerve roots.

Few, if any, of the analgesic drugs have more than a transitory effect. When patients have this very severe pain it is unwise to advise amputation and they should be told that it is extremely unlikely that removal of the limb will affect the intensity in any way. Those who have elected to have the amputation despite this warning have found difficulty in using the prosthesis because the pain has had an inhibitory effect.

This type of pain should not be confused with the dull ache which many patients experience in the shoulder due to the weight of the unsupported flail limb. If this is relieved when the whole limb is at rest or when the shoulder is passively elevated then amputation is more than likely to afford complete relief of the ache.

Patients' comments

A year or more after some of the patients elected to have the paralysed limb amputated and, where indicated, the shoulder arthrodesed, they were sent a detailed questionnaire requesting information about the value or otherwise of the amputation and prosthesis. Of the 80 forms sent out, 77 were completed and returned – 90 per cent of the patients wore the prosthesis at work and, of these, 63 per cent said it was either essential or of considerable benefit. A few wore the limb purely for dress purposes and although it had no functional value for them they would not venture out of doors without it on.

To one question: 'Knowing the alternative was keeping a paralysed arm, are you now glad you had an amputation?' all but one patient replied in the affirmative. The one who regretted losing his arm chose amputation assuming it would rid him of his pain! He maintained that he had never been told the pain was likely to persist. Even *he* made practical use of the prosthesis.

The following are some comments made in answer to the above question.

Left below-elbow amputation and arthrodesis of shoulder: 'There can be no other alternative but to have the arm amputated as it is useless, whereas an artificial arm can be used.'

Right above-elbow amputation and arthrodesis of shoulder: 'Yes, the arm as it was, was a nuisance. It got in the way and looked unsightly. It would not hesitate in recommending to another person with the same injury to have the operation.'

Right above-elbow amputation and arthrodesis of shoulder: 'Yes, most definitely. A "dead" or paralysed limb is completely useless. It acts only as a hindrance. After keeping the useless limb for 2 years I am very glad I decided to have it removed; I have never regretted this.'

Left above-elbow amputation, shoulder ankylosed: 'Very glad, a paralysed arm is useless. With an artifical arm there are very few, if any, things I cannot do. If I had kept my arm I would not have been able to continue my job and I don't know that I am wearing an artificial arm. I am very pleased I took the *right* decision.'

Left above-elbow amputation and arthrodesis of shoulder: 'Definitely yes. After the amputation I had a sense of freedom from a burden. Speaking impartially from experience it is my belief the decision I made to part with my useless arm was one of the best decisions I ever made.'

Right above-elbow amputation and arthrodesis of shoulder: 'Very glad. I can do jobs at work and home far more easily with the help of my artificial arm. I also feel more contented in my own self.'

Right below-elbow amputation and arthrodesis of shoulder: 'Very definitely yes. With a paralysed arm it is always noticeable and can be unpleasant, whereas the artificial hand is very seldom noticed. It is also far more comfortable not to have a useless limb which only gets in the way.'

The occupations of these amputees are many and varied and they range from clerical to motor mechanic. Many are trained welders, some are engineering draughtsmen and the list includes spray-painters, panel beaters, crane driver, taxi driver and butcher. An electro- and stereotyper is referred to on page 354.

Pastimes include sports (for which the prostheses are removed), field games, athletics and swimming. For these activities there is far more freedom of movement after the amputation. Many of the patients have found the prosthesis to be useful for photography, sailing (*Figure 7.11*), fishing, gardening and house decorating.

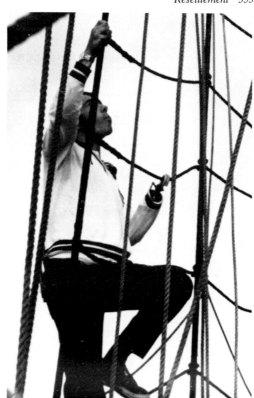

Figure 7.11   Patient with below-elbow amputation and an arthrodesis of the shoulder (following a lesion of the left brachial plexus), climbing the rigging of the 'Sir Winston Churchill' training ship

RESETTLEMENT

Rehabilitation is a continuous process and it is the aim of those treating the amputee to endeavour to restore him to his original estate.

Early in his treatment one must ascertain the possibility of his returning to his former employer, who may need convincing that the patient will be capable of performing his original occupation, or other suitable alternative work, in the same industry.

The patient may not wish to return to his former job, and so consideration must be given to vocational assessment with a view to arranging suitable vocational training. Liaison with the disablement resettlement officer, of the appropriate area, is essential. The medical officer concerned with the prescription of the prosthesis, and the patient's training in its use, is the person most involved and accepts this responsibility, for it is he who will be seeing the amputee for many years to come. For as long as a prosthesis is worn it will be necessary for the amputee to attend the nearest artificial limb and appliance centre (or limb fitting centre) periodically for a check on his stump, the prosthesis and any repairs or refitting which may be necessary. The patient may also wish to discuss certain aspects of his work, pastimes or other activities and many welcome the opportunity of these visits where problems may be discussed and often overcome.

Case histories

Case 7.1.   This patient sustained a traumatic forequarter amputation. Extensive skin grafting was necessary to provide cover for the chest wall but after being fitted with a prosthesis he returned to his former occupation as a telephone engineer with the Post Office. His work involved intricate soldering of numerous wires situated in confined spaces and whilst in the Arm Training Unit at Roehampton he soon mastered the necessary technique on equipment loaned by the then GPO. One-handed wire strippers proved to be a great asset.

Case 7.2.   A young national serviceman on an overseas tour was involved in a road traffic accident which resulted in the loss of both arms, above the elbow. He was admitted to Queen Mary's Hospital (Roehampton) and attended the limb fitting centre. The two establishments started him on a course of intensive rehabilitation which began with stump exercises and the fitting of leather gauntlets to initiate independence. He was subsequently fitted with a pair of prostheses with a split hook on each. He learnt to wash, shave, dress (including the fastening of buttons) and put on his prostheses. He progressed from eating out of a 'floating' spoon to using ordinary eating utensils. Writing and handling a telephone, together with other office work, were quickly mastered. The most difficult task was fastening the top button of his shirt and tying a tie which was achieved only after telling him that it was *possible* but that *he* would never manage it!

On completion of his rehabilitation he returned to his pre-Service occupation in a solicitor's office and has now qualified as a solicitor. He is completely independent and passed a driving test at the first attempt on a three-pedal car with floor change gear lever and no conversions. Having succeeded in overcoming the difficulty with his tie, he married and now lets his wife do the tying!

Case 7.3.   A young married woman was involved in a train accident in which she lost her left arm above the elbow and her right arm below the elbow. There were other injuries which delayed the fitting of prostheses but eventually she was fit enough to have the limbs and her chief worry was managing her young baby. Although she was managing well with a pair of split hooks they were considered to be dangerous when nursing the infant. It was decided safer to train her to handle the child using bare stumps, which proved quite successful. The prostheses were made so that they could be worn over clothing for quick application and removal and this allowed the patient to attend to her housework and the infant without much difficulty. Not only does this woman look after her own house and shopping but she decided to take a course in shorthand and gained a teacher's diploma in the subject.

Figure 7.4.   A teenage motor-cyclist, right hand dominant, sustained a traction lesion of his left brachial plexus resulting in permanent paralysis of the limb. He was sent to Roehamptom Limb Fitting Centre to ascertain whether it would be possible for him to continue his apprenticeship in the printing industry. He had been training for electro- and stereotyping and his indentures had been cancelled. He was prepared to have the limb amputated if this would mean a return to his chosen career. Following visits to his firm and representations to the apprenticeship committee, the chairmen of which were most helpful and sympathetic, the patient was advised to have an above-elbow amputation. Following the fitment and training with the prosthesis he underwent a special and rather rigorous test in the printing industry, as a result of which his indentures were restored. He completed his apprenticeship and gained the highest prize in his final year – a tribute to his perseverance and the confidence shown by the chiefs of the industry.

REFERENCES AND BIBLIOGRAPHY

Battye, C. K., Nightingale, A. and Whillis, J. (1955). The use of myo-electric currents in the operation of prostheses. *Journal of Bone and Joint Surgery* **37B,** 506

Bottomley, A. H. and Cowell, T. K. (1964). An artificial hand controlled by the nerves. *New Scientist* **21,** 668

Bottomley, A. H., Kinnier Wilson, A. B. and Nightingale, A. (1963). Muscle substitutes and myo-electric control. *Journal of the British Institution of Radio Engineering* **26,** 439

Fletcher, I. (1969). Traction lesions of the brachial plexus. *The Hand* **1,** 129

Langdale Kelham, R. D. (Ed.) (1957). *Artificial Limbs in the Rehabilitation of the Disabled.* London: HMSO

London, P. S. (1970). Upper limb amputation. *British Journal of Hospital Medicine* **4,** 590

Robertson, E. (1978). *Rehabilitation of Arm Amputees and Limb-deficient Children.* London: Baillière Tindall

The Rheumatoid Hand 8

Unlike traumatic conditions in the hand, rheumatoid arthritis poses quite different problems because the disorder is unpredictable, constantly changing and involves many joints and systems.

The effect on function of involvement of joints in the hand may depend as much, even more sometimes, on affection of shoulders or elbows and the necessity of using sticks or crutches due to disease in joints of the lower limb.

It is therefore essential to take an overall view of the patient and one cannot consider the hand in isolation. Moreover, the extent to which function may be affected depends on many factors other than the precise disease process. The social and domestic background, the psychological make up of the patient and his reaction to the disease are of the greatest importance.

The cause of the disease is still unknown. Modern views support the idea of an abnormal immune response to an antigen – possibly a virus – but why the disease affects some people rather than others, being rare in eastern countries, and why it should vary so much in its effects are mysteries. It is a systemic disorder and most clinicians speak of rheumatoid disease rather than rheumatoid arthritis.

The obvious clinical feature is the involvement of the small joints of the hands and feet but medium-sized joints are commonly affected. To illustrate the wide ranging involvement of the body which can be seen in this disease, *Table 8.1* presents the common systemic manifestation.

There are a variety of modes of onset. The disease can start explosively with swelling of the metacarpophalangeal and proximal interphalangeal joints of hands and feet, with much pain and disability, fever and malaise. Or it can creep up insidiously on the patient, with gradually increasing stiffness in the joints, fatigue and malaise taking weeks or months before obvious joint swellings are seen. Jacoby, Jayson and Cosh (1973) reported that, of 100 patients followed up, 23 initially had transient myalgia, 'fibrositis' and mild swelling of one or more joints as mini-attacks months before the overt disease picture developed.

A third mode of onset is the development of swelling in one joint – often the knee or ankle or one metacarpophalangeal or proximal interphalangeal joint – and the

Table 8.1   Systemic manifestation of rheumatoid disease

Skin and subcutaneous tissues	Nodules Bursitis
Tendons	Tenosynovitis Nodules Trigger finger Tendon rupture, due either to intrinsic disease or to attrition on diseased bone (e.g. over ulnar styloid)
Blood	Raised erythrocyte sedimentation rate Anaemia Rheumatoid factor (abnormal globulin)
Lungs	Nodules Diffuse interstitial fibrosis Pleural effusion
Vascular system	Vasculitis Necrotic ulcers Splinter haemorrhages
Nervous system Peripheral nerve involvement	(1) Pressure on nerves – ulnar nerve at the elbow due to effusion in the elbow joint; median nerve in the carpal tunnel due to flexor tenosynovitis; lateral popliteal nerve at the knee due to effusion in the knee joint (2) Digital sensory neuropathy – patchy involvement of digital nerves in the fingers or toes (carries a good prognosis) (3) Mononeuritis simplex or multiplex, one or more nerves being affected by rheumatoid vasculitis (4) Diffuse systemic polyneuritis affecting hands and feet with wasting and sensory loss (carries a poor prognosis)
Central nervous involvement	Pressure on the cervical cord due to atlantoaxial subluxation following rheumatoid synovitis of the joint of the odontoid peg and stretching of the capsule. This presents with paraesthesiae in the hands and pyramidal signs in the legs. It can be confused with bilateral compression of the median nerves in the carpal tunnel; electromyography will distinguish the two
Renal tract	Amyloid in long-standing disease causing nephrotic syndrome Effect of drugs in treatment – gold, phenacetin, penicillamine
Bone	Generalized osteoporosis Effect of treatment with steroids → vertebral collapse
Eye	Iritis Scleromalacia Cataract (steroid treatment) Sjögren's syndrome (dry eye and dry mouth)

disease may be so confined for many months. Sometimes there is symmetrical involvement of the larger joints – knees, ankles, elbows, wrists – sparing for a long time, perhaps always, the small joints of hands and feet.

Finally there is the interesting variety known as palindromic rheumatism in which the patient suffers repeated attacks of swelling in the soft tissues over the dorsum of the hand or foot or in one particular joint. The attacks last a few days only and a cyclic pattern is quite common, in which it takes 48 hours for the swelling to reach its peak.

The swelling remains for 3 days and then subsides in the same period of time it took to build up – hence the term palindromic. This may continue for years and then cease or, in one-third to one-half of patients, typical rheumatoid arthritis develops.

It is natural for both patient and doctor to want to predict the likely pattern that the disease will take. Only 10–15 per cent are likely to become severely crippled, 10–15 per cent will suffer a single attack and have no residual deformity or disability, while the other 70 per cent pursue a fluctuating course of remissions and relapses over many years with variable degrees of structural damage being left with each flare-up. Because a great deal can be done to minimize the amount of joint damage caused by a flare-up and modern surgery has so much to offer both prophylactically and in the field of reconstruction, it is important to follow up patients with care for an indefinite period and to reassess their general and joint status at regular intervals. Although it is difficult to predict the outcome in an individual case, general trends can be discerned.

Fleming and colleagues (1976) have reported on studies of the early manifestation of the disease and the subsequent outcome. They note that a bad prognosis is associated with the following features.

(1)   Early involvement of wrist and metacarpophalangeal joints.
(2)   Early involvement of hands and feet only.
(3)   Continued active joint swelling 1 year after onset.
(4)   Involvement of first and second metatarsophalangeal joints in patients who are seropositive.
(5)   Involvement of the larger joints in older patients who are seropositive.

In general, it is well recognized that an insidious onset of disease carries a worse prognosis than an explosive onset, and a high erythrocyte sedimentation rate, marked anaemia, positive rheumatoid factor with a high titre, presence of nodules and systemic involvement are all bad signs.

Conversely, favourable signs are asymmetry of joint involvement at onset and involvement of second to fifth metatarsophalangeal joints in younger people, negative Rose Waaler test, absence of anaemia, no systemic involvement, moderate rise in erythrocyte sedimentation rate and an explosive onset.

MANAGEMENT OF THE ACUTE STAGE

Inflamed painful joints must be rested; if several joints are involved, it is best if the patient is rested in bed. Ideally, admission to hospital will bring the quickest relief. One is constantly amazed at how the whole condition settles with as little as a few days' rest, and undoubtedly much suffering and disability could be prevented if there were sufficient hospital beds available, for patients will not or cannot rest adequately at home. There are splints available for resting inflamed joints in a variety of materials. We favour either a simple plaster of Paris splint or Plastazote. The splint extends from mid-forearm to the finger tips so as to rest the wrist, metacarpopha-langeal and proximal interphalangeal joints (the terminal interphalangeal joints rarely being involved), the wrist in neutral position, the metacarpophalangeal joints and the proximal interphalangeal joints slightly flexed and the thumb in half opposition.

These splints can be worn for 3–4 weeks at a time, and not only is there no need to remove them to give active or passive movement but any activity is positively contraindicated. The joints will not stiffen in this time and absolute rest means no movement.

Because one of the gravest complications of the disease is flexion deformity of the knees, one may be forgiven in a book on the hand for insisting that the splinting of the swollen knee is not more than 5 degrees' flexion, with ruthless refusal to allow pillows under the knees for comfort. The hip is splinted in neutral rotation; the ankle at 90 degrees; the shoulder in 30 degrees' abduction, 45 degrees' forward flexion and neutral rotation; and the elbow at 90 degrees' flexion and neutral rotation (*Figure 8.1*).

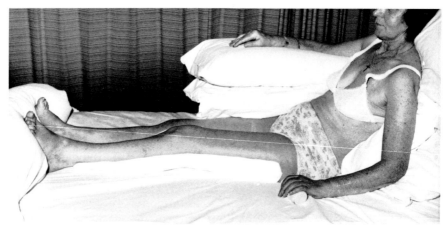

Figure 8.1   Position of function for rest in bed in acute stage of rheumatoid disease

During this stage the clinician will start drug treatment – at first with non-steroidal anti-inflammatory agents such as Naproxen, Benorylate or Propionic acid derivatives, later if necessary with Salicylates if no response is seen.
is seen within a few weeks.

If one fails to control inflammation by these means, gold or penicillamine is considered, for they do seem to affect the natural history of the disease though it is not known how either of the agents acts. Steroids are reserved by most clinicians now for patients who have failed to respond to all these measures or in whom the disease appears to be highly active, progressive and involving many systems, or if there is no other way to keep the patient active for work or household duties.

Once the inflammation has subsided, active exercises can be started and gentle passive movements given if the patient is too timid to risk a full range. It must be stressed that the joints have been inflamed and they need time to settle; too vigorous activity will cause a flare-up. Only a gentle, cautious and slowly progressive plan of exercises is advisable.

Similarly, too vigorous exercises to develop muscle power can be dangerous and it is wise to use static exercises only to redevelop power in the intrinsic muscles. Function will return best by using the hands in normal activities; it is one of the roles of the occupational therapist to guide the patient and spot which tasks present difficulty, tailoring treatment accordingly with regular discussions with the physio-therapist. Craft techniques that are useful include stool-seating, leather work, mosaic and thread sculpture.

Application of ice reduces swelling and is a potent means of relieving pain, thus allowing more active co-operation. We prefer ice to heat. Most patients with rheumatoid arthritis have variable periods of early morning stiffness and find great relief in soaking their hands in warm water for 10 minutes before starting the day.

ASSESSMENT

Rheumatoid disease being a generalized disorder, assessment of hand function must inevitably involve assessment of the whole patient; this means recording the range and muscle power of all the joints of upper and lower limbs.

Range is measured accurately with a goniometer recording limits of movement both actively and passively. Deformity is carefully described and clinical photographs taken for future comparison. A yearly photograph of hands and feet in standard positions is valuable. Muscle power is recorded both in the standard MRC 0–5 way and using strain gauges and dynamometers (page 29). Stamina is recorded by ability to continue with a task.

Functional capacity

There are almost as many hand assessment schemes as there are occupational therapy departments. It is virtually impossible to produce a satisfactory assessment form that will satisfy everyone; one needs a different approach for different diseases – almost for different stages of the disease, because much depends on other joint involvement, concurrent diseases, the patient's general health, the patient's home and work setting, and her attitude to disease. Harris (1969) has reported the most impressive effect of rehabilitation and he grades his patient quite simply:

0   No disability
1   Minor disability
2   Light work
3   No work but light housework
4   Restricted (e.g. in dressing)
5   Totally disabled

He showed the value of residential rehabilitation by comparing these grades before and after treatment in 988 patients over a 5-year period: 55 per cent were grade 4 or 5 on admission and this had dropped to 25 per cent on discharge; only 14 per cent could work on admission and this had risen to 57 per cent on discharge.

Pain and tenderness

This can be assessed either on the usual analogue scale 0–10 or on a 1–4 chart from mild through moderate and severe to very severe.

Swelling

The Mannerfelt measuring device is useful both for the quantification and for the comparison of swelling over time (*Figure 8.2*).

There are many advantages of admitting patients to hospital either in the initial stage of the disease or on the occasion of a relapse. First, the patient cannot escape the treatment – absolute rest (physical and mental) can be given and be seen to be given. Second, it allows all members of the rehabilitation team to study the patient in

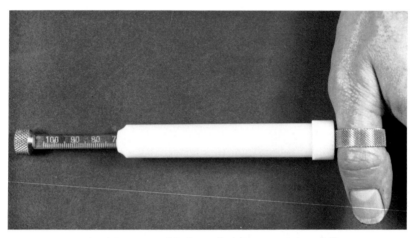

Figure 8.2   Mannerfelt device for measuring joint swelling

detail, both as a locomotor problem and as a person in relation to his social and economic background. Time spent getting to know the patient at the onset of what may be a lifetime's journey together is enormously valuable. The opportunity can be taken to meet the relatives and discuss with them and the patient the implications of the disease. The occupational therapist and the medical social worker can visit the home and make recommendations about aids to living. The patient has the opportunity of learning about his disease and acquiring good habits such as correct splinting, exercise, rest periods, use of walking aids and organization of the working day in the home.

Much fatigue can be avoided and the patient's energies best used by a work study of the home so that the various jobs in the home are spaced out evenly over the week and fit in with rest and exercise periods.

Much of the depression and anxiety that arise with rheumatoid arthritis can be prevented or mitigated by a frank discussion and clear explanation of what is known about the disease and how much can be done by physical means, drugs and surgery to alleviate symptoms and improve function.

Wright and Owen (1976) reported that, in 37 housewives with rheumatoid arthritis, 78 per cent suffered from anxiety, depression and frustration due to limitation of activity, 67 per cent suffered from feelings of being a burden to their relatives and 59 per cent felt a sense of guilt; 63 per cent suffered from not understanding the nature of the disease – a high proportion, for example, felt they had to 'work off' their stiffness and pain, thus damaging their joints further.

A period of assessment also allows an exact delineation of the cause of symptoms – for this may not be obvious.

An exacerbation of symptoms may be due to a variety of factors – it may be a true relapse of joint activity or a flare-up of general disease requiring full investigations with repeat of serological tests and further X-rays; it may be due to a mechanical cause – often pressure of synovitis on the median nerve in the carpal tunnel may be manifest as pain, not paraesthesiae, and the temptation may be to increase the drugs whereas careful clinical, functional and electrical testing will reveal the true nature of the symptoms.

An exacerbation may be due to reaction to agents such as aspirin, gold or steroids. It may be associated with a change in the social or domestic setting – a change of job putting more demands on the patient both physically and mentally, or a problem with children or misunderstanding between husband and wife. Husbands do not always understand the extent to which the disease puts a burden on the housewife; they can be surprisingly unsympathetic until a full explanation is given and their active co-operation enlisted. It may be due to a true depression, when an antidepressant can transform the situation.

Many people with rheumatoid arthritis live on their own and can just about cope with their disease. It may take only one 'straw' to break their spirit – the death of a friend, a change in a home help who has become a friend, some other medical condition such as osteoarthritis, circulatory disorder, diabetes, etc.

Only by careful assessment over some days can the whole complex of factors be unravelled. Finally, if active intensive treatment is required to improve locomotor function, it is often more effective as an inpatient, for long journeys in transport and long waits for return transport can be fatiguing and obviate the good effected by the therapy. Sometimes it is a break from routine that is needed and a holiday may need to be organized or, at the least, attendance at a day centre to meet other people and banish a sense of isolation and loneliness.

HAND DEFORMITIES

A bewildering variety of deformities can occur in the rheumatoid hand – not always symmetrical; thus ulnar drift can be pronounced on one side and minimal on the other, one finger can show a boutonnière deformity while the adjacent finger shows a swan neck deformity, or one thumb may be extensively deformed and the other normal. One cannot overemphasize the fact that a patient's ability to use the hand may be virtually normal despite a fearsome-looking hand – functional assessment is the only way of judging the importance of the deformity.

Subluxation of metacarpophalangeal joints and ulnar drift (*Figures 8.3* and *8.4*)

Some 50 per cent of patients attending hospital 5 years after onset of disease show subluxation of these joints. The earliest sign is lateral instability of the joints. If the metacarpophalangeal joints are flexed to 90 degrees, there should be virtually no lateral movement; when the ligaments are stretched by rheumatoid synovitis, lateral movement is easily produced.

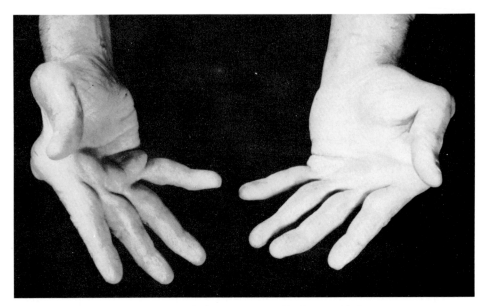

Figure 8.3   Ulnar drift in a patient with rheumatoid disease

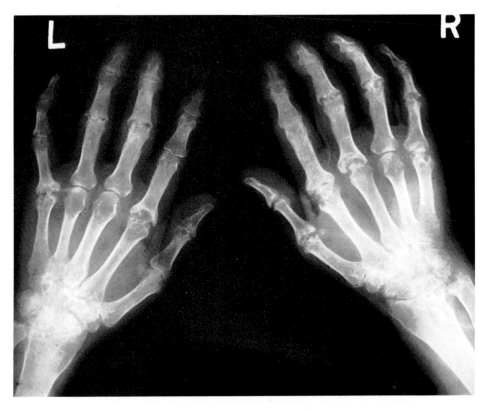

Figure 8.4   Typical X-ray appearance of rheumatoid disease affecting the metacarpophalangeal and proximal interphalangeal joints and wrist joints. (© Institute of Orthopaedics)

The next stage is that the joint is subluxed in an anteromedial direction, for, as the cartilage is destroyed by the pannus of inflammatory synovial tissue, the ligaments become relatively longer. The long flexors are stronger than the extensors and pull the fingers in a volar direction, while the extensor tendons become displaced and lie in the interosseus spaces or gutters. The tendency to ulnar drift is enhanced by the anatomy of the metacarpal head, the condyle being larger on the radial side, and the asymmetry of the collateral ligaments for the radial ligament runs obliquely, while the ulnar ligament is more vertical.

The disability consequent upon this deformity depends not just on the dislocation of the extensor tendons but also on the degree of pain and swelling in the metacarpophalangeal joints and coexisting trouble with the proximal interphalangeal joints. Ulnar drift in burned out disease and painless joints is compatible with excellent function. In our view there is no place for splintage either to try to prevent ulnar drift or to correct it. Treatment therefore depends on the amount of pain in the metacarpophalangeal joints and can be either by synovectomy removing the excess diseased tissue or by joint replacement.

Some years ago there was a vogue for early synovectomy in the belief that this would prevent joint damage, but long-term follow-up has not substantiated this. There is no doubt, however, that synovectomy will relieve pain because one mechanical impediment to joint movement is removed. This may be quite sufficient if the patient is not making many demands on his hands and there is little evidence of joint destruction. If there has been obvious joint destruction with erosions, subluxation, ulnar drift and tendon imbalance, and stability is required then joint replacement is advisable. After synovectomy, the hand is elevated for 48 hours and active exercise started. Stitches are removed at 7–10 days and intensive exercises to regain movement begin.

Joint replacement

In the past, arthroplasty was used to restore movement but this has been abandoned because instability followed and the deformities recurred.

There are three aims of replacing the metacarpophalangeal or proximal interphalangeal joints with artificial joints: mobility, relief of pain and provision of a stable joint. The earliest replacements used metal hinges but it was found that they eroded the soft rheumatoid bone and now flexible implants made of Silastic are used. They move slightly within the medullary cavity, do not erode bone and act as spacers rather than as true joints. In time the development of a false capsule is promoted. The choice of the various types of implant depends on individual preference – our team prefers the Swanson implant to the type with Dacron fixing the prosthesis, for the soft inflamed bone rejects rigid foreign substances under continued stress of joint use.

After Swanson implants there are two main regimens for postoperative rehabilitation.

Swanson (1977) starts active movements in a dynamic splint 3 days after operation. He splints the proximal interphalangeal joints in extension to bear a flexion force on the metacarpophalangeal joints and to prevent an extensor lag.

The other technique is to restrict metacarpophalangeal flexion to 30 degrees with a plaster cast for 2–3 weeks until the extensor expansion has healed and to allow interphalangeal joint flexion. At 7 weeks the patient is readmitted for intensive exercises – dynamic braces not being used. It is likely that the end-results are much the same. The difference lies in whether or not patients can be admitted for postoperative rehabilitation at 3 weeks; if shortage of beds and/or the lack of a rehabilitation service does not permit such a regimen, reliance is placed on the dynamic splinting.

Madden, DeVore and Arem (1977) have described their detailed postoperative programme. For 5 days a dorsal splint is used with the wrist in 15–20 degrees' extension, incorporating a brass rod outrigger with rubber bands and finger loops keeping the metacarpophalangeal joints of the index, middle and ring fingers in extension and slight deviation, the little finger being taped to the ring. At 6 weeks the splint is taken off by day but worn at night, for another 14 weeks. From the fifth day to the third week, daily passive range of movement is given for 10–15 times but no deviation is allowed. Active exercises are allowed at 6 days in the splint. At the fourth week the flexion band is arranged to give 15 degrees' radial deviation.

Madden and his colleagues insist on early maximum passive range of movement and prolonged dynamic splinting because they found that, without this and relying entirely on the patient's own efforts, there is a decrease in movement over the first 2–4 months postoperatively. They found in their study that the passive range of movement was the same after surgery as before, averaging 76 degrees, but that the arc of movement was changed with a shift towards extension; active movements averaged 43 degrees postoperatively and increased by 15 degrees 6 weeks after operation, a range that was maintained for 2 years.

Goldner and colleagues (1977) reported a similar average increase in active movements – by 14 degrees. They have a 6½ year experience of silicone–Dacron prostheses for metacarpophalangeal joint arthroplasty. Again, they use elaborate splinting with an extension night splint alternating with dorsiflexion splints. By day, a loop splint is used, supporting the proximal phalanges for up to 4 months. Active exercises start at 7–21 days. Our impression is that elaborate splinting may be the treatment of choice when, for various reasons, a supervised daily rehabilitation programme is impossible; if, however, rehabilitation facilities are available and the patient is admitted when active rehabilitation can start, the results are comparable.

Arthroplasty is rarely indicated in the thumb because stability is so important and arthrodesis is the commonest operation used.

Soft tissue involvement

Tendon involvement by rheumatoid synovitis is very common – it has been estimated that two-thirds of patients attending hospital have a tendon lesion at one time or another, which may precede joint involvement by months or years. Tenosynovitis of the long flexors can cause irritation of the median nerve in the carpal tunnel, producing the characteristic pins and needles in the median distribution – worse at night – with weakness of the thenar muscles and limitation of tendon excursion.

Soft tissue involvement may be the first indication of rheumatoid disease, and in our experience can appear 2 years or more before joint swellings appear. It is our practice to X-ray the hands and feet in all patients with symptoms of median nerve compression in the carpal tunnel, carry out screening tests for rheumatoid factor and follow up such patients to ensure that they are not developing rheumatoid arthritis.

Decompression and synovectomy comprise one of the most gratifying procedures for the rheumatoid patient. Pain is relieved, tendon function restored and tendon rupture prevented. The hand is elevated for 48 hours, the wrist is supported in a plaster slab for 3 days and active exercises are commenced, continuing until full extension and flexion are regained.

It is very common to see swelling of the flexor tendons over the volar surface of the metacarpophalangeal joints, causing pain on movement of the fingers. Passive range of movement is almost full and painless, indicating that the condition is due to soft-tissue disease, not joint involvement. The rheumatoid synovitis can extend all the way down the flexor tendon sheath in the palm and can be felt as tender doughy swellings. The middle and index fingers are the commonest to be involved. Often with partial rest these swellings subside spontaneously, and it is not uncommon to put such patients on the list for synovectomy only to find when their turn for admission comes that the condition has fully settled. Thus conservative treatment is advisable for 3 months at least, counselling the patient to avoid excessive use of the hands. Steroid injections into the tendon sheaths can be dramatically successful. We favour soluble preparations and not hydrocortisone because at subsequent operation, hydrocortisone particles can be found in the tendon and repeated injections can make surgery more difficult.

If conservative treatment has not been effective, synovectomy can be dramatic, relieving pain and restoring the normal gliding movement of the tendon. These are among the most grateful of patients. The arm is elevated for 48 hours and active exercises started at 10 days.

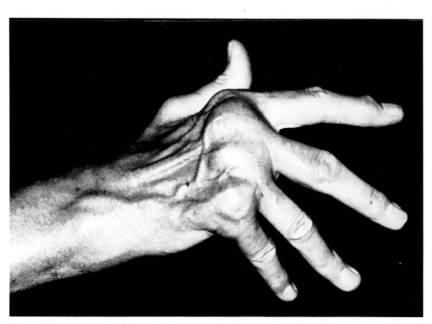

Figure 8.5 Rupture of the extensors of the middle, ring and little fingers in a patient with long-standing rheumatoid arthritis

Trigger fingers are common, with nodules forming usually at the entrance to the fibrous flexor sheath. These often subside spontaneously within 6 months; only if they do not and the finger is locking or painful on use, is surgery advised. Active exercises start 2 weeks afterwards, when the stitches are removed. After extensive synovectomy of the long flexors involving dissection in mid-palm and in no man's land, adhesions occur easily and it is important for the patient to bend the interphalangeal joints individually himself, supporting them at each joint for 5 minutes every hour of the working day. A block of wood in the palm with its distal end just proximal to the joint is useful in concentrating the movement.

Tendon ruptures

There are two mechanisms by which tendons rupture: either by attrition when rubbing over diseased bone – the extensor tendons are very vulnerable over the styloid process of the ulna; or by intrinsic disease by infiltration with rheumatoid tissue (*Figures 8.5* and *8.6*).

It is a common experience for a patient to notice that the little finger suddenly drops into flexion, followed within hours or a day or so by the ring finger and then the middle finger, the index often being spared. This constitutes an emergency, and surgical repair is undertaken as soon as possible. Repair is accompanied by excision of the ulnar styloid, if this is the cause, or by excision of the thickened synovial mass involving the tendons. Rupture of the extensor pollicis longus can occur due to erosions in the radial styloid damaging the tendon. Ruptures of the finger flexors are rarer and, as Brewerton (1957) has pointed, out they can be surrounded by extensive rheumatoid tissue yet have relatively normal function. After tendon repair, the hand is elevated for 48 hours and a plaster cast applied proximal to the interphalangeal joint. This prevents flexion of the metacarpophalangeal joints and protects the suture line. The metacarpophalangeal joints are immobilized in a few degrees of flexion, not in full extension. The plaster is removed at 3 weeks and active free exercises are begun. The occupational therapist can help re-establish functional patterns. Individual exercises for each tendon (as described on page 42 *et seq.*) are necessary because these tendons are normally weaker than the flexors.

Boutonnière deformity

Proliferative synovitis in the proximal interphalangeal joint may stretch the dorsal expansion and permeate through the extensor tendon, stretching it and causing the joint to flex. The lateral slips sublux laterally and shorten, and then extend the metacarpophalangeal joints, so the characteristic deformity of flexion at the proximal interphalangeal joint and hyperextension at the metacarpophalangeal joint is seen (*Figure 8.7*). This causes a considerable functional impairment, as the finger gets in the way. It is treated by synovectomy and relocation of the lateral slips. The hand is elevated for 48 hours and active exercises are started after a few days.

If the central slip is destroyed, Matev's procedure is favoured by our team. One lateral band is divided distally and one proximally over the middle phalanx. The

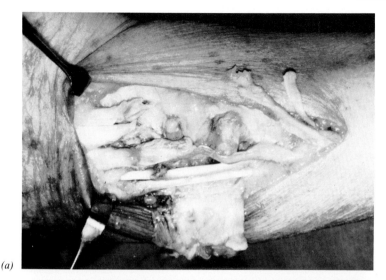

(a)

(b)

Figure 8.6   Appearances at operation in a patient with ruptures of the extensor tendons. (a) Top, tendon extensor indicis; below this, extensor communis to index; beneath this, the attrition and fraying of tendon to middle finger is well shown; beneath this, the ruptured tendons of those to the ring and little fingers are seen. Note the 'saw edge' of the inferior radioulnar joint. (b) Use of extensor communis to the index to motor the extensor. (Operation by Mr I. Bayley, FRCS)

shorter proximal portion is sutured to the extensor expansion, replacing the middle slip. The longer portion is sutured to the longer proximal portion, thus giving an elongated extensor to the metacarpophalangeal joint, for shortening of the extensor apparatus occurs in chronic cases.

After elevation for 48 hours, the finger is immobilized in plaster (which is prolonged to involve the forearm) in extension for 3 weeks. Active exercises begin at 3 weeks, resistance being delayed until 6 weeks.

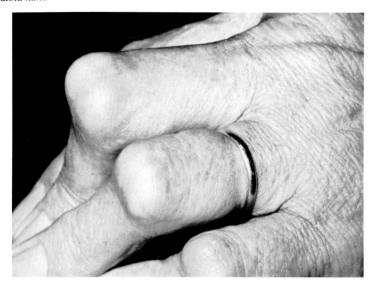

Figure 8.7   Boutonnière deformity in rheumatoid disease

Swan neck deformity

Brewerton (1957) found that 13 per cent of rheumatoid patients suffered from swan neck deformity. This is the reverse of the boutonnière deformity, the proximal interphalangeal joints being hyperextended and flexed at the metacarpophalangeal joints (*Figure 8.8*).

It is due to destruction of the proximal interphalangeal joint, involving the volar plate, and also to insufficiency of the sublimis, so that there is overaction of the proximal interphalangeal extensors as the lateral bands migrate dorsomedially. The result is inability to flex the interphalangeal joints. The flexors may not be able to flex the joints further than 180 degrees. If the proximal interphalangeal joint is mobile, release of the lateral bands may be all that is required, though sometimes a tenodesis of one extensor slip is added. If the deformity is fixed, then arthrodesis in flexion is the only effective treatment.

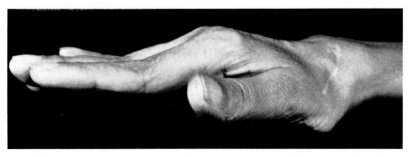

Figure 8.8   Swan neck deformity in rheumatoid disease

THUMB

Inflammation of the metacarpophalangeal joints leads to collapse of the thumb into flexion with hyperextension of the interphalangeal joint. In extreme cases the metacarpophalangeal joint can be flexed to 90 degrees and the interphalangeal joints extended to 90 degrees. This flail thumb makes any precision activities impossible. Patients still retain a strong adduction key grip but lack the most sensitive opposing surfaces of the pulps of the index finger and thumb, for rotation is completely lost. If the ligaments are significantly stretched, the thumb becomes unstable laterally and power is lost.

There is really no solution to the problems of unstable weak thumbs other than arthrodesis in the position of function, using a Kirschner wire kept in for 6 weeks and giving supervised progressive active exercises until full power and function are restored.

WRIST

The wrist is the key joint for hand function. It is commonly affected in rheumatoid disease – a painful wrist effectively stops hand function. The joint is swollen, hot and tender, and attempts at movement cause pain. It can be affected without any involvement of the finger joints but the restricted use of the hand will cause secondary stiffness in the metacarpophalangeal and interphalangeal joints. Usually, though, there is coexistent affection of the small joints of the hand.

Not only does the synovitis limit wrist function, it also causes erosion of the styloid processes of the radius and ulna, with the possibility of tendon ruptures. In many cases, rest to the joint in splints will settle the inflammation in a matter of weeks and, like synovitis elsewhere in joints or tendons, completely resolve; there is thus no call for radical measures until the patient has been watched over a period of time. In the early stages the wrist is splinted in plaster or a polyethylene slab until the inflammation has subsided. During this time the unaffected joints are used normally.

At first the splints are removed by day and gentle activity allowed, being worn at night or when any heavy work is requested.

Some patients have chronic ache in the wrists, not sufficiently severe to warrant surgery, and these are well controlled by a light splint such as the Futura (*Figure 8.9*). They can be worn when there is an exacerbation of pain or when using the wrist for activities likely to cause pain. Persistent synovitis not responding to prolonged rest or medical treatment can be treated by synovectomy and appropriate excision of bone such as the terminal 2.5 cm of the ulna. The wrist is splinted for 3 weeks and gentle mobilization instituted thereafter. Vigorous activity is avoided for 6 weeks.

When the joint is destroyed, with pain and serious limitation of movement, arthrodesis is indicated. (A trial period in plaster will decide if this is the treatment of choice.)

The joint is then stable and pain free. If both joints have to be fused, one should be fused in slight flexion to allow toilet activities. If the shoulder and elbow are very stiff, arthrodesis of the wrist may seriously impair function.

The wrist is kept in plaster for 8 weeks after fusion and the unaffected fingers are used to the full meanwhile. Usually, no formal rehabilitation is required.

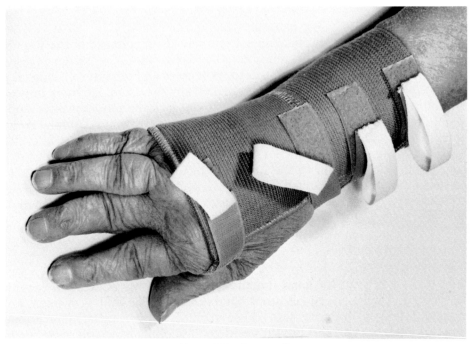

Figure 8.9   Futura splint

ELBOW

The elbow is commonly involved in rheumatoid arthritis. Most patients with long-standing disease will be found to have limitation of full extension by 30 degrees. This is not of functional significance in itself. If the joint becomes inflamed and painful, the whole function of the upper limb is jeopardized.

Rest in a plaster slab will settle the inflammation and one intra-articular steroid injection is often dramatically successful in relieving pain. The elbow is a peculiar joint and dislikes being moved passively. Consequently, rehabilitation of the stiff elbow joint must be by active exercises only, with the help of ice to relieve pain and swelling, and hydrotherapy to encourage maximum movement.

When there are erosive changes in the head of the radius and chronic synovitis in the joint with continued pain and stiffness (*Figure 8.10*), excision of the head of the radius and synovectomy comprise a most rewarding procedure. Rotation often improves considerably but not extension. The operation is done primarily for pain and, as such, can transform the patient's life.

Following operation the arm is immobilized in a plaster of Paris back splint with the elbow at 90 degrees and in mid-forearm rotation. The Redivac drain, if used, is removed at 48 hours and, if the wound allows, assisted active exercises are commenced. This can be delayed, though, if there is much pain. Once active control of the elbow is established and the skin sutures are removed (between 10 and 14 days), the patient is discharged to continue supervised physiotherapy for a further 3–4 weeks.

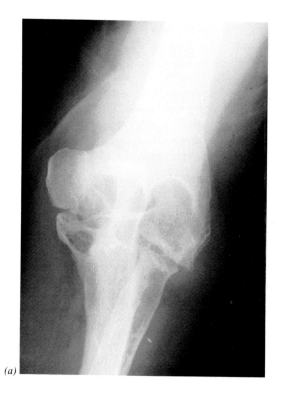

(a)

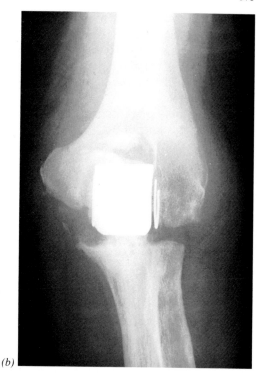

(b)

Figure 8.10   (a) Typical X-ray appearance of rheumatoid disease affecting the elbow joint. (b, c) Joint replacement

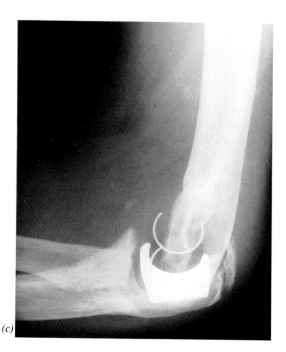

(c)

There is often some loss in range of movement as compared with the preoperative mobility, but this is usually not significant and the pain relief afforded by the operation more than compensates.

Many surgeons have had gloomy experiences with elbow replacements but recently Scales, Lettin and Bayley (1977) have reported promising results with the Stanmore elbow prosthesis.

Immediately after operation a plaster of Paris back splint is applied with the elbow at 90 degrees and in mid-rotation. The Redivac drain is removed at 48 hours; at this time the wound is inspected, for wound healing can be a problem since many patients have been on steroids. Any deep haematoma noticed at this stage requires evacuation; in practice, this is seldom necessary.

Following removal of the drain the plaster back splint is reapplied until removal of sutures at 2 weeks.

Supervised assisted active, as opposed to passive, mobilization is then started and, again, proceeds according to the patient's progress. Mobility is usually regained fairly rapidly although there is often a loss of full extension.

The length of stay in hospital following operation generally averages 3–4 weeks. On discharge, the patient is encouraged to continue his own mobilization with normal use.

In 30 elbow replacements (in 24 patients), results were assessed according to five criteria: relief of pain, restoration of function, stability, mobility and patient's reaction. Pain was assessed as severe, moderate, mild or none. Operation was reserved for those in severe pain.

All patients improved by at least one grade and most by two or more grades. Function was greatly improved in 80 per cent. The average increase in flexion–extension was 35 degrees and pronation–supination 40 degrees. All but two patients said they would have the operation again (Scales, Lettin and Bayley, 1977).

SHOULDER

Both the soft tissues and the joint are involved. Rotator cuff lesions and capsulitis are common, causing marked limitation of movement and pain. Steroid injections can be dramatic, up to three being given over a 6-week period. There is little place for vigorous exercises in rheumatoid shoulder disorders.

In the acute stage it is essential to rest the shoulder; the arm is placed in a sling with the hand elevated to prevent oedema, and the fingers are given regular exercise. In the chronic stage, hydrotherapy and exercises with, sometimes, one intra-articular steroid injection can be successful.

In severe chronic painful joints, total shoulder replacements have proved their worth. Although it is unlikely for there to be a dramatic increase in range, one can expect relief of pain and therefore a most welcome improvement in function of the whole upper limb.

In Kessel and Bayley's (1979) series over 5 years, 24 shoulders were replaced in 23 patients, 17 being for rheumatoid arthritis. Of these 17, 14 shoulders were pain-free or virtually so after operation; in 11 function was improved and in 12 movement was increased.

Immediately after operation the arm is immobilized in a collar and cuff and constrained using a crêpe bandage body spica. As soon as the patient is co-operative, the bandage can be removed. This usually coincides with removal of the Redivac drain at 48 hours. At that time the arm is held abducted in neutral rotation in a roller towel and supervised elbow flexion can be instituted.

On removal of sutures, a programme of assisted active mobilization is commenced and can proceed as fast as the patient's progress permits, bearing in mind that external rotation should not be forced.

Inpatient stay following operation is usually of the order of 3 weeks. This is then followed by continued outpatient physiotherapy, probably for a further 3–4 weeks.

REHABILITATION

Perhaps the most important aspect of rehabilitation of the patient with rheumatoid disease is the careful assessment of exactly what the functional disability is and how the patient's environment can be adapted to compensate for this.

We have already spoken of the importance of careful assessment by the occupational therapist of the exact cause of disability. In multiple joint involvement it may be difficult, indeed impossible, to decide in the clinic whether the major factor is finger deformities, wrist involvement or stiff and painful elbows and shoulders. We like to admit our patients for a few days for a comprehensive look at the overall problem. Each patient can be studied at leisure during several days and observed at all the various tasks of daily living in the home and at work. It will become clear then which are the priorities for surgery. If the patient is independent on crutches or sticks, restoration of painless wrists may be the most important factor. If dressing, toilet and eating are difficult, it may be wise to tackle the elbow first.

Simple measures such as supportive splints can be tried first or the effect of an arthrodesis mimicked by splintage or plaster.

Most occupational therapy departments have realistic kitchen and bathroom mock-ups where assessment can be made and a trial undertaken of aids and gadgets. At Stanmore we have the Graham Hill Assessment Unit (page 299), where patients actually live on their own or with relatives, and shop, cook and generally fend for themselves while the rehabilitation team study each problem as it arises and provide necessary solutions. At the same time home visits are made to study the exact environment to which the patient will return. Once it is clear that the patient's disability has not responded to drug treatment or is unsuitable for surgery, aids and appliances can be provided (*Figure 8.11*).

Dressing

Stiff joints make dressing lengthy and tiring. Button hooks, Velcro fittings for weak hand muscles, long-handled shoe-horns, stocking aids and toilet aids for patients with stiff shoulders are standard supply.

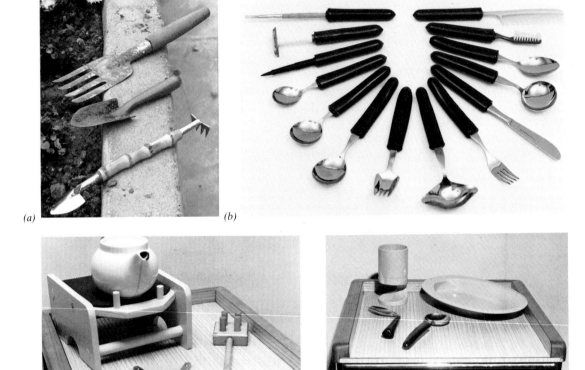

(a)   *(b)*

(c)   *(d)*

Figure 8.11   Aids to daily living. (a) Adapted gardening tools. (b) Special cutlery and writing and toilet equipment (reproduced by courtesy of the Editor of Modern Medicine*). (c) Teapot tipper and aids to open taps and bottles, on a trolley, which is at the same level as kitchen equipment. (d) Special cutlery, plate and mug*

Bathroom

For the patient with multiple joint handicap, taking a bath can be a formidable performance. Sometimes it is such a problem and so exhausting for the patient that providing a shower may be the best answer. The patient's hands and wrists may be so weak and painful that he cannot support himself on grab rails when transferring to the bath. Long-handled flannels are very useful when shoulders and elbows are stiff, and toilet aids with angled wipers are invaluable.

Kitchen

Ideally, all working surfaces should be at the same level, to save lifting objects on and off, and, of course, simplify wheelchair life. Special tap-turners, teapot or kettle tippers, jar openers, padded cutlery all take the strain off weak and painful joints.

Manoy mugs make drinking easier and plates are available with a lip for one-armed feeding.

A trolley with a shelf at the same level as the oven allows easy transfer of food and also acts as a walking aid.

Communication

Padded pens make writing easier when joints are stiff. An electric typewriter may be the answer if writing is slow and painful; in Britain this can be provided cheaply through the local authority if the patient is a registered disabled person.

In severe disability when both upper and lower limbs are severely affected, a POSSUM link system is invaluable. Then the patient, with minimal effort, can control the front door, television, lights, telephone, heaters and radio. If the hands are so severely affected that driving a conventional geared car is impossible, automatic gears are substituted or a padded steering wheel provided.

Hobbies must always be considered; for example, there is available a whole variety of gardening tools specially designed for patients with stiff joints in the upper limb.

The disablement resettlement officer or, when available, the hospital rehabilitation officer will liaise with the patient's employer and recommend appropriate alterations to the work situation – alteration of level of working, adaptation of tools – or will indicate to the surgeon what degree of movement or power is necessary for successful work. The close collaboration of surgeon and rehabilitation officer will allow a realistic surgical programme to be outlined. It is impossible to assess the patient's requirements at home or at work at an outpatient clinic. No surgical programme is ever undertaken in our unit without a full functional assessment by occupational therapist and/or rehabilitation officer, for it may be found that a simple adjustment to the work environment or a gadget or appliance will be all that is necessary. It is not unusual for the report to indicate that what might seem the reasonable operation to improve function (e.g. arthrodesis of the wrist to increase power) may be quite wrong, leading, for example, to inability to propel a wheelchair through lack of wrist flexion.

Finally, one cannot overemphasize the changing nature of the disease. Regular follow-up and assessment at least 6-monthly, however static the disease may seem, is vital. The disease may relapse and require revision of medication; mechanical pressure on nerves or tendon dysfunction may be causing increasing pain and disability and require surgery; the patient's home or work situation may have changed and demand reassessment of aids and appliances; degenerative changes may be superimposed on old inflammatory disease and stabilization procedures or joint replacement be required.

Only by regular review by clinician, therapists, rehabilitation officer and medical social worker acting as a team will the best management be offered to unfortunate patients with this disease.

REFERENCES AND BIBLIOGRAPHY

Brewerton, D. A. (1957). Hand deformities in rheumatoid disease. *Annals of the Rheumatic Diseases* **16**, 183–196
Fleming, A., Crown, J. A. and Corbett, M. (1976a). Incidence of joint involvement in early rheumatoid arthritis. *Rheumatology and Rehabilitation* **15**, 92–96

Fleming, A., Crown, J. M. and Corbett, M. (1976b). Early rheumatoid disease – onset. *Annals of the Rheumatic Diseases* **35,** 357–360

Fleming, A., Benn, R. T., Corbett, M. and Wood, P. H. N. (1976). Early rheumatoid disease – patterns of joint involvement. *Annals of the Rheumatic Diseases* **35,** 361–364

Goldner, J. L., Gould, J. S., Urbanic, J. R. *et al.* (1977). Metacarpophalangeal joint arthroplasty with silicone-Dacron prostheses (Nieubauer type): six and a half years experience. *Journal of Hand Surgery* **2,** 200–211

Hall, M. R. P. (1976). Barthel's index. The assessment of disability in the geriatric patient. *Rheumatology and Rehabilitation* **15,** 59–63

Harris, R. (1969). Rehabilitation. In *Arthritis and Physical Medicine*, p. 48. Ed. by S. Licht. New Haven, Conn: E. Licht

Jacoby, R. K., Jayson, M. I. V. and Cosh, J. A. (1973). Onset, early stages and prognosis of rheumatoid arthritis. A clinical study of 100 patients with 11-year follow-up. *British Medical Journal* **2,** 96

Kessel, L. and Bayley, I. (1979). Prosthetic replacement of shoulder joint. Preliminary communication. *Journal of the Royal Society of Medicine* **72,** 748–752

Madden, J. W., DeVore, G. and Arem, A. J. (1977). A rational postoperative management program for metacarpophalangeal joint implant arthroplasty. *Journal of Hand Surgery* **2,** 358–366

Scales, J. T., Lettin, A. W. F. and Bayley, I. (1977). The evolution of the Stanmore hinged total elbow replacement. In *Joint Replacement in the Upper Limb*, pp. 53–62. London and New York: Institute of Mechanical Engineering

Sheik, K., Smith, D. S., Meade, T. W., Goldenberg, E., Brennan, P. J. and Kinsella, G. (1979). Activities of daily living index in studies of chronic disability. *International Journal of Rehabilitation Medicine* **1,** 51–57

Swanson, A. (1977). In *Operative Surgery: The Hand*, pp. 297–337. Ed. by R. G. Pulvertaft. London: Butterworths

Wright, V. and Owen, S. (1976). The effect of rheumatoid arthritis on the social situation of housewives. *Rheumatology and Rehabilitation* **15,** 156–166

Resettlement 9

This chapter deals with the resettlement of patients with severe loss of function. It is an essential part of medical treatment to ensure that the patient who cannot return to his old job, because of severe disability, is found a different job commensurate with his abilities.

Since the end of World War II, a great deal has been done for the needs of the disabled person. Anyone reviewing the varied nature of the services available will realize that it is not primarily more money or more services that are now required, but a better knowledge of their existence and a more efficient use of them.

As the Piercy Report, paragraph 42, mentioned in 1956, consultants and general practitioners are still slow to consider the rehabilitation needs of their patients, and they still require education in the scope, nature and potential of rehabilitation.

Randle (1972) stated that 'The present services for the disabled could be vastly improved by better communication and co-operation between all the services involved, whether they be those of Central Government, Local Authority or Voluntary Society'.

All disabled people require the best possible advice and facilities for satisfactory resettlement, and in none is this more important than in the patient with a severely affected hand.

In the first part of this chapter the various services, both national and voluntary, will be reviewed in detail, and the type of resettlement clinic that has proved successful in practice will be discussed. In the second part of the chapter, specific problems in the resettlement of those with hand injuries will be analysed.

NATIONAL FACILITIES (GREAT BRITAIN)

In 1944 the Disabled Persons' Employment Act was passed, being the first big step in providing facilities for disabled persons. Two years later the National Health Service was introduced, and in 1948 the National Assistance Act made provision for the welfare of handicapped persons; thus the employment, treatment and welfare needs of disabled persons were all catered for in considerable detail within a period of 3 years of the end of World War II. Since then a number of acts have been passed modifying the original act, culminating in the Chronically Sick and Disabled Persons Act 1970. This Act makes mandatory on local authorities a number of functions which were previously permissive under the National Assistance Act of 1948. Among these are a requirement to determine the incidence of disability in their area, and an annual debate in Parliament to discuss advances in technology to help the disabled.

Disablement resettlement officer (DRO)

The main backbone of the service for the disabled is the disablement resettlement officer. Recruited from Employment Service Division (MSC) staff, his statutory duties are to advise the disabled on employment problems, and to make liaison with employers for the satisfactory employment of disabled people. A register of disabled persons is kept at every Employment Exchange, and it is essential that a disabled person be registered before he can obtain all the available facilities. At present there are nearly half a million people on the register.

The definition of a disabled person is one who, through injury or disease, is substantially handicapped in obtaining employment. Normally, medical evidence is required before the DRO can register a patient as a disabled person. When the hospital consultant refers a patient, this evidence is given on form DP.1. This is not for a medical history but is a method of estimating the patient's functional abilities.

These forms are now subdivided into DP.1 (H) for use by hospitals, DP.1 (R) used by regional medical officers, DP.1 (U) for psychiatric patients and DP.1 (E) for epileptics.

If the disablement is obvious – for examples, loss of a limb – medical evidence need not be sought.

Once registered, the patient is given a card which he can present at any Employment Exchange in Great Britain and be sure of receiving the advice and help of the DRO.

Apart from his work at the Employment Exchange, advising patients who come to him and making liaison with employers, he has a statutory duty to visit hospitals and medical institutions where there are patients requiring his advice. The frequency of visits is arranged between the DRO and the appropriate institutions. In some hospitals there is a regular resettlement clinic (described in detail later). In some, the DRO visits only when needed; in too many he is not invited to visit at all.

Initially, patients are put on the register for a period of 1–5 years. Two months before the end of this period the patient is reviewed by the DRO, who will decide whether he should remain on the register. In case of doubt, the problem is referred to the Disablement Advisory Panel.

There are various ways in which the DRO can help the patient to get employment. Whenever possible, he visits local industries in order to maintain an up-to-date knowledge of the type of work available and, of course, the vacancies that exist. By an Act of Parliament, those employing more than 20 work people must have a 'quota' of their employees as registered disabled persons. The present figure, which the Secretary of State can alter, is three. It is an offence for an employer to engage able-bodied workers if his disabled quota is not up to strength.

It is wise, if possible, to resettle the patient into the same sort of job he was doing before his disability, but if this is impossible there may well be many different jobs that he can do in the same firm. Close liaison between the DRO and the personnel management staff will result in satisfactory placing. Obviously the more intimate rapport that exists between the DRO and the employers, the easier it should be to resettle a patient. This takes time and it means that the DRO has to be away from his office, but experience has shown that this is by far the best way of getting results.

There is room for considerable research into the types of jobs that can be done by disabled persons, and there is a need, too, for an intermediary between the medical staff looking after the patient and the employers, who can advise on suitable work positions, alteration of machinery, rest periods, and so on. This will normally be done in large firms by the industral medical officer, but his job is often difficult, as there is room for better appreciation of the problems of the disabled person in industry. This problem will be discussed later in greater detail.

Government training scheme

If a patient requires resettlement in a new trade, the government training scheme is used. There are now 67 skill centres in Great Britain, providing training in a wide range of different trades specifically for the disabled person. The centres are run on factory lines – classes range from 8 to 16 trainees so that personal attention can be given by the instructor. The instructor must have had at least 5 years' postapprenticeship experience and a special course of instruction at one of the Department of Employment's training colleges.

When a patient requires training in a subject not covered by the scheme, arrangements can be made with outside organizations or with individual employers. In such cases the State will finance the organization or employer direct. The skill centres are situated in the following areas.

England
Basildon, Billingham-on-Tees, Birmingham (2), Blackburn, Bradford, Bristol, Charlton, Coventry, Darlington, Doncaster, Dudley, Durham, Enfield, Felling-on-Tyne, Gloucester, Hindley, Hull, Killingworth, Kirby in Ashfield, Leeds, Leicester, Letchworth, Liverpool, Long Eaton, Manchester (3), Maryport, Medway, Middlesbrough, Milton Keynes, North Staffs, Norwich, Perivale, Peterborough, Plymouth, Poplar, Portsmouth, Preston, Reading, Rochdale, Runcorn, St Helens, Sheffield, Slough, Southampton, Twickenham, Waddon, Wakefield, West Sussex, Wolverhampton.

Scotland
Bellshill, Dumbarton, Dundee, Dunfermline, Edinburgh, Glasgow (3), Irvine, Port Glasgow.

Wales
Cardiff, Llanelli, Port Talbot, 'West Gwent' Newport, Wrexham.

The courses are usually for 6 months, though some, particularly watch and clock repairing, are for 1 year. The list of trades taught is too large to reproduce here, but it includes all sections of the building trade, engineering, draughtsmanship, fitting, welding, boot and shoe making and repairing, electrical servicing, motor repair, radio and television servicing, display painting, surgical appliance making, and watch and clock repairing. Application for enrolment at one of these centres is made by the DRO when the patient has been registered as disabled.

For most courses, a test and an interview are required before acceptance. In draughtsmanship, for example, a test involving algebra and simple trigonometry is given and the patient's industrial background reviewed by a committee. The object of this interview is to ensure that only those who have a sound chance of completing the course and being successful tradesmen are accepted as trainees.

Apart from the financial aspects of wasted training, if a disabled person fails at the end of a course, it is liable to have a severe psychological effect on him and may make his future employment extremely difficult.

There are both residential and non-residential centres; if a patient wishes to attend a non-residential centre but lives too far away for daily travel, the DRO will help him to obtain accommodation.

The Employment Service Division will also subvent courses at some residential training centres run by voluntary societies – for example at Finchale Training College, Durham; Portland Training College, Mansfield; Queen Elizabeth's Training College, Leatherhead; and St Loye's College, Exeter. These colleges provide places for 600 patients. Further education is available at all skill centres.

COURSES PROVIDED AT RESIDENTIAL TRAINING CENTRES

Commercial

Audio/copy typing; calculating machine operating; clerk/book-keeper; clerk – builders' quantities; clerk – general office practice; computer programming; punch card operating; shorthand and typing.

Construction

Carpentry (bench)

Engineering

Draughtsmanship; electrical/electronic wiring and assembly; instrument fitting and machining; light electrical servicing; light precision engineering; welding – electric and oxyacetylene.

Other trades

Cooking; gardening; radio and television servicing; spray painting; storekeeping (industrial); telephone switchboard operating; typewriter repairing; watch and clock repairing.

In addition, disabled people can train in ordinary commercial and technical colleges and in individual firms with State support during training.

Training in the skill centres is free and patients receive certain allowances. An unmarried trainee aged 20 years or over receives £25.70 (1978) per week and fares and free lunches. A trainee with a wife, and two children under the age of 19 years, receives £39.20 (1978) per week with fares and lunches. If they are resident the rates are slightly lower. A lodging allowance is payable for those living in lodgings, and a travel allowance is available. In cases of real hardship, a grant may also be allowed from the Supplementary Benefits Commission to supplement the essential financial requirements of the household.

On completion of the course, the patient is considered to be a semiskilled person; he is then offered a position in the appropriate industry as near to his home as possible. The placing of trainees is the responsibility of the DRO, and it must be emphasized that there is no direction of labour. The patient is free to refuse jobs if he wises, within reason.

A trainee does not receive full union rates of pay during the first 18 months of employment because he is not considered to be a fully skilled person.

During training, regular tests are held to assess the patient's progress and to prevent those who are obviously not going to complete the course from wasting further time.

The patients work hard at these centres, the hours are those of a full working day, and the standard of training is extremely high.

Only in special cases is medical treatment provided, though all are under the observation of a medical officer throughout training.

There is a gymnasium attached to Queen Elizabeth's Training College and a remedial gymnast is in attendance.

It is possible, in exceptional cases, to allow a patient daily treatment, but his course is then extended by 3 months or more. In the main, these centres are designed for patients who have reached medical or surgical finality.

Of the disabled patients invalided from the RAF rehabilitation centres, about one-third have been trained at one or other of the centres. This high figure is to be expected most among the younger age-groups, and many, of course, have not received any training before joining the Service. In the type of patient seen in civil hospitals, the figure is much lower.

Wherever possible the patient is encouraged to return to his previous employment, or to a modification of it; retraining is indicated only where absolutely necessary. Finance is one of the major obstacles to a patient taking up retraining.

Although payment of allowances is made during training, many patients cannot afford to meet their various financial commitments, among which, these days, are hire-purchase repayments; this is a difficult problem. Very special effort is made to persuade young people to forego easy money immediately and take the long-term view by becoming skilled tradesmen. It is a great temptation for a young person to engage in many types of unskilled labour, as the immediate wage is high. The prospects of such employment, however, are never as good as for a skilled man; furthermore, the best resettlement for a disabled person is into the most skilled job that he can perform. Not only will this give satisfaction and enable him to conquer the disability, but the more highly skilled the less likely he is to lose the job in times of economic stress.

Before applying for enrolment at a skill centre, care should be taken to ensure that there are adequate openings in the particular trade in which the patient is being trained near his home. It is usually impossible, due to the housing shortage, for him to move to any district where the appropriate work is available. The patient usually chooses a trade in which he can find employment near his own home.

Designated employment scheme

There are two occupations which are open only to registered disabled persons; these are car park attendant and passenger lift operator. It is not the government's intention to increase the number of occupations under this scheme.

Employment rehabilitation centres

There are at present 25 employment rehabilitation centres, and they are situated in industrial areas: Bellshill, Billingham, Birmingham, Bristol, Cardiff, Coventry, Dundee, Edinburgh, Egham, Felling-on-Tyne, Garston Manor, Glasgow (Hillington), Hull, Killingworth, Leeds, Leicester, Liverpool, Long Eaton, Manchester, North Staffs, Perivale, Plymouth, Port Talbot, Sheffield and Waddon. Their function is to assess a patient's capabilities for employment and, by an intensive course of work, to restore confidence and prepare him for the rigours of industrial life after long spells in hospital.

The maximum time that is spent in these employment rehabilitation centres is 12 weeks; most patients spend 8 weeks there. There is room for 200 at Egham, which is the only residential unit, and 100 at each of the others. The pay structure is the same as at skill centres.

The staff of a rehabilitation unit includes a doctor, an occupational psychologist, a social worker, a DRO and a chief occupational supervisor. Patients are under the control of a rehabilitation officer who is not a doctor.

Functional and educational assessment and psychological testing are aimed to help the patient decide on the trade appropriate to his abilities. Many patients will therefore go on to a government training centre from the employment rehabilitation centre. The activities are graded so that the atmosphere of a modern industrial factory is gradually created. There are woodwork, assembly and engineering sections. The work is all productive and patients receive a weekly payment similar to those in skill centres. A remedial gymnast is in attendance and there is a close liaison between the unit medical officer and local consultant. The unit medical officer must have had previous experience of industrial medicine before appointment.

One of the employment rehabilitation centres, Garston Manor, is now a combined medical rehabilitation unit and industrial rehabilitation unit. We have discussed already the great value of having workshops which can be used for work assessment as well as vocational guidance, and one hopes that the integration of industrial and medical rehabilitation will develop further.

There is, of course, a hard core of difficult patients at such units and this, together with the difficult employment situation, explains why about 40 per cent of people attending these units are still unemployed 3 months after discharge. However, of the 14,221 who entered IRUs (now ERCs) in 1970, 42 per cent were employed at follow-up and 16 per cent were in training.

There is no doubt that these centres serve a useful purpose in special cases. Better and more enlightened use of occupational therapy departments for assessment of function would lead to less need for patients to be transferred to employment rehabilitation centres. Indeed, there is great scope for occupational therapists in the careful assessment of function, and there is no doubt that modern occupational therapy has a great deal to offer in this connection. Departments are becoming more orientated towards functional assessment, the provision of aids to daily living and adaptation of tools for disability, in place of the somewhat useless craftwork as a quasi-diversional activity. It is hoped that doctors will make the most use of the modern approach to occupational therapy.

Some hospitals have solved the problem of resettlement of severe injuries by appointing a rehabilitation officer. Usually this person is basically an engineer who has become interested in the problems of disabled people. His job is to effect a close liaison between the medical staff of the hospital and the patient's employer. He sees the patient from the earliest stages of treatment and right at the beginning of treatment he visits or contacts the employer to determine the type of work the patient was doing prior to his injury. He discusses with the employer and his staff the likely possibility of when the patient will return to work and what function the patient will probably have. In many cases it is possible for the patient to return to work at a very early stage of treatment, which is the ideal form of rehabilitation – especially to return to his own job and to earn a full wage. This is not always feasible, but modifications of the work may be possible if there is understanding and goodwill between the rehabilitation officer and the employer.

It is clear that the calibre of the rehabilitation officer is of supreme importance. There is no doubt that more of these people would be of tremendous value to rehabilitation of the disabled. It is equally clear that the co-operation of the trade unions is essential and this can again be effected by a tactful and understanding approach by the rehabilitation officer. It is, of course, an enormous help if the rehabilitation officer has himself been an engineer, or worked in a factory, thereby having an understanding of the peculiar problems of industry (Brewerton and Daniel, 1969).

It is felt, however, that many more patients could be assessed and helped to an early return to work by graduated activity through better use of the rehabilitation facilities in hospitals than by sending them to employment rehabilitation centres. Furthermore, some of the difficult problems are not solved by the transfer of a patient to a different doctor who has not had the experience of this particular patient and his personal reactions to the disability.

Sheltered workshops

Sheltered workshops have been opened for the very seriously disabled patients who cannot earn their living in open competitive industry, and further workshops under an organization known as Remploy have been opened up where such patients can work at a slower rate. These workshops are especially useful for those with such diseases as epilepsy, organic nervous diseases, respiratory tuberculosis and muscular dystrophy. Selected cases of recovery from pyschiatric breakdown also do well. Each employee is reviewed medically at least once every 6 months.

Remploy is a public company, receiving government loans to cover expenditure. It operates at a loss which is met through public funds. There are 88 factories in government buildings at present employing 8300 severely disabled persons and 55 sheltered workshops with 5000 eployees. These sheltered workshops do not come under the direct authority of Remploy and are often sponsored by the local authority. As it is essential that there be some reasonably able-bodied persons to fill some of the posts in the factories, a campaign is organized to recruit some 15 per cent of this staff from the less severely disabled. The work undertaken includes book binding, leather work, the manufacture of cardboard boxes, furniture, surgical appliances, and so on. London rates of pay are around £52 per week, with a bonus incentive scheme related to productivity in most factories.

Employment rehabilitation centres can be used to assess the suitability of all patients for Remploy. Each year some 250 Remploy workers leave the factories to take up work in outside industry. Although the scheme operates at a loss and, as the Piercy Committee (Report, 1956) pointed out, it is unreasonable to expect such a scheme to operate without a loss, the humanitarian aspect is outstanding. Even from the economic point of view, it is better for severely disabled patients to be able to make some contribution towards production rather than none at all.

Professional grants

Under a special education and training scheme, grants were available to ex-servicemen who wished to take up a professional training. This scheme has now lapsed and applies only to disabled patients.

When a patient cannot be satisfactorily placed in employment by the DRO, either directly through the Employment Exchange or through the government training scheme, a grant of money is payable in special cases for patients to take up professional training. The patient must show evidence that he intended to continue his vocation before disability. Grants are made by the Department of Education and full fees for training and maintenance can be claimed. Under this scheme patients have been trained as school teachers and have taken courses at many of the universities. Two of our patients with hand disabilities made use of this scheme; one trained to be a school teacher and the other as a geologist at a university.

If a patient can show that it is impossible for him to work with other people, a grant may be made for the setting up of his own business; for example, one patient has had a workshop built in his garden, fully equipped, to enable him to repair boots and shoes. These grants can be substantial in amount. Under Section 29 of the National Assistance Act 1948, local authorities may make provision for structural adaptations, such as the widening of doors, raised toilet seats, and so on. Full use should be made of these facilities, which are now mandatory by the Chronically Sick and Disabled Persons Act 1970.

Disablement advisory committees

These committees exist to advise the Employment Service Division on a local basis. There are some 250 committees attached to main Employment Exchanges. They consist of an independent chairman, who is usually a person of some local standing, an equal number of employers' and workers' representatives, and other persons chosen for their knowledge of the problems of the disabled, some of whom are members of voluntary organizations and welfare societies. There is also a medical member, nominated by the Employment Service Division (MSC) and who is banned from acting as a medical member of a panel.

The committees advise on problems in the areas and make recommendations to the head office of the Manpower Services Commission. Other executive functions are to recommend on specific matters connected with the registration of disabled persons and any other matters that may arise in the area. A committee sometimes appoints a panel, the members of which need not necessarily be members of the full committee. Usually it consists of an independent chairman, employers' and workers' representatives, a doctor, and a person with experience of problems of disabled persons. Both these organizations serve a useful function but are not widely enough known; it is certain that their services can be better used.

One of the criticisms of the present scheme for the disabled is that too many organizations are concerned with the disabled person, and there is not enough liaison. It has been suggested that there should be a ministry set up to deal with all the problems of the disabled, but this was not accepted by the Piercy Committee (Report, 1956), who recommended that better liaison between the various persons concerned with the disabled would solve the problems.

One fact has emerged quite clearly in our experience in resettlement – a closer relationship between the DRO and the doctor solves almost all the problems that are likely to arise. For this reason it is felt that the resettlement clinic is the best place to tackle the problems; it is here that the doctor and the DRO can come to close liaison on any given case so that in time the doctor learns a good deal about industrial employment, and the DRO improves his knowledge on the medical problems of the disabled.

Cooksey (1960) pointed out how important it is to integrate the various facilities required in the rehabilitation and resettlement of a disabled person. He made it clear that the necessary services are well represented in a sizable community, but these are often geographically widely separated, and the various personnel involved in helping a patient often have no opportunity of meeting. He suggested the establishment of a medicosocial centre for an area, in the general hospital. This would provide accommodation for the various people concerned, such as the general practitioner, senior health visitor, senior welfare officer, local housing officer, DRO, medical technical officer from the regional appliance centre and limb fitting centre, based on the industrial rehabilitation workshop. This would mean that there would be much closer liaison between the various people concerned and an interchange of ideas. Certainly, anything that can help in the integration of these facilities and the speeding up of the whole rehabilitation and resettlement process, is to be encouraged.

Resettlement clinics

Special clinics have been organized in some hospitals and rehabilitation centres to deal with all the problems confronting the disabled person, and we are convinced that this is the ideal way to cope with the resettlement of the disabled. The clinic meets as often as necessary, and not less than once a week. The members are the patient, the doctor in charge, the DRO, medical social worker or appropriate equivalent (welfare officer in the Services), an occupational therapist, and anyone else who may be able to give advice on a particular problem. A full industrial and social history is compiled which includes any problems associated with accommodation, finance, transport, education, and so on, for discussion before the patient is brought to the clinic.

At the clinic the doctor presents a brief outline of the medical history, including the prognosis; the occupational therapist gives her observations on the patient's abilities, his reaction to work and the ability to handle tools; the medical social worker or welfare officer discusses any social or domestic problems that may arise. The DRO will then advise the patient on training facilities and employment prospects, or take steps to find out about such matters for discussion at the next meeting at the clinic. The object of the first attendance is to show the patient all the various facilities that exist for his resettlement, and to give him confidence and encouragement. It is beneficial to introduce the patient to the clinic at an early stage of rehabilitation, even though he may not be taking up employment for many months. It is essential that the patient be assured that everything possible will be done to find him satisfactory work, or that he will be retrained in a new trade; he can then participate in all the rehabilitation activities with a calm mind.

As soon as a patient has decided on one or perhaps a number of trades, the next step is to give him a trial period of work. It is an advantage if the patient can be given the opportunity of trying out a chosen trade for himself.

The following three questions require to be answered in such circumstances.

(1) Is the patient physically fit for the job? The only way to ascertain this is for the patient to try out the job for himself.
(2) Does the patient like the job? Patients may be attracted to a particular job for a variety of reasons. They may well change their minds when they actually get down to the job itself. We have found that some patients, in theory, feel that they would like to take up watch repair, for example, but they soon find that the close attention to detail and the endless patience required does not suit their temperaments. Some, on the other hand, are in error as to the nature of the work. One patient was emphatic in his desire to be a draughtsman but quickly changed his mind when he discovered that the job was not drawing beer in a public house!
(3) Does the instructor or supervisor feel that the patient is likely to make a success of the job?

Once these questions are answered, a patient can confidently be advised to take up the employment chosen, with or without training as the case may be. Sometimes, it requires only an afternoon or a day to solve these problems, but in other cases it may take much longer.

We were fortunate at Chessington in establishing a close liaison with a nearby skill centre who allow us the facilities to have patients tested at their chosen trades. When possible it is eminently desirable that patients should combine part-time retraining and rehabilitation; this gives the patient a goal to work for which lessens the time in which he will be out of work. It will be seen that this scheme dispenses with the necessity of sending the patient to an employment rehabilitation centre in all but the most difficult cases.

This is in no sense meant to be a criticism of these centres, but it is obvious that the sooner a patient's future is decided, the better, and by making use of the occupational therapy department, their workshop facilities or the rehabilitation centre, a great deal can be done to help the patient decide on his future.

Where such facilities are not available, or when the patient's problems cannot readily be solved in this way, the employment rehabilitation centres are very often ready to offer their advice by interviewing and assessing patients for 1 or 2 days. It is often not necessary to have to admit a patient for the full course at such a centre; a day or so may be all that is necessary. Certainly, on this basis, the employment rehabilitation centres should be used more by the resettlement clinics for assessment of a patient's abilities.

The atmosphere of the resettlement clinic is very important. The patient should be encouraged to talk freely and explain his problems, and it must always be remembered that what is obviously straightforward to the doctor and the staff may be very different to the patient.

Several attendances at the clinic are recommended throughout the period of treatment. Each attendance may be for only a few minutes, merely for the DRO to convince the patient that he is actively engaged in arrangements for his future, or in discovering additional useful information, and this may be very important to a patient who is naturally worried about what is going to happen.

The ability to talk about his problems and to receive the advice and opinions of a number of people with different points of view is of tremendous help to the patient in making up his mind. Time spent at these clinics is never wasted for it may prevent a patient from taking up the wrong sort of employment, or from drifting into unskilled labour with all the serious implications for his disability that this holds.

Granville (1956) was the first to report on the use of paid work in rehabilitation. At a suitable stage in the patient's treatment he will be employed in a workshop undertaking subcontract work as part of his rehabilitation. This work produces income to offset the cost of administration of the rehabilitation centre, and the subcontractor providing the work is brought into the rehabilitation scheme. A rehabilitation association was formed, based on the area covered by the regional hospital board. Its objective is to crystallize the relationship between the hospital and rehabilitation staff and the employers in the area. A large number of interested employers have joined the scheme to provide details of the types of work available in their factories, and close liaison is made between the hospital and the employers with the aim of finding out exactly what type of adaptations or modifications of tools, working conditions and so on, will be required on the patient's return to work. It also helps the patient's confidence and this is instrumental in getting the employer to accept the patient back at an earlier stage of treatment than would otherwise be possible.

In many cases an employer may have to be persuded that a disabled person is perfectly able to carry out a full day's work, provided the right type of work is chosen for his disability. This needs patient explanation and personal contact. It has been found that once an employer has placed a disabled person in the right sort of employment, that worker gives such loyal and conscientious service that the employer is anxious to have more disabled people on his staff.

The organization of the resettlement clinic is devised so that the ultimate person in charge is the doctor. Any resettlement organization that is not so constituted is liable to fail in the last resort because only a doctor can appreciate the possible fluctuation of a disability (such as rheumatoid arthritis) and assess the ways in which employment may affect the patient and his condition.

In a rehabilitation centre, facilities usually exist for deciding on the sort of employment most suited to a patient's disability, and the machinery of the clinic will indicate at the earliest possible stage the likelihood of employment in the patient's home area, or the training facilities available. In really difficult cases, such as extensive loss of function in the hands, it may take months to discover the right type of job for that patient. Consequently, the sooner the patient is brought before the clinic, the better.

There are certain general principles which are at the basis of all satisfactory resettlement. First, the patient must understand his disability. This means that the doctor should take great care to explain in simple language the exact nature of the condition and the prognosis. This should include advice on the sort of conditions to be avoided; for example, extremes of heat and cold. He should be warned of any sensory loss in the hand and given advice on the precautions to be taken in cold weather, and in such matters as moving machinery.

Second, the patient should be encouraged to make the most use of his abilities. Those who have experience of the severely disabled know just how much potential waiting to be realized there is in most people. This is particularly true in patients with poliomyelitis. Perhaps the most dramatic of all patients we have seen was one who was paralysed below the neck, but despite this learnt to pain with a brush between his teeth and is now earning his living by this means. The aim should be for the patient to be in a more skilled occupation than before his disability.

Third, resettlement should be started as early as possible during treatment, and the various aspects such as vocational guidance, retraining, provision of gadgets for work, self-help devices and invalid transport should be dovetailed to cover the least period of time. Much can be done by using the existing facilities of an ordinary hospital and adapting these to specific requirements.

Fourth, there should always be personal contact between the doctor and the DRO.

Compensation problems

O'Malley at a meeting at the Royal Society of Medicine in 1957 stated that 15 per cent of patients in a civil rehabilitation centre are compensation cases. He compared the treatment times in a group of compensation cases and non-compensation cases. The total treatment time was just double for the compensation cases; the great majority of this increased time was spent at the hospital.

The problem of a patient awaiting settlement of a compensation claim is a very real one, and while a complete solution cannot be offered here, certain aspects of the problem must be discussed.

In 1948 new legislation on compensation laid down that an injured worker could claim in two ways for the consequence of his injury. First, the National Insurance (Industrial Injuries) Act 1965 provides payment for the degree of disablement. The Act is administered by the Department of Health and Social Security, quite distinct from the Law Courts. In cases of dispute, the workman has a right of appeal to the Local Appeal Tribunal, consisting of a chairman and two other members, one the trades union representative, and one the representative of the employers' organization.

A special hardship allowance is payable for loss of earning, in such conditions as when the patient has had to change his regular occupation.

This Act replaced the old Workman's Compensation Act, removing the unfair bias that existed whereby a skilled man with a mild injury might be worse off than an unskilled man with a severe injury.

Second, an injured workman can claim for damages at Common Law.

Before 1948 it was not possible to claim for both. Now, irrespective of whether the injured person is claiming in the Courts or not, he receives his Supplementary Benefit. The claimant has to satisfy the Court that someone was to blame for the injury. Damages are awarded as a lump sum to compensate the patient for loss of wages, expenses, pain and suffering, and possible disability in the future.

If a patient is a member of a trade union, the legal department will deal with the claim; otherwise this is done through a private solicitor.

Before the claim is settled, a long time elapses during which various medical examinations are made, reports are taken by the insurance company and employers, offers may be made and rejected, and the patient becomes possessed more often than not of a compensation neurosis; on the one hand he is being persuaded to return to work by his wife, and he himself finds that he is losing money by being unemployed; on the other hand there may be pressure from the trade union to go on with the case lest it creates a precedent by a less adequate settlement than he deserves. It is true to say that the aim of the injured man's advisers is to get him as much money as possible and conflicts with the aim of the defending insurance company to minimize the damages. This means that a long time elapses between injury and eventual settlement.

Medical advice is invariably in favour of an early settlement, and if a round table conference between all interested parties can be called in the early stages and liability agreed, the patient can concentrate on getting back to work quickly. Whereas the majority of workmen return to work as soon as they are fit, there is a significant minority who do not do so in the hope of obtaining a substantial sum of money. If the greatest amount of money is to be awarded in damages, it is difficult for the patient not to get into the habit of making the most of his disability. There is a widespread belief among workers that a return to work before the claim is settled may reduce the amount of damages awarded. This is not so, for the majority of the legal profession trying such cases are favourably impressed by patients' attempts to return to work as soon as possible.

The real core to this problem lies in the attitude of the injured man and the relations between him and his employers. If the patient can be made to realize how important it is that his rehabilitation should be started as early as possible, and if the employer has a reputation for fair dealing, difficulties arise much less frequently.

In the last resort, the difficulties of compensation problems will be substantially overcome if there is a closer understanding between all the interested parties, and a realization that all concerned should have as their main goal the speedy rehabilitation of the patient and his return to work. Consequently, the doctor has a vital part to play in representing to both sides the importance of these points.

The best way to avoid, or at least minimize, compensation neurosis is to provide a background of interest in getting the patient back to work, and it may well be that all the resources of a rehabilitation department will have to be used to encourage the patient to forget his disability and to work to regain function as quickly as possible.

It has been suggested that if liability were admitted in the early stages of litigation and the question of the amount of damages left for subsequent negotiations, this would go a long way towards solving the problems.

Above all, it is vital that the patient should not be encouraged to spend a period of inactivity unless it is absolutely necessary, and the doctor can do a great deal to persuade the patient to return to work if he takes the trouble to explain the possible complications and limitations that may arise in the future.

VOLUNTARY ORGANIZATIONS

There are an enormous number of voluntary organizations which help disabled persons in a variety of ways. Some are concerned with specific disabilities such as deafness, blindness, loss of limbs, spasticity, poliomyelitis, and many others. Two directories of such organizations are that compiled by Darnbrough and Kinrade (1977) and that from King's Fund (1979).

It is very important that all persons connected with the resettlement of the disabled be fully aware of the various societies and organizations – both national and voluntary – that exist to help the disabled person. There are virtually no patients whose problems are so difficult that one or another of the organizations cannot materially help.

SPECIFIC RESETTLEMENT OF PATIENTS WITH HAND DISABILITIES

General remarks

As each patient presents a different problem, and the resettlement of a particular patient depends on so many other factors besides his physical disability, only a general indication of resettlement can be given here.

The aim of rehabilitation of all hand disabilities is to obtain the best possible function. This may take many months, but in most cases if it is at all possible for the patient to have treatment for the period of time needed, every effort should be made to give it. If, for example, a man sustains an injury to the median nerve at the wrist, and he is a skilled workman, such as a motor mechanic, it is essential that he should be rehabilitated back to his skilled occupation. While he can well return to some form of work quite soon after nerve suture, he will be most unlikely to earn anything like the amount he was getting in his skilled occupation. Consequently, such a patient is advised to remain under full-time treatment until the best possible result is obtained. If, after the appropriate time has elapsed, it is clear that function is not going to be adequate for his skill, then is the time to consider a change of job or retraining.

Where possible, resettlement should be devised to utilize the patient's experience and knowledge. Thus, a bench fitter whose disability prevents him from carrying out the fine work required, can, if he is in other ways suitable, be employed as an inspector or supervisor. In large firms and organizations these problems are fairly easily solved, but in the smaller firms such a patient may be impossible to assimilate, and, unless retraining is advised, the best prospect of satisfactory resettlement is in the personal contact of an enlightened DRO with local firms. At the other extreme is the case of an engine driver who was able to return to work within a few weeks after secondary suture of the median and ulnar nerves at the wrist, attending daily for physiotherapy (Glanville, personal communication).

Cases where disability is permanent and static, such as paralysis following poliomyelitis or residual impairment after paralysis, fractures, burns and so on, present few problems that cannot eventually be overcome with the organization and help described in this chapter. Patients in the paralysed stage of nerve injuries, or during an extensive programme of reconstructive surgery, can be more difficult, but here resettlement is best postponed until the ultimate result is seen, or at any rate is going to be obvious. The main difficulty with such patients is that they will be unemployed and drawing Supplementary Benefit for a long time. In large firms, where there are rehabilitation workshops, patients can return to productive work, but this is impracticable for patients in small firms.

The ideal organization for these patients would seem to be some form of productive workshop conveniently situated near a local industry, and near a hospital, where patients can carry out part-time useful productive work devised, where possible, to promote active recovery for their disability, and be paid at agreed rates. It might not be possible to arrange the work specifically to increase the range of movement in the stiff joints and redevelop weak muscles. Following surgery for a severe injury there may be little that a patient can do with that hand for some months. He can, however, carry out a multitude of useful jobs with the good hand, and even coarse movements with the affected hand improve the circulation.

There are many difficulties in the way of providing temporary employment for a disabled person, and the setting up of such workshops, carefully supervised by the medical staff of the hospital, might provide the answer.

There is certainly a great need for some organization that will allow a patient with a severe hand disability or, indeed, any disability that is going to take time to improve, to carry out some useful work and be paid for it. Otherwise there is a great temptation for such patients to take up unskilled work, which may militate against their recovery, in order to make ends meet.

Furthermore, the therapeutic value of productive work cannot be overstressed. The longer a patient remains away from his work, the more difficult it is for him to acclimatize himself on his eventual return. The most difficult of all cases are those in which the disability is remittent and liable to flare up at unpredictable intervals, a good example of this being rheumatoid arthritis. All that has already been said about the principles of good resettlement apply even more to this condition.

A very special effort must be made to explain to employers the liability of the patient to have relapses from time to time.

Each case presents its own problems but much can be done to help the patient if the employer will consider altering chairs, benches and so on, to suit the individual deformity, and fixing larger operating handles or grips to industrial tools.

Fortunately, the function is usually much better than the deformity would seem to allow, and it is not so much the hand disability as the general condition of the patient that causes him to miss work.

There is clearly no easy answer to these problems. Close co-operation between the doctors and employment officials leading to an understanding of the difficulties of patients offers the best hope. For many cases sheltered employment is the only course open. In others, the patient may at some times be able to work normally and at other times unable to work at all, and it is in this type of case in particular that regular review at the resettlement clinics is of special value.

PRINCIPLES OF RESETTLEMENT IN PARTICULAR HAND DISABILITIES

Those with most experience of assessing and placing disabled persons in industry are agreed that the main subdivision of trades to be considered is into clerical and non-clerical.

Whenever educational standards allow, a person with an imperfect hand is encouraged to take up clerical work. The Employment Service Division (MSC) on the advice of its units, is able to arrange for clerical training either at a skill centre or at a residential or technical college.

In the case of the master hand being unaffected, all clerical duties are possible, the affected hand being used as a support. So many industrial activities require use of both hands at some stage, whether for fine work or coarse power, that a patient with an imperfect hand is much more likely to achieve satisfactory resettlement in a clerical grade.

Clerical work is divided into commerical and industrial. Commercial work comprises such activities as book-keeping and typing. Industrial clerical work includes store-keeping, store-checking and telephone operating. All these activities command reasonable pay and offer, in most cases, long-term security – an important consideration with disabled persons.

If educational standards are low and manual industrial work is impossible, such work as time-keeping, where integrity of character and reliability are demanded, responsible messenger work, security, checking and inspection are well worth consideration.

Patients with artistic abilities wishing to employ them in commercial art, dress designing, and so on, should be dissuaded whenever possible on setting their hearts on such a future. The prospects of placing are very poor and experience of ERCs and DROs in general shows that they very rarely do well. If a patient is keen on interior decorating, for example, it is better to advise him to take a course in painting and decorating. This ensures him a livelihood and may lead later to an artistic opening.

If clerical work is not possible, through lack of background, employment or physical disability, placing in industry is then considered.

Industrial trades are divided into skilled, semi-skilled and unskilled. The skilled worker who meets with a severe hand disability is always easier to resettle than the unskilled man. He is more able to learn compensatory tricks at his job and can deploy his experience and intelligence to overcoming difficulties as he meets them. The innate adaptability which is a main feature of a skilled worker sees him over many of the hurdles throughout the period of rehabilitation. A patient, for example, with engineering ability and experience whose disability prevents him from performing the many skilled movements of the upper limb required in engineering trades is well resettled in the drawing office if his mathematics are or can be up to the required standard.

It is essential to effect a proper liaison between the future employer or training centre and the patient and his medical advisers early on in rehabilitation. Patients can then be guided into the right channels of preparatory work – the embryo draughtsman can study trigonometry, the radio enthusiast circuit diagrams. Patients must be strongly advised against wasting time on correspondence courses which they have taken up on their own initiative, as too often their trade rules may not allow them employment. There are very few areas in Great Britain where commercial and technical colleges are not available for part-time study. It is incumbent on the patient's doctor to advise him in the strongest terms of the benefit in preparing himself for his future. If, indeed, it is not feasible so to do, at the least the patient can improve his general education and general knowledge by reading, attending evening classes, intelligent and selective listening and viewing.

It cannot be overemphasized how much a positive approach to the future and using enforced time off work to best advantage promote recovery.

Above all, resettlement should never be hurried; the more skilled the worker, the more important for his future happiness, and the country's good, that he should return to as skilled work as possible. Long-term rehabilitation should be accepted as ultimately the most economic answer to severe disablement.

The three major considerations in assessing a patient's abilities for industrial work are fine finger control, sensibility and power of grip.

Although each patient must always be treated as an individual and as a unique problem, and some patients through courage and perseverance are capable of surprisingly skilled work with severe disability, for the general run of people the following principles apply.

Loss of control

Loss of fine finger control and loss of sensation go together. A patient with a motor palsy of the ulnar nerve and one with sensory loss in the median nerve are equally handicapped for fine work. Such patients cannot carry out high-class assembly work – they are incapble of holding one part of a machine steady while manipulating other parts. Repairs and watch and clock repairing are impossible, as are instrument making and repairing. They may, of course, be able to carry out the majority of processes in a task involving coarse grip and movements, but the fine work such as insertion of small screws and split pins proves impossible.

Loss of sensation

Loss of sensation in the hand generally rules out all the electrical trades, and those trades where extremes of heat and cold are unavoidable. It must be remembered that cold as well as heat is dangerous to a person with loss of sensation, and such activities as refrigeration engineering are contraindicated. Coarse fitting, however, is possible, as the affected hand can be used as control, or for follow-through action. Drills can be operated and much automatic machine work is possible.

Loss of movement of fingers

Any fine work is difficult if there is loss of movement in the finger joints. Manipulation of tweezers, delicate work in watch and clock repairing, radio repair and assembling, all demand virtually full movement in the interphalangeal joints.

Following tendon grafting, movement in the distal interphalangeal joint may sometimes be limited, but the patient may be able to bring his finger down to the palm. This movement is essential for gripping such machines as presses and drills, and is therefore to be encouraged despite lack of progress at the terminal joint.

Loss of movement and power in the little finger seriously restricts the gripping of tools such as hammers. The little and ring fingers are vital for the general balance of the hand.

Loss of grip

Loss of grip is a serious disability. If fine finger control and sensation are present, the disability is less serious, and patients can be resettled fairly easily if they have the capacity to be skilled workers. Such activities as draughtsmanship, light assembly work, even some types of instrument making, are possible.

Loss of grip with loss of dexterity, or loss of grip in an unskilled worker, considerably restricts placing. Efforts must be made to adapt machinery by the use of springs or power operated devices to minimize the force necessary on the part of the operator to work the machine. Here again a wide field of research is open in the adaptation of machinery to the disabled patient in industry.

Stiff hand

When the hand is stiff – for example, after crush injuries, severe burns, long-standing oedema – machinery can be altered to accommodate the restricted movement of the hand. Such patients can pull presses with a hook action, can grip handles (particularly if the size of handle can be altered) and can indulge in spray painting and electric welding.

Patients with stiff hands can often operate simple types of machine; in such cases assessment by a competent engineer used to disabled people is invaluable.

Electric weldng is a trade that can successfully be performed with a gross degree of hand damage. In fact, patients with only one arm, and some with no hands, have been satisfactorily placed as electric welders.

Loss of digits

Loss of the index finger or thumb, or both, restricts activity to coarse grip or use of the hand to guide and control. Such patients can press, drill, weld, engrave, and paint and decorate (hanging the paint pot over the affected arm). However, a person with any degree of damage to the hand should not be allowd to work on heights. Without the control and balance given by the hand the danger of falling is ever present.

Rheumatoid arthritis

The rheumatoid hand presents grave problems; much depends on associated joint involvement and the general state of health. Patients with severe degrees of rheumatoid involvement of the hands have successfully managed trades which include scientific glass blowing (where the hands are used only for control and turning the glass), clerical and stores work, light drilling, light machine work and manipulation of machinery by foot presses.

The attention to the individual problems and the exercise of ingenuity to adaptations to machinery are all-important in this disease.

In industrial placing of the disabled in general, staged resettlement is most useful. If a patient is incapable of fine work or machine operating, it may be that some months working in the factory on simpler activities may lead to development of ability to cope with more complex activities. (Assembly work may lead gradually to machine operating.) This may be due to natural remission of disease, regaining of confidence by the patient, actual improvement in the physical state by the work itself or the effect in general of work on the disability. This is somewhat neglected by doctors, but industrial medical officers vouch for the remarkable therapeutic effects of gainful employment on physical disability.

Wilkinson (personal communication) is impressed by the effect of work on diminishing relapses in rheumatoid arthritis, epilepsy, head injury and organic nervous diseases.

Spastic hand

Patients with a spastic hand cannot operate machines requiring turning, nor are they capable of skilled work with the affected hand. Usually the affected hand can be used as a support, though tremor may be a drawback – fine movements are impossible. They can often undertake simple work such as sandpapering or sweeping. Much depends on associated brain damage with mental effects and speech disability, and it must not be forgotten how greatly the emotional handicap of fear of losing a job may aggravate symptoms. A sense of security is thus vital in employment of such patients.

In conclusion, it cannot be overstressed that, as resettlement is an integral part of rehabilitation and as the doctor is the overall director of the team, his must be the ultimate responsibility for seeing that his disabled patients resume their rightful place in society.

REFERENCES AND BIBLIOGRAPHY

Brewerton, D. A. B. and Daniel, J. W. (1969). Experiences of a hospital rehabilitation officer. *British Medical Journal* **2**, 240–242

British Medical Association (1968). *Aids for the Disabled.* London: BMA

Central Office of Information (1975). *Care of Disabled People in Britain.* London: HMSO

Charities Digest (annual). London: Butterworths/Family Welfare Association

Cooksey, F. S. (1960). Progress and problems in the rehabilitation of disabled people. *Proceedings of the Royal Society of Medicine* **53**, 707–711

Darnbrough, Ann and Kinrade, Derek (Compilers) (1977). *Directory for the Disabled. A handbook of information and opportunities for disabled and handicapped people.* Cambridge: Woodhead–Faulkner, in association with RADAR

Department of Employment (1973). *Sheltered Employment for Disabled People; a consultative document.* London: DoE

Department of Health and Social Security (1976) *Health and Personal Social Services Statistics for England 1975 (with summary tables for Great Britain).* London: HMSO

Department of Health and Social Security (1978). *On the State of the Public Health for the Year 1977.* London: HMSO

Glanville, H. J. (1956). A unit for early rehabilitation in a general hospital. *Annals of Physical Medicine* **3**, 101–104

Glanville, H. J. (1977). *What is Rehabilitation?* Southampton: University of Southampton

Greaves, Mary and Massie, Bert (1979). *Work and Disability*, 2nd edn. London: RADAR

Industrial rehabilitation 1970–71 (1971). *Department of Employment Gazette* December

King's Fund (1979). *Directory of Organisations for Patients and Disabled People.* London: King Edward's Hospital Fund for London

MacMorland, B. (1977). *ABC of Services and Information for Disabled People*, 3rd edn. London: Disablement Income Group Charitable Trust

Memorandum of Evidence submitted to the Council of the British Medical Association to the Interdepartmental Committee (1954). *The Rehabilitation and Resettlement of Disabled Persons.* London: BMA

Randle, A. H. (1972). Rehabilitation and society. *Proceedings of the International Congress on Physical Medicine* 1972

Report (1956). *Report of the Committee of Inquiry on the Rehabilitation. Training and Resettlement of Disabled Persons* (The Piercy Report). London: HMSO

Return to the community physiotherapy (1972). *Physiotherapy,* January

Aids for the disabled are on display at:

Disabled Living Foundation, 380 Harrow Road, London W9 2HU

Royal Association for Disability and Rehabilitation, 25 Mortimer Street, London W1

Index